MANAGING MANAGED CARE
QUALITY IMPROVEMENT IN BEHAVIORAL HEALTH

Margaret Edmunds, Richard Frank, Michael Hogan,
Dennis McCarty, Rhonda Robinson-Beale,
and Constance Weisner, *Editors*

Committee on Quality Assurance and Accreditation Guidelines
for Managed Behavioral Health Care

Division of Neuroscience and Behavioral Health

Division of Health Care Services

INSTITUTE OF MEDICINE

NATIONAL ACADEMY PRESS
Washington, D.C.   1997

NATIONAL ACADEMY PRESS • 2101 Constitution Avenue, N.W. • Washington, DC 20418

NOTICE: The project that is the subject of this report was approved by the Governing Board of the National Research Council, whose members are drawn from the councils of the National Academy of Sciences, the National Academy of Engineering, and the Institute of Medicine. The members of the committee responsible for the report were chosen for their special competences and with regard for appropriate balance.

This report has been reviewed by a group other than the authors according to procedures approved by a Report Review Committee consisting of members of the National Academy of Sciences, the National Academy of Engineering, and the Institute of Medicine.

The Institute of Medicine was chartered in 1970 by the National Academy of Sciences to enlist distinguished members of the appropriate professions in the examination of policy matters pertaining to the health of the public. In this, the Institute acts under both the Academy's 1863 congressional charter responsibility to be an adviser to the federal government and its own initiative in identifying issues of medical care, research, and education. Dr. Kenneth I. Shine is president of the Institute of Medicine.

Support for this project was provided by the Center for Substance Abuse Treatment of the Substance Abuse and Mental Health Services Administration, U.S. Department of Health and Human Services. Any opinions, findings, conclusions, or recommendations expressed in this publication are those of the author(s) and do not necessarily reflect the view of the organizations or agencies that provided support for the project.

Library of Congress Cataloging-in-Publication Data

Managing managed care : quality improvements in behavioral health /
    Margaret Edmunds . . . [et al.], editors ; Committee on Quality
    Assurance and Accreditation Guidelines for Managed Behavioral Health
    Care, Division of Neuroscience and Behavioral Health [and] Division
    of Health Care Services, Institute of Medicine.
          p. cm
          Includes index.
          ISBN 0-309-05642-X
          1. Managed mental health care—United States—Quality control.
    2. Managed mental health care—Accreditation—United States.
    I. Edmunds, Margaret. II. Institute of Medicine (U.S.). Committee
    on Quality Assurance and Accreditation Guidelines for Managed
    Behavioral Health Care.
          [DNLM: 1. Mental Health Services—organization & administration—
    United States. 2. Managed Care Programs—organization &
    administration—United States. 3. Quality Assurance, Health Care—
    standards—United States. WM 30 M2666 1997]
    RC480.5.M325   1997
    362.2'00973—dc21
    DNLM/DLC
    for Library of Congress   97-20004
                                                                CIP

The serpent has been a symbol of long life, healing, and knowledge among almost all cultures and religions since the beginning of recorded history. The image adopted as a logotype by the Institute of Medicine is based on a relief carving from ancient Greece, now held by the Staatlichemuseen in Berlin.

COMMITTEE ON QUALITY ASSURANCE AND ACCREDITATION GUIDELINES FOR MANAGED BEHAVIORAL HEALTH CARE

*Member, Institute of Medicine.

CONSTANCE WEISNER, Senior Scientist, Alcohol Research Group, Western Consortium for Public Health and School of Public Health, University of California at Berkeley, Berkeley, CA

Institute of Medicine Staff

MARGARET EDMUNDS, Study Director
CARRIE INGALLS, Research Associate
THOMAS WETTERHAN, Project Assistant/Research Assistant
AMELIA MATHIS, Project Assistant
TERRI SCANLAN, Administrative Assistant
EUGENE LEE, Student Intern
MOLLA DONALDSON, Senior Program Officer, Division of Health Care Services
CONSTANCE PECHURA, Director, Division of Neuroscience and Behavioral Health

Preface

Introducing a report that addresses such a complex and dynamic issue as managed behavioral health care is a daunting task. The charge to the Committee on Quality Assurance and Accreditation Guidelines for Managed Behavioral Health Care was to develop a framework to guide the development, use, and evaluation of performance indicators, accreditation standards, and quality improvement mechanisms. The framework could then be used to assist in the purchase and delivery of the most effective managed behavioral health care at the lowest appropriate cost for consumers of publicly and privately financed care.

There were numerous challenges in addressing this charge. The committee was operating in a rapidly changing environment in which multiple efforts by accreditation organizations, government agencies, consumer groups, and other interested parties were under way to develop report cards, performance indicators, and other measures of behavioral health care quality. The committee members chose to take an evidence-based approach to their task, but they found that the research base and the development of quality assurance and accreditation standards are far less advanced in behavioral health care than in other areas of health care.

Discussions among committee members clearly indicated a great diversity in opinions and experiences. The committee, however, believed that its charge to create a framework for assessing quality assurance and accreditation guidelines was best served by the development of recommendations broad enough to allow various stakeholder groups to make them more specific to their own needs and circumstances, as appropriate. This report fulfills this charge and provides a framework that will be useful and enduring. In addition, this report—possibly for the first time—weaves together in a single place the many complex issues, concepts, and challenges involved in assuring quality in behavioral health care in a way that is accessible to a broad audience.

To accomplish its task, the committee began by developing the Statement of Principles included in Chapter 1 of the full report. These principles served to guide and unite the committee and are the outcome of intensive discussion and consensus-building across a rich diversity of views and perspectives.

As a primary care physician listening to the workshop presentations and deliberations, it was sometimes unclear to me whether or not mental health and substance abuse problems really presented unique challenges. For example, many of the presentations and discussions emphasized the importance of viewing mental health and substance abuse problems as chronic, relapsing conditions that do not differ significantly from other health problems, such as diabetes and heart disease. Other presentations, however, emphasized key differences, such as greater needs for integration of services, a large percentage of substance abuse problems being dealt with in the publicly funded Medicaid system, and the emergence of so-called "carve-out" companies providing behavioral health care, among other examples. Thus, the committee has tried throughout the report to underscore a critical distinction between the unique aspects of the *structure of behavioral health care delivery* and the *nature of the disorders themselves*, which are not unique, but can range from a single episode of illness to chronic, recurrent, and disabling conditions.

From early on in its deliberations, the committee was determined to be scrupulous in separating evidence-based research results from information based on current clinical strategies or best practices. Thus, the body of the report includes findings that were rigorously grounded in the research literature. However, the committee felt that this report could not go forward without expressing the strong clinical judgments that this is an exciting time in research, that rapid progress is being made in the diagnosis and treatment of behavioral health conditions, and that there is an increasing recognition of the importance of continuing care as a way to prevent or ameliorate relapses.

Although the report covers a wide range of topics and issues in this field, it might be useful to highlight some of the issues that the committee could not address fully and that will require ongoing consideration by federal and state agencies, as well as a number of other stakeholder groups. Four key areas seem to be important areas for further work by others. First, there are complex and often overlapping systems of regulation and accreditation, which result in different data requirements, specifications, and timetables. In addition, there are compelling needs to ensure the quality and integrity of the various measures used by many different organizations. This complexity presents real challenges to purchasers, consumers, providers, and practitioners of behavioral health care. This report describes the complexity and presents general recommendations to be considered by the variety of regulatory agencies and accreditation organizations (e.g., the utility of external audits and quality improvement mechanisms). Whether or not the current system requires modification and how such modification should be approached, however, was beyond the scope of our work.

The second key area involves questions regarding the analysis and reporting of the many different types of quality assessment (e.g., report cards, patient satisfaction measures, and other evaluations) and, further, how to use such measures to develop accurate and appropriate case-mix and risk adjustment models. To address these questions, the committee believes that further development of analytical tools is necessary and that this evidence base needs to be expanded before detailed recommendations can be made. In addition, development of such tools will require collaboration among various components of the public and private sectors. The public- and private-sector entities involved might find it fruitful to consider ways to foster these collaborations.

Third, there is a general need to develop strategies to address the complexities of the Medicaid population, particularly as they relate to people with mental health and substance abuse problems and to the devolution of responsibility for this population from the federal government to the states. A comprehensive survey of the states and an analysis of the specific needs of the mental health and substance abuse segment of Medicaid-covered health care—and the variety of needs across states—were beyond the committee's charge. Yet, this theme was expressed at many of the committee's workshops and in its deliberations, and further work seems necessary to understand the complex needs of this population, particularly as they relate to strategies to integrate services across social services agencies and health care providers.

The fourth area relates to the variety of health care practitioners, often working simultaneously, who are involved in treating mental health and substance abuse problems. Clearly, tensions exist among some of these groups of practitioners, but there is also a great need to integrate care across the various disciplines when a patient is being treated by a team of practitioners. This situation is an excellent example of a systemic problem that contributes importantly to the fragmentation of services discussed in the report and that this committee could not solve. However, the variety of practitioners involved also presents special problems for measuring quality in managed behavioral health care, and these problems could benefit from further research to design specific approaches to handle the tensions and to address the need for integration of treatment services.

The entire health care system is changing rapidly, and behavioral health care is no exception. During the spring and summer months of 1996 when the committee met, Congress deliberated and then passed a compromise mental health parity bill, consumer groups challenged the capacity of accreditation organizations to measure quality, and researchers reported that psychotherapy had been found to produce changes in brain function similar to those seen with medications. While the report was being reviewed, President Clinton announced the formation of a federal advisory commission on the quality of health care. Thus, the issues considered by the committee are timely and seem to reflect some fundamental policy questions, some of which will continue to be debated over the next decade and, possibly, longer.

As one who has been fortunate to participate on a number of Institute of Medicine committees, I must close with a personal statement. The subject matter, the committee and its generous participation in lively and informative meetings as well as in writing the report, and the IOM staff—particularly the study director, who kept the work on track and synthesized and balanced the multiple streams of input—have made this effort one of the most satisfying in which I have participated in the past 15 years.

Jerome Grossman, M.D., *Chair*
Committee on Quality Assurance and
Accreditation Guidelines for
Managed Behavioral Health Care

Acknowledgments

The committee would like to acknowledge the contributions of many individuals and organizations to the committee's work.

The committee expresses deep appreciation to all the individuals and groups who contributed to the public workshops. The speakers in the workshops were Don Austin, John Bartlett, Linda Bresolin, Ray Bridge, Catherine Brown, Reginald Cedar Face, Robert Cole, William Dennis Derr, Elizabeth Edgar, Robert Egnew, Michael Faenza, Daniel Fisher, Julia Puebla Fortier, Ann Froio, Donald Galamaga, Susan Goldman, Sybil Goldman, Sarah Gotbaum, Elizabeth Hadley, Laura Lee Hall, Judith Hines, Michael Jeffrey, Linda Kaplan, Randall Madry, Ron Manderscheid, David Mee-Lee, Raphael Metzger, Margaret O'Kane, Peter Panzarino, Mark Paris, Mark Parrino, Geoffrey Reed, Gwen Rubinstein, Paul Schyve, Tim Slaven, Golnar Simpson, Sarah Stanley, Tom Trabin, Robert Valdez, Rita Vandivort, and Grace Wang. Many individuals who were not speakers also participated by asking the workshop speakers questions, and they are listed in Appendix D.

The committee thanks Don Steinwachs and Thomas McLellan and his colleagues Mark Belding, James McKay, David Zanis, and Arthur Alterman for contributing their papers, which were used by the committee in preparing this report and which appear as Appendixes to this report.

The committee expresses appreciation to Don Detmer and Ed Perrin, who served, respectively, as liaisons to the Institute of Medicine (IOM) Board on Health Care Services and the National Research Council's Committee on National Statistics (CNSTAT).

The committee is particularly grateful to the members of the liaison panel, who raised many questions for the committee's consideration and helped to identify materials for the committee's review. All of the members are listed in Appendix E. The members who were especially active in responding to requests for information were Linda Bresolin, Peggy Clark, Judith Emerson, Elizabeth Hadley, Judith Hines, Linda Kaplan, Anne Kilguss, Yvonne Lewis, Mark Paris, Mark Parrino, Clarke Ross, Gwen Rubinstein, Paul Schyve, Claire Sharda, Tom Trabin, Jeanne Trumble, Margaret Van Amringe, and Robert Valdez. Organizations that submitted written comments for the committee's review are listed in Appendix F.

The committee is grateful to several individuals who provided technical comments on preliminary drafts of sections of the report. They include Gary Chase, Peggy Clark, Denise Dougherty, Lynn Etheredge, Joe Frisino, Susan Goldman, Judith Katz-Leavy, Kathleen Lohr, Hal Luft, David Mactas, Ron Manderscheid, Clarke Ross, Hector Sanchez, Eugene Schoener, Paul Schyve, Claire Sharda, Lisa Simpson, and Tim Slaven.

The committee could not have accomplished its task without the insightful and tireless support of the study director, Margo Edmunds. Dr. Edmunds' extraordinary skills in planning and managing the study, imaginative guidance of the committee's activities, and writing or editing numerous sections of the report provided an anchor for the committee throughout the study.

Other members of the IOM professional staff also provided invaluable help. Constance Pechura developed the idea for the study with the sponsor and provided guidance throughout, including descriptions of the IOM process and identification of resources and materials. Molla Donaldson attended committee meetings and reviewed draft sections of the report. Marilyn Field was responsive to many questions and reviewed draft sections of the report. Linda Bailey and Jane Durch helped to coordinate this study with the IOM study on public health performance monitoring, as did Jeff Koshel, study director for the CNSTAT effort on performance partnership grants.

The professional staff were supported by the efforts of Carrie Ingalls, research associate; Thomas Wetterhan, project assistant/research assistant; Amelia Mathis, project assistant; Terri Scanlan, administrator; and Eugene Lee, a summer student intern from the Massachusetts Institute of Technology. Other IOM and National Academy of Sciences staff who were helpful at a variety of stages include Carolyn Fulco, Carlos Gabriel, Kate-Louise Gottfried, Linda Kilroy, Lauren Leveton, Catharyn Liverman, Luis Nunez, Dan Quinn, Mary Lee Schneiders, and Andrea Solarz. During report review, Claudia Carl and Mike Edington provided valuable direction and technical assistance. The extensive commentary and suggestions made by the copy editor, Michael Hayes, are gratefully acknowledged.

Finally, support for this study was provided by the U.S. Department of Health and Human Services, Substance Abuse and Mental Health Services Administration (SAMHSA), and its three centers: the Center for Substance Abuse Treatment (CSAT), the Center for Mental Health Services (CMHS), and the Center for Substance Abuse Prevention (CSAP). David Mactas, the Director of CSAT, the lead agency for the study, described the sponsor's goals for the study at the committee's first meeting. For their helpful responses to the staff's inquiries and requests throughout the study, the committee thanks Mady Chalk, Director of Managed Care Initiatives at CSAT and the government's project officer; Eric Goplerud, Director of SAMHSA's Managed Care Initiative; Jeff Buck, Acting Director of the CMHS Office of Policy and Planning; Nancy Kennedy, Managed Care Coordinator for CSAP; and Ron Manderscheid, Chief of the Survey Analysis Branch for the CMHS Division of State and Community Systems Development.

Contents

ACRONYMS   xviii

SUMMARY   1

1   INTRODUCTION   15
    Terminology Used in This Report, 21
    Consumers and Families, 22
    Practitioners, 25
    Purchasers, 27
    The Managed Care Industry, 29
    Statement of Principles, 33
    Organization of the Report, 36

2   TRENDS IN MANAGED CARE   40
    The Changing Health Care System, 41
    Concerns with Managed Care in the Public Sector, 47
    Behavioral Health in the New Marketplace, 49
    Health Care Quality, 53
    Quality Improvement and Quality Assurance, 61
    Ethical Issues in Managed Behavioral Health Care, 67
    Summary, 71

3   CHALLENGES IN DELIVERY OF BEHAVIORAL
    HEALTH CARE   76
    Extent and Impact of Behavioral Health Problems, 77
    The Role of Primary Care, 87
    Special Issues for Quality in Behavioral Health Care, 89
    Developments in the Private Sector, 93
    Quality and Consumer Protection Challenges, 95
    Variability at the State Level, 95
    Historical Perspective on Systems, 96
    Summary: System Integration, 115

4   STRUCTURE   122
    Practitioner Issues, 123
    Medicaid, 128
    Medicare, 130
    Substance Abuse Service Systems, 131
    Mental Health Treatment, 135
    Wraparound Services, 136
    The Managed Behavioral Health Care Industry, 141
    Workplace Services, 142
    U.S. Department of Defense and U.S. Department of Veterans Affairs, 148
    Care and Services for Children and Adolescents, 152
    Care and Services for Seniors, 156
    Indian Health Service, 157
    Cultural Competence, 159
    Rural Health and Managed Care, 162
    Summary of Structural Issues, 163

5   ACCESS   168
    Importance of Assessing Access, 169
    Measures of Access, 171
    Need and Access, 174
    Needs of Special Populations, 175
    Measuring Access to Services Within Managed Care Organizations, 178
    Summary, 179

6   PROCESS   184
    Quality and Accountability, 184
    Quality Management in Behavioral Health Care, 189
    Performance Measurement in the Public Sector, 199
    Accreditation, 203
    Information Infrastructure for Quality Measurement, 217

Role of Government in Quality Assurance, 218
Summary, 223

7   OUTCOMES   226
Definitions of Success, 226
General and Specific Measures of Outcomes, 228
Links Among Structure, Process, and Outcomes, 232
Performance Indicators as Outcomes Measures, 233
Efficacy and Effectiveness, 234
Outcomes and Quality Improvement, 234
Criteria for Evaluating Outcomes Measures, 235
Summary, 238

8   FINDINGS AND RECOMMENDATIONS   241
   1.   Structure and Financing, 242
   2.   Accreditation, 243
   3.   Consumer Involvement, 247
   4.   Cultural Competence, 248
   5.   Special Populations, 249
   6.   Research, 249
   7.   Workplace, 250
   8.   Wraparound Services, 251
   9.   Children and Adolescents, 251
   10. Clinical Practice Guidelines, 252
   11. Primary Care, 253
   12. Ethical Concerns, 254

GLOSSARY   255

APPENDIXES
A   Committee Biographies   263
B   Commissioned Paper: Can the Outcomes Research Literature
    Inform the Search for Quality Indicators in Substance Abuse
    Treatment?, *A. Thomas McLellan, Mark Belding, James R. McKay,*
    David Zanis, and Arthur I. Alterman   271
C   Commissioned Paper: Consumer Outcomes and Managed
    Behavioral Health Care: Research Priorities, *Donald M. Steinwachs* 312
D   Public Workshop Agendas and Participants   336
E   Liaison Panel Members to the Committee   349
F   OrganizationsThat Submitted Written Materials to the Committee   355

INDEX   357

LIST OF TABLES, FIGURES, AND BOXES

TABLES

Table 1.1   Estimated Annual Prevalence of Behavioral Health Problems in the United States (Ages 15–54), 16
Table 1.2   U.S. Health Insurance Data (in millions), 1992–1995, 29
Table 1.3   Utilization of Services for Behavioral Health Problems, 30

Table 2.1   Types of Managed Care Organizations, 43
Table 2.2   Ecology of Consumer Protection: Current Context, 55

Table 3.1   Estimated Annual Prevalence of Behavioral Health Problems in the United States (Ages 15–54), 78
Table 3.2a Sample of Estimated Annual Prevalence of Behavioral Health Problems in Children and Adolescents, 79
Table 3.2b Estimated Annual Prevalence of Drug Use Among Children and Adolescents, 1995, 80
Table 3.3   Estimated Annual Economic Costs of Substance Abuse, 1990 (millions), 81
Table 3.4   Estimated Annual Economic Costs of Mental Disorders by Disorder, 1990 (millions), 82
Table 3.5   Estimated Annual Costs of Illness for Selected Diseases and Conditions (billions of dollars), 83
Table 3.6   Uses of Funds for Mental Health and Substance Abuse: United States, 1990, 92

Table 4.1   Profiles of U.S. Practitioners in Behavioral Health Care, 124
Table 4.2   Medicaid and Medicare Total Populations and Number Enrolled in Managed Care (MC) Plans, 1991–1995, 130
Table 4.3   Types of Care in Substance Abuse Treatment, 132
Table 4.4   Mental Health Treatment Settings, 137
Table 4.5   Comparison of Public and Private Sectors of Care in Mental Health, 138
Table 4.6   "Wraparound" and "Enabling" Services, 140

Table 6.1   Cross-Comparison of Managed Behavioral Health Care Performance Indicators, 192
Table 6.2   Cross-Comparison of Selected Accreditation Organizations in Managed Behavioral Health Care, 206
Table 6.3   Selected Regulatory and Consumer Protection Models, 220
Table 6.4   Desirable Attributes of a Quality Assurance Program, 223

Table 7.1   Substance Abuse-Specific Outcomes Objectives by Level of
             Treatment, 229
Table 7.2   General Outcomes Measures for Substance Abuse and Mental
             Health Populations, 230
Table 7.3   Performance Indicators Based on Outcomes Research, 233

FIGURES

Figure 1.1   Number of HMO enrollees, 1976–1995, 32
Figure 1.2   Framework for quality assessment, 34
Figure 7.1   Model for research on the quality of mental health services, 231

BOXES

Box 1.1   Terminology Used in This Report, 23
Box 2.1   National Demonstration Project on Quality Improvement
             in Health Care: Applications and Implementation, 63
Box 3.1   The Case for Treatment of Mental Disorders and Addiction, 86
Box 3.2   Historical Perspective on the Development of Behavioral
             Health Systems, 97
Box 5.1   Sample Access Standards and Measures for Behavioral
             Health Care, 172

Acronyms

AA	Alcoholics Anonymous
AAAHC	Accreditation Association for Ambulatory Health Care
AAAP	American Academy of Addiction Psychiatry
AAFP	American Academy of Family Physicians
AAHP	American Association of Health Plans
AAMFT	American Association of Marriage and Family Therapy
AAPCHO	Association of Asian Pacific Community Health Organizations
ABA	American Bar Association
ABMS	American Board of Medical Specialties
ABPN	American Board of Psychiatry and Neurology
ACPM	American College of Preventive Medicine
ADAMHA	Alcohol, Drug Abuse, and Mental Health Administration
AFDC	Aid to Families with Dependent Children
AHCPR	Agency for Health Care Policy and Research
AIDS	Acquired Immune Deficiency Syndrome
AMA	American Medical Association
AMBHA	American Managed Behavioral Healthcare Association
AMTA	American Methadone Treatment Association
ANA	American Nurses Association
APWA	American Public Welfare Association
ASAM	American Society of Addiction Medicine
ASI	Addiction Severity Index
ASTHO	Association of State and Territorial Health Officials

CAC	certified addiction counselor
CARF	Rehabilitation Accreditation Commission, formerly the Commission on Accreditation of Rehabilitation Facilities
CASSP	Child and Adolescent Service System Program
CCMC	Committee on the Costs of Medical Care
CD	chemical dependency
CDC	Centers for Disease Control and Prevention
CHAMPUS	Civilian Health and Medical Program of the Uniformed Services
CHAMPVA	Civilian Health and Medical Program of the Veterans Administration
CMHC	Community Mental Health Centers
CMHS	Center for Mental Health Services
CNSTAT	Committee on National Statistics, part of the National Research Council
COA	Council on Accreditation of Services for Families and Children
CONQUEST	Computerized Needs-Oriented Quality Measurements Evaluation System
COSSHMO	National Coalition of Hispanic Health and Human Services Organizations
CQI	continuous quality improvement
CSAM	California Society on Addiction Medicine
CSAP	Center for Substance Abuse Prevention
CSAT	Center for Substance Abuse Treatment
CSP	Community Support Program
DHHS	Department of Health and Human Services
DOD	Department of Defense
DUF	Drug Use Forecasting
EAP	employee assistance program
EAPA	Employee Assistance Professional Association
ECA	epidemiologic catchment area
EPSDT	early and periodic screening, diagnosis, and treatment
ERISA	Employee Retirement Income Security Act
FACCT	Foundation for Accountability
FDA	Food and Drug Administration
FFS	fee-for-service
HCFA	Health Care Financing Administration
HEDIS	Health Plan Employer Data and Information Set, developed by NCQA
HIAA	Health Insurance Association of America
HIV	human immunodeficiency virus
HMO	health maintenance organization

HRSA	Health Resources and Services Administration
IBH	Institute for Behavioral Healthcare
IHS	Indian Health Service
IOM	Institute of Medicine
IPA	Independent Practice Association
JCAH	Joint Commission on Accreditation of Hospitals
JCAHO	Joint Commission on Accreditation of Healthcare Organizations
LAAM	levo-alpha-acetylmethadol
MBHC	managed behavioral health care
MBHO	managed behavioral health care organization
MC	managed care
MET	motivational enhancement therapy
MHSIP	Mental Health Statistics Improvement Program
MOS	Medical Outcomes Study, conducted by the RAND Corporation
MR/DD	mentally retarded and developmentally disabled
MSO	management services organization
NA	Narcotics Anonymous
NAADAC	National Association of Alcoholism and Drug Abuse Counselors
NACCHO	National Association of County and City Health Officials
NACMBHD	National Association of County Managed Behavioral Health Directors
NAHDO	National Association of Health Data Organizations
NAIC	National Association of Insurance Commissioners
NAMI	National Alliance for the Mentally Ill
NARSD	National Association for Research on Schizophrenia and Depression
NASADAD	National Association of State Alcohol and Drug Abuse Directors
NASMHPD	National Association of State Mental Health Program Directors
NASW	National Association of Social Workers
NBCH	National Business Coalition on Health
NCHS	National Center for Health Statistics
NCQA	National Committee for Quality Assurance
NDATUS	National Drug and Alcohol Treatment Unit Survey
NDMDA	National Depressive and Manic Depressive Association
NEC	National Empowerment Center
NFSCSW	National Federation of Societies for Clinical Social Work
NGA	National Governors' Association
NIAAA	National Institute on Alcohol Abuse and Alcoholism

NIDA   National Institute on Drug Abuse
NIH   National Institutes of Health
NIMH   National Institute of Mental Health
NMHA   National Mental Health Association
NTIES   National Treatment Improvement Evaluation Study
PACT   Program in Assertive Community Treatment
PBGH   Pacific Business Group on Health
PERMS   Performance-Based Measures for Managed Behavioral
              Healthcare Program, developed by AMBHA
PHO   physician hospital organization
PHS   Public Health Service
PO   physician organization
POS   point-of-service plan
PPO   preferred provider organization
RTI   Research Triangle Institute
SAIC   Science Applications International Corporation
SAMHSA   Substance Abuse and Mental Health Services
              Administration
SAODAP   Special Action Office for Drug Abuse Prevention
SEC   Securities and Exchange Commission
SMHRCY   State Mental Health Representatives for Children and Youth
SSDI   Social Security Disability Insurance
SSI   Supplemental Security Income
TASC   Treatment Alternatives for Special Clients, formerly
              Treatment Alternatives to Street Crime
TB   tuberculosis
TCA   Therapeutic Communities of America
TEDS   Treatment Episode Data Set
UFDS   Uniform Facility Data Survey
UM   utilization management
UR   utilization review
URAC   Utilization Review Accreditation Commission
URICA   University of Rhode Island Change Assessment
VA   Department of Veterans Affairs, formerly Veterans
              Administration
WBGH   Washington Business Group on Health
WFMH   World Federation for Mental Health

MANAGING MANAGED CARE
QUALITY IMPROVEMENT IN
BEHAVIORAL HEALTH

Summary

With great speed and a considerable amount of controversy, managed care has produced dramatic changes in American health care. At the end of 1995, 161 million Americans—more than 60 percent of the total population—belonged to some form of managed health care plan. Health maintenance organizations (HMOs), preferred provider organizations, point-of-service plans, and other forms of managed care networks differ in organizational structures, types of practitioners and services, access strategies, payment for practitioners, and other features. Their goals, however, are similar: to control costs through improved efficiency and coordination, to reduce unnecessary or inappropriate utilization, to increase access to preventive care, and to maintain or improve the quality of care.

The movement into managed care has been especially rapid for treatment of mental health and substance abuse (alcohol and drug) problems, also known as *behavioral health*. Behavioral health problems are common: every year, an estimated 52 million Americans have some kind of mental health or substance abuse problem. At the end of 1995, the behavioral health benefits of nearly 142 million people were managed, with 124 million in specialty managed behavioral health programs and 16.9 million with benefits managed within an HMO.

Both private-sector employers and public-sector agencies (Medicaid and state mental health and substance abuse authorities) have turned to managed behavioral health care companies to control costs and improve quality and access for mental health and substance abuse care. Purchasers share with responsible managed care organizations a unifying goal of a more responsive health care delivery system, one that is both more efficient and more effective. Several approaches have been developed to assess the quality of care: accreditation, licensing and certification, credentialing and privileging, and the use of practice guidelines, performance measures, report cards, and other means. Thus, the array of quality improvement approaches resembles a complex patchwork, reflecting the fragmented system that delivers the care and the wide variety of evidence and opinions about quality of care.

TECHNICAL APPROACH

In the spring of 1995, the Center for Substance Abuse Treatment (CSAT), part of the Substance Abuse and Mental Health Services Administration (SAMHSA), asked the Institute of Medicine to convene an expert committee that would consider issues related to quality assurance and accreditation in managed behavioral health care. The charge to the committee was to develop a framework to guide the development, use, and evaluation of performance indicators, accreditation standards, and quality improvement mechanisms. The framework could then be used to assist in the purchase and delivery of the most effective managed behavioral health care at the lowest appropriate cost for consumers of publicly and privately financed care. The 17 members of the committee were chosen for their expertise with national accreditation processes and procedures, public and private managed care organizations, employee assistance programs, corporate and public purchasing of mental health and substance abuse services, public and private medical administration, and health services research. The committee also included individuals who had experience as direct consumers of behavioral health care or who were family members of consumers.

The committee met five times between February and July 1996. To gather information to assist in their deliberations, the committee convened two public workshops. In addition to these workshops and presentations, liaison panels were formed with more than 150 representatives of national accreditation groups, national professional associations, consumer and advocacy groups, managed care industry groups, and federal and state agencies.

Many interested parties are using a variety of methods to protect consumers and improve the quality of care in this environment of rapid change. The charge and focus of this committee is on managed care, although the committee recognizes that other issues such as licensure of practitioners and state inspection and certification of provider agencies play critical roles in consumer protection. Furthermore, in its focus on managed care, the committee has been particularly concerned with two prominent strategies: accreditation of managed care entities and the use of performance measurements. At the same time, it has considered complementary strategies that can aid in consumer protection and quality improvements, such as consumer choice of health plans, better integration of research and practice, and especially, reducing the flaws in the organization of behavioral health care.

To provide a framework for the study, the committee adapted the work of

Avedis Donabedian, who has described three interrelated ways to understand and measure quality: structure, process, and outcomes. Structural measures of quality include the types of services available, the qualifications of practitioners, staffing patterns, adherence to building and other codes, and other administrative information. Process measures of quality focus on procedures and courses of treatment, such as the numbers of individuals served; on the appropriateness of the care; and on ongoing efforts to maintain quality, such as practice guidelines and continuous quality improvement activities. Outcome measures of quality include health status changes after treatment and consumer satisfaction with the care provided, as well as short-term or intermediate outcomes.

CHALLENGES TO DELIVERY OF BEHAVIORAL HEALTH CARE

The most unusual aspect of the care and financing system for behavioral health care services is the presence of a distinct and substantial publicly managed care system that serves as a safety net. Thus, public services are available for those with public insurance as well as for those with private insurance. Public services are funded through a large number of categorical programs administered by different agencies, creating both duplication and gaps in service, and these programs almost always have different eligibility requirements. Fragmentation in funding leads to fragmented service delivery.

Another challenge is that much of behavioral health care, perhaps as many as half of all episodes of care, is provided in primary care settings, not in specialty programs. Despite clinical practice guidelines, continuing education courses, and other training programs, primary care providers tend to underdiagnose depression, substance abuse, and other behavioral health problems. This is changing, but there is a great need to improve the quality of behavioral health care delivered in primary care settings and to better coordinate the care delivered in primary care and specialty sectors.

In addition, a significant portion of the public care system for individuals with the most disabling conditions extends beyond health care services to rehabilitative and support services, including housing, job counseling, literacy, and other programs. The coordination of these services requires collaborative and cooperative relationships among many agencies, including public health, mental health, social services, housing, education, criminal justice, and others. Most of these services are not covered by private insurance and have not been developed by most private behavioral health care companies.

The dynamics of the three interrelated sectors—privately funded primary and specialty care and public systems—are complex and also highly idiosyncratic from state to state, community to community, and plan to plan. Any approach to reform of behavioral health care services or to the problem of accountability must reckon with these factors, which are not simultaneously present in any other substantial sector of the health care system.

STRUCTURE

Analysis of the structure of the behavioral health care service system requires a review of the public and private service systems for both substance abuse and mental illness. The behavioral health care delivery system involves a complex combination of public and private financing as well as public and private practitioners of care. Public-sector services are financed either with state and federal appropriations or through Medicaid and Medicare coverage and are delivered in a wide variety of treatment settings. Private systems of care have different structures but coexist and often overlap with public sector services. Workplace service systems (e.g., employee assistance programs) and managed behavioral health care strategies have had a stronger influence in the private sector, but they are beginning to develop linkages with public agencies.

Federally supported service systems developed by the U.S. Department of Defense and the U.S. Department of Veterans Affairs share characteristics of both the private- and public-sector systems of care but represent separate and distinct service systems. In addition, service systems also exist for distinct populations: children, seniors, and Native Americans. The existence of a large number of independent service delivery systems serving different populations through different funding streams complicates the assessment of quality and can inhibit the development and implementation of comprehensive standards to improve the quality of care.

ACCESS

Managed behavioral health care organizations define access and accessibility using utilization (e.g., penetration rates and the use of specific services) and telecommunication (e.g., on-hold time and call abandonment rates) measures. Purchasers, however, may prefer to view access more broadly and include reductions in barriers to care and improvements in benefits (e.g., reductions in copayments, increases in hours of service, reductions in travel time, and expanded eligibility for specific services or populations).

The nature of managed care and the nature of mental illness and substance abuse combine to make access a most critical issue. Well-developed public and private health care and behavioral health care plans will promote access to mental health and substance abuse services. Enrollees that access care promptly and early in their illness episode may require less intensive care, and with appropriate continuing support they may be less likely to experience relapses.

Measures of access, however, should go beyond telephone answering time and begin to reflect the real and perceived barriers to care including cultural differences, geographic distance, inconvenient locations and times, and care that is less intensive than needed. Moreover, the purchasers of health care plans and the plan administrators must begin to assess the adequacy of their current access. Information on the ambient level of need in the health plan is required to truly assess the adequacy of the plan in meeting the demand and need for care.

PROCESS

In broad terms, measurement of the quality of health care is driven by different forces in the private and public sectors. In the private sector, quality measurement is a reflection of the requirements of the accreditation process and is increasingly a response to the demands of employers and other purchasers through contracting, report cards, and other means. In the public sector, performance measurement is the primary tool of accountability for spending public funds on health care.

Many methods are used to assess quality: accreditation, licensing and certification, credentialing, auditing, peer review, performance monitoring, contracts, clinical standards and guidelines, consumer satisfaction surveys, and report cards. Some private payers have developed their own standards for HMOs and other managed care organizations that provide care and are also urging contracted organizations to collect and publicly report information on their performance. Public agencies are also developing performance standards.

The interest in quality is reinforced by consumer demand and empowerment, professional ethics, legal and regulatory interpretation of citizens' rights, and attempts by businesses to satisfy and keep customers in a competitive health care marketplace. For public purchasers who are accountable for public funds, it is important to demonstrate that health care has good value and is worth the investment.

OUTCOMES

In the committee's view, outcomes research is vitally important to improve the base of evidence related to treatment effectiveness. Outcomes research is needed to provide explicit direction in identifying performance indicators associated with good outcomes for different patient characteristics, types of treatment programs, and types of managed care organizations. In their current forms, performance indicators are not specific for particular treatment characteristics (organizational and clinical), and there is a lack of consensus of clinical judgment with regard to the relationship to outcome.

Public interest in quality of care is keen, and purchasers are not waiting for conclusive outcomes research to help them make decisions on the value and effectiveness of different managed care options. However, much needs to be done to link findings from outcomes research with the development of practice guidelines, performance measures, and accreditation approaches. Future methods of quality assessment will need to bridge the domains of research and practice and will need to provide more direct input into the development of accreditation and other assessment strategies.

HIGHLIGHTS OF FINDINGS AND RECOMMENDATIONS

Federal, state, and local governments, accreditation organizations, managed care organizations, purchaser coalitions, consumers groups, professional organizations, and the media are actively involved in quality assessment. Some of these efforts are collaborative, but some are competitive. Overall, the picture is incomplete, inconsistent, and inadequate for making truly informed health care purchasing decisions. To those who are responsible for purchasing care, the absence of consensus on quality measurements is a challenge.

The committee developed a set of findings and recommendations in 12 areas: structure and financing; accreditation; consumer involvement; cultural competence; special populations; research; workplace; wraparound services; children and adolescents; clinical practice guidelines; primary care; and ethical concerns. Chapter 8 of this report contains all of the findings and recommendations. Only the recommendations are presented in this Summary.

1. STRUCTURE AND FINANCING

Recommendations

1.1   The reform of systems of care financed by states and counties must: (1) recognize current aspects of private health care in those states and counties and (2) consider the design and development of mechanisms to inhibit cost-shifting.

1.2   Payment arrangements that reduce incentives to underserve individuals with behavioral health conditions should be encouraged.

1.3   The reform of state and local systems through the use of managed care should incorporate a recognition of and responsiveness to the unique needs of consumers served by public systems.

1.4   Accreditation organizations, when appropriate, and purchasers should develop criteria and guidelines that: (1) recognize and measure dumping, skimming, and cost-shifting; and (2) specify rewards for organizations, groups, and individuals that provide appropriate care and penalties for those that do not.

1.5   Purchasers should ensure continuity of care for consumers when managed care contracts are awarded to different provider organizations.

2. ACCREDITATION

Recommendations

Monitoring Quality of Care

2.1   Public and private purchasers, consumers, providers, practitioners, behavioral health care plans, and accreditation organizations should continue to monitor and assess the quality of care in the following ways:

2.1.1   Quality improvement should be a priority, and principles and methods of improving quality should be adopted.

2.1.2   Accreditation and review processes must be reliable and valid and must be continuously reviewed and improved.

2.1.3   Domains relevant to the effective treatment and prevention of behavioral health problems must be emphasized in accreditation processes. These include practitioner training, consumer education, improvements in consumer self-care, and the presence of a continuum of services, including wraparound services such as housing assistance, child care, and transportation.

2.1.4   Accreditation processes must focus on areas of managed care in which there may be a risk of quality problems: (1) variability in utilization review; (2) inconsistent or inappropriate precertification processes; (3) vulnerable groups and those who are unfamiliar with managed care processes; and (4) conditions that occur frequently and are treated by many practitioners, giving opportunities for variation in treatment practices.

2.1.5   Performance measures must be relevant to treatment processes and outcomes.

2.1.6   Data must have demonstrable integrity. External, independent audits can help to validate data quality.

2.1.7   Stakeholder consensus and consumer satisfaction measures must be included in the tools used to monitor quality of care.

2.1.8   Outcomes measures should increasingly be based on evidence from research.

Contracting

2.2   Quality of care should be clearly addressed in contracts between purchasers and providers.

2.2.1   When plans contract or subcontract for the management and delivery of behavioral health care services (e.g., health maintenance organizations contracting with carved-out managed behavioral health care firms), purchasers can benefit from independent audits of the contractor regarding the level of adherence to prespecified standards of performance with respect to quality.

2.2.2   Purchasers can benefit from carefully constructed contract language to ensure the quality, accessibility, and effectiveness of behavioral health plans. Contracts should also specify the ways in which the quality and effectiveness standards will be monitored and enforced, including conditions for applying positive incentives for meeting or exceeding the standards and penalties for substandard performance.

Role of the Federal Government

2.3   The federal government should play a role in consumer protection in managed care by:

2.3.1   Promoting the improvement and use of performance measures for managed care.

2.3.2   Monitoring and studying the use and effectiveness of quality assurance, accreditation, performance measures, and outcomes measurements.

2.3.3   Establishing minimum standards for accreditation organizations to achieve deemed status (i.e., when the government, in its role as purchaser of managed care services, accepts accreditation as a measure of adequate quality and consumer protection).

Role of State Governments

2.4   The role of state governments in consumer protection should include the following:

2.4.1   Support the development of consumer protection standards for managed behavioral health care by state mental health and substance abuse agencies, state Medicaid agencies, state insurance departments, state licensing boards, state hospitals, and state child welfare agencies. State consumer groups, such as the chapters of the National Mental Health Association (NMHA), National Depressive and Manic Depressive Association (NDMDA), National Association for Research on Schizophrenia and Depression (NARSD), and National Alliance for the Mentally Ill (NAMI), should be included in the development of standards.

2.4.2   Maintain the minimum necessary regulatory standards, including the use of accreditation, to assure consumer protection while encouraging innovations in the delivery of care.

2.4.3   Consider offering deemed status to specific accreditation organizations that meet state-defined standards for quality of managed behavioral health care services.

Roles of All Levels of Government

2.5   Both federal and state governments should:

2.5.1   Encourage the development of report cards or other similar materials to help inform consumers and families about specific plans and the quality of care.

2.5.2   Include all stakeholders (accreditation organizations, employers, state agencies, consumers, families, providers, and practitioners) in the development, implementation, and use of standards.

Provider Inclusion

2.6   Because managed care methods are increasingly applied to public systems, accreditation bodies and managed care plans should evaluate the inclusion of a variety of types of practitioners, including substance abuse counselors and mental health workers, in provider panels; collect information on practitioner effectiveness; and remove any practitioners from networks only for performance reasons (e.g., poor outcomes and poor consumer satisfaction).

2.6.1   The Substance Abuse and Mental Health Services Administration (SAMHSA), Agency for Health Care Policy and Research (AHCPR), Health Resources and Services Administration (HRSA), and National Institutes of Health (NIH) (National Institute on Alcohol Abuse and Alcoholism [NIAAA], National Institute on Drug Abuse [NIDA], and National Institute of Mental Health [NIMH]) should cosponsor research to evaluate the components of treatment that are most effective in providing behavioral health care, including strategies used by psychiatrists, psychologists, social workers, counselors, and primary care practitioners.

2.6.2   The Substance Abuse and Mental Health Services Administration (SAMHSA), Agency for Health Care Policy and Research (AHCPR), Health Resources and Services Administration (HRSA), and National Institutes of Health (NIH) (National Institute on Alcohol Abuse and Alcoholism [NIAAA], National Institute on Drug Abuse [NIDA], and National Institute of Mental Health [NIMH]) should cosponsor research to evaluate the cost-effectiveness of using different practitioner types to provide behavioral health care, including individual psychiatrists, psychologists, social workers, counselors, primary care practitioners, and teams with different practitioner combinations.

3. CONSUMER INVOLVEMENT

Recommendations

3.1   Health care purchasers must be responsive to consumers and families and should develop means of ensuring their meaningful participation in treatment decisions, measurement of satisfaction, and measurement of treatment effectiveness.

3.2   Accreditation bodies should evaluate the extent of inclusion of consumers and families in treatment decisions and program planning.

3.3   The activities that are used to develop and review quality measures should include all stakeholders, including consumers, families, practitioners, and researchers.

4. CULTURAL COMPETENCE

Recommendations

4.1   Health plans and programs should be responsive to community demographics and to the cultural needs of the populations that they serve.

4.2   Practitioners of alternative and innovative treatments without an accepted research base should not arbitrarily be excluded from health plans. If these treatments are used, their effectiveness should be studied so that standards of quality improvement can be developed.

4.3   Health plans should have an explicit mechanism for evaluating new and innovative techniques and types of practitioners.

5. SPECIAL POPULATIONS

Recommendations

5.1   Research is needed to identify incentives for plans to serve vulnerable populations. The Substance Abuse and Mental Health Services Administration (SAMHSA) should work with other federal agencies to develop a plan to conduct such research.

5.2   Plans that serve distinct populations should measure and evaluate the needs of those groups through reviews of research literature, consumer surveys, and other appropriate mechanisms.

5.3   All plans should meet the same core standards. Supplemental standards can be developed for special populations, whether they are in stand-alone programs or in mainstream plans, for example, for a child of an employed person with family coverage.

6. RESEARCH

Recommendations

6.1   The committee recommends continued development of collaborative health services research in substance abuse and mental health, and encourages the Agency for Health Care Policy and Research (AHCPR), Centers for Disease Control and Prevention (CDC), Health Resources and Services Administration (HRSA), National Institutes of Health (NIH) (National Institute on Alcohol Abuse and Alcoholism [NIAAA], National Institute on Drug Abuse [NIDA], and the National Institute of Mental Health [NIMH]), and Substance Abuse and Mental Health Services Administration (SAMHSA) to maintain, to evaluate, and, where necessary, to expand programs and initiatives that support collaborative health services research.

6.2   The agencies mentioned above should support further research on the effectiveness of different treatment strategies for a variety of practitioner types and for consumers with different needs.

6.3   Researchers should become more involved in studies carried out in managed care organizations and community-based settings and in other clinical outcomes research used to develop standards and performance measures.

7. WORKPLACE

Recommendations

7.1   Employers should investigate the benefits of wellness activities, employee assistance programs, and health risk reduction initiatives that enhance prevention, early intervention, access, and treatment adherence for health and behavioral health problems.

7.2   The Substance Abuse and Mental Health Services Administration (SAMHSA) should identify models of successful behavioral health programs in the workplace and increase public awareness of these models.

8. WRAPAROUND SERVICES

Recommendations

8.1   Further research is needed to prioritize the essential components of a treatment regimen that can address adequately the complex behavioral aspects of recovery from alcoholism and other drug addictions.

8.2   To maximize full functioning for individuals with severe and persistent mental illness, and to optimize conditions supporting recovery for individuals with chronic substance abuse problems, wraparound services such as social welfare, housing, vocational, and rehabilitative services should be available and should be coordinated.

8.3   For children and adolescents with severe emotional disturbances, educational and home environment-family support services should be coordinated and integrated with mental health care.

8.4   Accreditation systems must address the social and rehabilitative aspects as well as the medical aspects of comprehensive treatment for addiction and severe and persistent mental illness.

9. CHILDREN AND ADOLESCENTS

Recommendations

9.1   The Substance Abuse and Mental Health Services Administration (SAMHSA), National Institutes of Health (NIH) (National Institute on Alcoholism and Alcohol Abuse [NIAAA], National Institute on Drug Abuse [NIDA], and National Institute of Mental Health [NIMH]), and the Health Research and Services Administration (HRSA) should identify exemplary models of coordinated systems of care for children and adolescents.

9.2   The Substance Abuse and Mental Health Services Administration (SAMHSA), National Institutes of Health (NIH) (National Institute on Alcoholism and Alcohol Abuse [NIAAA], National Institute on Drug Abuse [NIDA], and National Institute of Mental Health [NIMH]), and the Health Resources and Services Administration (HRSA) should identify exemplary models of linking behavioral health treatment and prevention programs for children and adolescents to address suicide, substance abuse, and other areas.

9.3   The Substance Abuse and Mental Health Services Administration (SAMHSA), National Institutes of Health (NIH) (National Institute on Alcoholism and Alcohol Abuse [NIAAA], National Institute on Drug Abuse [NIDA], and National Institute of Mental Health [NIMH]), and the Health Resources and Services Administration (HRSA) should support research to identify the elements of developmentally appropriate treatment that should be available to adolescents who are abusing alcohol or drugs or who have mental health problems.

9.4   The public and private systems must make efforts to develop service capabilities to meet the needs of adolescents who are abusing alcohol or drugs and adolescents who have mental health problems.

10. CLINICAL PRACTICE GUIDELINES

Recommendations

10.1   The development of clinical practice guidelines should be linked to outcomes research, performance standards, and accreditation.

10.2   The Agency for Health Care Policy and Research (AHCPR), Substance Abuse and Mental Health Services Administration (SAMHSA), and other agencies and organizations that develop guidelines should sponsor additional research that examines the successful implementation of guidelines and identifies successful implementation models.

10.3 Practitioners and consumers should be included in the development of practice guidelines.

11. PRIMARY CARE

Recommendations

11.1 This committee endorses the view of the Institute of Medicine (IOM) Committee on the Future of Primary Care, which recommended "the reduction of financial and organizational disincentives for the expanded role of primary care in the provision of mental health services" and "the development and evaluation of collaborative care models that integrate primary care and mental health services more effectively. These models should involve both primary care clinicians and mental health professionals" (IOM, 1996, p. 137).

11.2 This committee recommends that the above recommendation include alcohol and other drug abuse problems as a defined area of expertise.

12. ETHICAL CONCERNS

Recommendations

12.1 Managed care organizations should be able to demonstrate that they recognize and have concern for the ethical risks created by managed care systems. Additionally, they should substantiate the use of safeguards that protect and maintain ethical standards and practices. These would include the following:

- a clear description of a plan, its benefits, and grievance procedures,
- accessible and responsive grievance, complaint, and appeals procedures,
- effective strategies to maintain confidentiality while meeting the needs of practitioners to coordinate care,
- culturally appropriate and gender-specific service practitioners in the network,
- consumer surveys and measures of consumer satisfaction,
- consumer representation on policy development and grievance resolution,
- continuous improvement protocols to promote better outcomes, and
- no contractual or other limitations for physicians and other practitioners concerning the discussion of clinically appropriate treatment options with patients and families.

12.2 A careful review of ethical issues in various settings, for example, managed care organizations, networks, and fee-for-service settings, is needed. The Substance Abuse and Mental Health Services Administration (SAMHSA), Health Care Financing Agency (HCFA), and Agency for Health Care Policy and Research (AHCPR) should develop a plan to examine ethical issues.

REFERENCE

IOM (Institute of Medicine). 1996. *Primary Care: America's Health in a New Era.* Washington, DC: National Academy Press.

1

Introduction

With great speed and a considerable amount of controversy, managed care has produced dramatic changes in American health care. At the end of 1995, 161 million Americans—more than 60 percent of the total population—belonged to some form of managed health care plan (HIAA, 1996a). The movement into managed care has been especially rapid for the treatment of mental health and substance abuse (alcohol and drug) problems, also known as *behavioral health*. Behavioral health problems are common: every year, an estimated 52 million Americans have some kind of mental health or substance abuse problem (see Table 1.1). At the end of 1995, the behavioral health benefits of nearly 142 million people were managed, with 124 million in specialty managed behavioral health programs and 16.9 million in an HMO (Open Minds, 1996).

Health maintenance organizations (HMOs), preferred provider organizations (PPOs), point-of-service plans, and other forms of managed care networks, such as managed behavioral health care organizations, differ in their organizational structures, types of practitioners and services, access strategies, payment for practitioners, and other features. Their goals, however, are similar: to control costs through improved efficiency and coordination, to reduce unnecessary or inappropriate utilization, to increase access to preventive care, and to maintain or improve the quality of care (IOM, 1996a; Miller and Luft, 1994).

Both private-sector employers and public-sector agencies (Medicaid and state mental health and substance abuse authorities) have turned to managed behavioral health care companies to control costs and improve quality and access for mental health and substance abuse care. Traditionally, mental health and substance abuse care benefits have been more limited compared with benefits for

15

TABLE 1.1 Estimated Annual Prevalence of Behavioral Health Problems in the United States (Ages 15–54)

Behavioral Health Problems	Prevalence (percent)	No. of People (millions)
All behavioral health problems (i.e., mental disorders, alcoholism, and drug addiction)	29.5	52
Any mental disorder	22.9	40
Any substance abuse or dependence (i.e., alcohol and illicit drugs)	11.3	20
Both mental disorder and substance abuse or dependence	4.7	8

NOTE: Prevalence data have been collected from the National Comorbidity Survey (NCS), a Congressionally mandated survey designed to study the comorbidity of substance use disorders and nonsubstance use-related psychiatric disorders in the United States. The survey was administered by the staff of the Survey Research Center at the University of Michigan between 1990 and 1992. NCS surveyed 8,098 noninstitutionalized participants with a structured psychiatric interview conducted by lay interviewers using a revised version of the Composite International Diagnostic Interview (CIDI). CIDI is a structured diagnostic interview based on the National Institute of Mental Health's (NIMH's) Diagnostic Interview Schedule, which can be used by trained interviewers who are not clinicians (Kessler et al., 1994).

SOURCE: Kessler et al. (1994) and SAMHSA (1995).

physical health, and for mental health and substance abuse care there also have been few alternatives to hospitalization. In the late 1980s, the majority (70 percent) of mental health funds spent by Medicaid and private insurance went for inpatient care, leading many researchers, clinicians, and advocates to question the imbalance and to search for policy changes. Only the introduction of managed care arrangements has led to a significant shift away from costly and often unnecessary inpatient stays to a more appropriate range of outpatient and community-based care. In sum, behavioral health care offers purchasers the potential to spread existing resources farther by paying for less intensive (and less expensive) treatment strategies that can return patients to a reasonable level of functioning, such as being able to return to work or school (England and Vaccaro, 1991).

The controversies in managed care are less about the goal of cost reductions and are more about the ways in which cost reductions are achieved. Methods of cost control include authorizing only certain practitioners who are under contract to provide services to an enrolled population, reviewing treatment decisions, closely monitoring high-cost cases, reducing the number of days for inpatient hospital stays, and increasing the use of less expensive alternatives to hospitalization (Iglehart, 1996; Shore and Beigel, 1996).

In the committee's view, managed care strategies are not inherently harmful and can be appropriate and helpful, as in the shift from inpatient to outpatient care, the additional supervision for complex cases, and applications of standards based on best practices. However, certain activities of companies that provide behavioral health care, such as limiting or denying services that are considered to be needed, adding barriers to access to care such as increased copayments for outpatient visits, and adding gatekeepers who change the practitioner-patient relationship, are viewed as having an adverse impact on the quality of care (Mechanic et al., 1995).

The overall impact of managed care on the quality of health care is difficult to determine. Managed care has many structures, making comparisons across organizational forms (e.g., HMOs vs. PPOs) difficult. In addition, the quality of health care is difficult to measure and define because of the complexity of health care. The Institute of Medicine (IOM) has defined quality of care as "the degree to which health services for individuals and populations increase the likelihood of desired health outcomes and are consistent with current professional knowledge" (IOM, 1990a, p. 21).

Definition of Quality of Care

The degree to which health services for individuals and populations increase the likelihood of desired health outcomes and are consistent with current professional knowledge (IOM, 1990a, p. 21).

Adopting this definition would suggest an array of health services research based on the variations of each component: health services (e.g., primary care and specialty drug abuse, alcoholism, and mental health treatment in different practice settings, including hospital-based and office-based practices and health centers), individuals (e.g., differences among children, adolescents, adults, and seniors, as well as gender differences), populations (e.g., cultural differences and differences between rural and urban populations), and outcomes (e.g., cure, relapse prevention, and return to functioning). The combinations are virtually unlimited.

Public interest in quality of care is keen, and purchasers are not waiting for conclusive outcomes research to help them make decisions on the value and effectiveness of different managed care options. HMO ratings, adapted from product and service rating systems such as those developed by *Consumer Reports*, are published in national magazines such as *Time*, *U.S. News and World Report*, and *Newsweek* and in national newspapers including *The Wall Street Journal*, *The New York Times*, and *USA Today*. Report cards and ratings are produced by managed care organizations, governments, purchaser coalitions, and trade organizations, emphasizing consumers' satisfaction with their care and the services that they have received.

The challenge of accountability studies is how to build report cards that report consistent, credible, and verifiable data back to the patients and the people who are trying to pick which HMO or PPO they're going to join.

Randall Madry
Utilization Review Accreditation Commission
Public Workshop, May 17, 1996, Irvine, CA

When these new measures of health care quality are added to the traditional approaches, primarily accreditation and licensure of practitioners and facilities, quality assessment becomes a complex patchwork of mechanisms. Federal, state, and local governments, accreditation organizations, managed care organizations, purchaser coalitions, consumer groups, professional organizations, and the media are actively involved in providing information on the quality of health care. Some of these efforts are collaborative, but some are competitive. Overall, the picture is incomplete, inconsistent, and inadequate for making truly informed decisions about the quality of health care services. To those who are responsible for purchasing care, the absence of consensus on quality measurement makes decisions more difficult.

In the spring of 1995, the IOM was asked by the Substance Abuse and Mental Health Services Administration (SAMHSA) to convene a committee to examine quality assurance and accreditation guidelines for managed behavioral health care. The committee's charge was to provide a framework to guide the development, use, and evaluation of performance indicators, accreditation standards, and quality improvement mechanisms in managed behavioral health care (i.e., services related to mental health, alcohol abuse, and drug abuse). In carrying out this task, the committee operated on a clear premise: the ultimate goal of the work was to improve the quality of care for people with behavioral health problems.

Although many of the committee's concerns about the quality of behavioral health care are unique, any study of accreditation and other quality assurance strategies also has relevance to the general health care system. The processes of accreditation and quality assurance are fundamentally the same in the primary care and specialty sectors, and the role of primary care practitioners contributes to the evaluation and delivery of behavioral health care. Furthermore, all sectors of the health care delivery system are responding to the same demands from policymakers and the public for accountability and cost-effectiveness.

> When you think about it, every organization—be it a
> managed care organization, an insurer, a hospital, an
> integrated delivery system, whatever—has huge financial
> systems that literally aggregate and track hundreds if not
> thousands of financial transactions. On the quality side, we
> pull 10 charts and do a review.
>
> *John Bartlett*
> *American Managed Behavioral Healthcare Association*
> *Public Workshop, April 18, 1996, Washington, DC*

Six themes emerged from the committee's review of the research and industry literature. The themes were echoed and amplified in the testimony from individuals from the managed behavioral health care industry, accreditation organizations, professional associations, and advocacy groups; consumers; and health policy analysts. They are as follows:

1.   Behavioral health problems include a wide range of conditions whose effects may be short-lived or lifelong and that may be mildly distressing or profoundly disabling. Many conditions are chronic and relapsing. Most can be effectively treated and respond to appropriate and ongoing care.

2.   Treatment is most successful when it matches an individual's needs and includes an array of integrated services, including primary care, specialty mental health and substance abuse care, and community-based care, such as social support programs.

3.   Behavioral health care is changing rapidly and profoundly, stimulated primarily by the introduction and evolution of managed care and by the discovery of new and effective medications and other treatments.

4.   The influence of managed care will continue to grow. Administered appropriately, it can provide quality care at reasonable cost. Without careful attention, it can result in the undertreatment and neglect of some of the most vulnerable individuals.

5.   The complex patchwork of quality measures and accreditation mechanisms has yet to produce significant progress in the effort to improve the quality of care, but it is laying a foundation of performance measures and accreditation standards that may ultimately serve that purpose.

6.   Differences in perspectives and differences in the timing of and strategies for treatment make it difficult to find a set of measures of the quality of behavioral health care services that all stakeholders can agree on.

> If we really focused on patient/client-driven, assessment-based, clinically-driven treatment in the most efficient and effective way, based on accountability and data, that would take care of costs.
>
> *David Mee-Lee*
> *American Society on Addiction Medicine*
> *Public Workshop, April 18, 1996, Washington, DC*

This final point must be emphasized. A combination of factors—including the expected outcome, the time at which treatment effects are measured, and the perspective of the individual consumers and practitioners—can produce dramatically different conclusions. Confronted with a patient with suicidal depression, for example, a psychiatrist might judge treatment as high quality if that patient no longer has suicidal thoughts after a week in the hospital. The patient's mother, on the other hand, may be disappointed with the hospitalization even if she is pleased that her son was released so soon and denies suicidal thoughts. She may feel that the resident psychiatrist was inexperienced, that the attending psychiatrist doubted her account of the potential reasons for her son's crisis, and that the underlying causes of his problem were not addressed. This same set of circumstances could occur in both fee-for-service and managed care settings, although the next steps for reviewing the treatment decisions might be very different.

Despite such challenges, the committee believes that all of the stakeholders—consumers, practitioners, public and private purchasers, managed care companies, accreditation organizations, and other citizens and groups with a stake in the quality of care—can and must work together to reach a coordinated, collaborative, and consensus approach to quality measurement and treatment. The committee believes that efforts to achieve consensus, both on definitions and on measures of quality, are a valuable investment in the effort to provide the best possible treatment at the lowest appropriate cost.

The development of consensus on quality is particularly important in the field of behavioral health for a variety of reasons that will be discussed throughout this report. Both the complexity of health care and the number of stakeholders have grown extremely rapidly. In the field of behavioral health, the growth in complexity can be attributed to at least four factors:

1.   Increased scientific knowledge about the effectiveness of treatment and the proliferation of new treatment methods give both primary care and specialty practitioners an opportunity to treat these problems.

2.   More publicity, greater public understanding, availability of insurance, and less stigma associated with behavioral health conditions result in increased

numbers of people seeking treatment and give purchasers new incentives to control their costs.

3.   Differences in the structure of insurance coverage for behavioral health care compared with that for physical health care, including the continued application of lifetime and annual limits and other restrictions, have drawn the attention of state and federal lawmakers, businesses, lobbies, and advocacy groups that seek parity for behavioral and physical health care coverage.

4.   The immense growth in managed care in general and in carve-outs (independent, specialty managed care organizations for behavioral health treatment) changes purchasers' choices and prompts new consumer actions.

What makes the health care system succeed or fail in providing high-quality treatment is the interaction between groups of stakeholders and their views on the system's structure, access to care, outcomes, costs, and other factors. Throughout the committee's deliberations, the perspectives of different stakeholders— consumers and families, practitioners, purchasers, and the managed care industry—were discussed. Different stakeholders provided their perspectives, and each must be considered to provide a context for the committee's observations and recommendations.

Will accreditation markedly change the quality of patient care? It may make the system better. It may make the system appear more efficient. But the principal question is, what happens to the patient?

Mark Parrino
American Methadone Treatment Association
Public Workshop, April 18, 1996, Washington, DC

TERMINOLOGY USED IN THIS REPORT

Managed care takes a philosophical approach different from traditional fee-for-service health care, and its terminology has influenced discussions about quality of care in health economics, public policy, and the media. In these contexts, the term *consumer* is used to refer to an individual who receives care, who purchases care directly, or who selects among health plans purchased on his or her behalf by an employer or by another entity, such as a professional association or union (the selection is also known as "consumer choice"). Consumer protection and consumer satisfaction, originally applied in the context of industry products, now can refer to quality assurance and quality improvement in the health care system.

The use of the term consumer is sometimes controversial in primary care and medical specialties, particularly psychiatry, and also in the mental health specialties of psychology, social work, marriage and family therapy, and counseling. Many clinicians view the term as placing undue emphasis on the purchase of health care rather than on the relationship with a practitioner who delivers the care. For example, the 1996 report of the IOM Committee on the Future of Primary Care used the term *patient* and did not refer to consumers. As Iglehart has described (1996), the application of managed care principles means that practitioners begin to share clinical decisionmaking with payers, insurance plan managers, as well as with consumers, and this is difficult for many practitioners.

In the course of its deliberations, this committee used the term *patient* in the context of a therapeutic relationship while an individual is receiving care from a clinician, but used the term consumer more broadly to refer to individuals in most circumstances, including individuals who are making purchasing decisions, who are evaluating report cards, or who have already had treatment and are in recovery. This usage is consistent with that of the U.S. Department of Health and Human Services, including the Agency for Health Care Policy and Research, Health Care Financing Administration, and SAMHSA. This usage is also consistent with that of four of the accreditation organizations whose activities and standards were reviewed for this report.

The term *behavioral health*, used throughout this report, is a creation of the managed care industry. The term was developed in private-sector managed care companies in the mid-1980s to describe mental health and substance abuse (abuse of alcohol and other drugs). This term also is controversial, on the grounds that a variety of treatment modalities (e.g., behavioral, cognitive, and psychodynamic modalities) are used, and also on the grounds that the disorders themselves may be physiological or organic rather than simply behavioral manifestations of dysfunction.

Box 1.1 summarizes the terms used in this report. The committee recognizes and respects the variety of uses of these terms, including those used by other IOM committees. In the rapidly changing health care environment, these terms seemed to this committee to be the most applicable for this study of quality assurance in managed behavioral health care.

CONSUMERS AND FAMILIES

Consumers are the ultimate end users of the health care system. The committee defines consumers as individuals who are, have been, or may in the future be receiving care or services (see Box 1.1). In the field of behavioral health care, the term consumer applies to those who are experiencing or have experienced behavioral health problems and illnesses as well as the family members or others who have financial or legal responsibility for their care. Also included are those who are or could be at risk for behavioral health problems and could need care in the future.

BOX 1.1
Terminology Used in This Report

Behavioral health: managed care term applied to mental health and substance abuse care and services.

Client: an individual who is being treated for mental health or substance abuse problems in a social or rehabilitation setting (e.g., a residential treatment program), or in the private practice of a psychologist, social worker, marriage and family therapist, or counselor.

Clinician: an individual who uses a recognized scientific knowledge base and has the authority to direct the delivery of personal health services to patients (IOM, 1996a, p. 33). The term is typically applied in medical settings.

Consumer: an individual who is, has been, or may in the future be receiving care or services.

Patient: an individual who is cared for by a clinician for purposes of diagnosis, treatment, or preventing illness or for maintaining recovery from illness. The term is usually applied in primary care and specialty medical settings, including psychiatric practice.

Practitioner: an individual who delivers clinical, rehabilitation, or psychosocial treatment to individuals in medical, clinical, or social settings.

Provider: a program, facility, or organization that delivers health care.

Purchaser: a group—such as an employer, unit of government, association, or coalition—that negotiates for and buys health care on behalf of a specified group, generally to cover specific benefits and services at reduced prices.

Stakeholders: individuals and groups for whom the cost, availability, accessibility, or quality of care hold direct implications, including individuals who receive care and their families, practitioners, public and private purchasers, managed care companies, accreditation organizations, and policymakers.

Behavioral health problems are more frequent than is generally realized (see Table 1.1), and their estimated costs to society are far greater than the costs of treatment (see Chapter 3, Challenges in Delivery of Behavioral Health Care). In the past decade, people with behavioral health problems have made great strides in their efforts to increase access to care and to influence the quality of treatment. Patients and families have grown increasingly sophisticated about scientific advances in treatment and about the types of behavioral health care practitioners, such as knowing which practitioners can prescribe medications. In addition to sponsoring regular meetings of support groups, consumers have taken their cause to legislators in state capitols and the U.S. Congress.

The result has been unprecedented change. For example, for the first time, consumers are working as active partners with practitioners to ensure that their causes are addressed by state and national legislative proposals. One such effort was the proposal by Senators Pete Domenici and Paul Wellstone for parity between physical health and mental health coverage. The original proposal was an amendment to the bill cosponsored by Senators Nancy Kassebaum and Edward Kennedy that was passed by the U.S. Senate in the spring of 1996. The final, compromise version of the bill passed in the fall of 1996 did not mandate any services, required parity only with regard to existing lifetime or annual limits for medical or surgical services, and exempted small businesses. However, advocates view the national discussions about parity as a landmark achievement, and many are actively involved in state parity legislation as well.

At the same time that public awareness of behavioral health issues has increased, the rise of managed care has changed the processes involved in obtaining appropriate treatment. After years of having limited insurance coverage but a selection of practitioners, many consumers now find that their health plan restricts their choice of practitioners and covers only a certain number of visits. Moreover, although a large number of people receive high-quality treatment in managed care plans, high-profile situations involving poor or devastating outcomes have attracted publicity or resulted in litigation.

Families and legal guardians are also concerned about managed care because they face tough and painful decisions when a loved one is or appears to be less willing or able to make rational choices. Caring for a child or other relative with severe mental illness leaves many families financially bankrupt and emotionally devastated. Alcohol and drug abuse also have severe consequences, including loss of family support and neglect of children. Thus, parents and other family members also have a stake in treatment decisions, the structure of care, and insurance coverage.

Advocacy groups have exercised an increasing influence on the structure and quality of care and have been vocal about the importance of client or patient satisfaction with care as a measure of its quality. For example, the Center for Mental Health Services (CMHS) has recently released a consumer-oriented report card for mental health services in a collaborative effort with many consumers and consumer groups (CMHS, 1996). Advocates are far better organized and influential in the mental health field than in the substance abuse field, where stigma and the fear of prosecution for using illegal substances are powerful deterrents to the open discussion of issues related to quality of care and where traditions of anonymity inhibit advocacy. Reflecting the current climate, in the spring of 1996 the U.S. Congress passed and President Bill Clinton signed legislation (P.L. 104-121, the "Contract With America Advancement Act of 1996"), to disallow Supplemental Security Income and Social Security Disability Insurance to individuals who are disabled only because of drug addiction or alcoholism, or both (i.e., without a disabling psychiatric or medical condition). These steps mean that these individuals will lose federally funded medical coverage as well.

We have always had managed care. Until now, we have had what I would call doctor managed care. We are shifting to corporate managed care. The third wave is what I call self-managed care, or self-determination, having a say in the important decisions of one's life.

Daniel Fisher
National Empowerment Center
Public Workshop, April 18, 1996, Washington, DC

Consumers of behavioral health care are tremendously diverse with respect to family and cultural backgrounds, the nature of their behavioral health problems, type of employment, type of insurance coverage, experiences with practitioners and treatment, philosophies and beliefs about treatment, and many other factors. Some consumers and advocates believe that family involvement in treatment is essential to its success, whereas others believe that involvement with the family will only prolong a person's distress and keep him or her from getting better. All these perspectives must be considered, and they all point to the importance of evaluating each person and family and taking all these variations into account in the development of treatment plans.

PRACTITIONERS

The variety of practitioners in the behavioral health care system adds complexity. In the behavioral health care system, the professional specialty practitioners include psychiatrists, clinical psychologists, psychiatric nurses, social workers, marriage and family therapists, and substance abuse counselors. Primary care physicians also play a significant role in treatment and referrals. In medically underserved areas (especially inner cities and rural and frontier areas), primary care practitioners include a large number of nurse practitioners and physician assistants. In addition, there is a long tradition of social support or self-help groups, starting with Alcoholics Anonymous in the mid-1930s. All these groups share the goal of reducing symptoms and improving the quality of life for individuals and families dealing with behavioral health problems, but the number of different treatment philosophies and strategies, many of which are conflicting and contradictory and which are recognized by insurers in varying degrees, is staggering.

In substance abuse treatment, counseling is traditionally provided by individuals who are in recovery from alcohol and drug abuse. State administrators and some national professional organizations are concerned that health plans may not view experiential counselors as essential practitioners by health plans and will not provide reimbursements for their services, despite their clinical and cost-effectiveness (NAADAC, 1996). Many states have a long history of supporting the social model programs or nonmedical programs in which these counselors predominate (Gerstein et al., 1994; IOM, 1990b).

A primary motivation for health care practitioners is to help their patients and clients to get better. Improvement can be measured in many ways, including a reduction in symptoms, the ability to return to work or school, improved quality of life, and improved relationships. Ideally, practitioners tailor treatment plans on the basis of a person's needs and preferences, the availability of appropriate services, and their judgments about what will bring the best results. The realities of health care financing, however, also mean that treatment plans will be developed on the basis of what is paid for by the person's insurance plan, whether it is a fee-for-service or managed care plan.

We have tensions between wanting to individually tailor services and the need for benefit packages.

Ann Froio
ComCare
Public Workshop, May 17, 1996, Irvine, CA

With managed care, treatment decisions are not only based on the private decisions of practitioners, clients or patients, and the clients' or patients' families. Managed behavioral health care companies in some cases approve a practitioner's treatment plans, so practitioners must disclose confidential information. Clinical protocols standardize treatment, and limitations can be imposed on the numbers and types of sessions, requiring approvals for additional sessions. Some companies emphasize medication management without counseling and psychotherapy, whereas others rely on nonphysician practitioners and use psychiatrists only when prescription medications or hospitalization are needed (Boyle and Callahan, 1993).

Arguably, the resistance to standardization of care is stronger in the behavioral health fields than anywhere else in the health care system. Treatment decisions are complicated by the great variability of conditions, and much remains to be learned about which treatments are most effective for which individuals at which time in the course of their treatment. Many clinicians resist the idea of standardizing care because of their belief in individual differences—no two people are alike, and the same person behaves differently during different episodes of treatment. The patterns of practice in psychiatry, psychology, psychiatric nursing, and social work include a large proportion of individuals in solo private practice, and they tend to view managed care as a threat to their autonomy and livelihood. The variations in practice, however, would seem to warrant standardization on the basis of evidence of treatment effectiveness.

In the vivid words of one commentator, behavioral health clinicians are sharply divided about whether "to wage a scorched-earth, take-no-survivors holy war against the 'great Satan' of managed care or to pursue a quality improvement strategy of making managed care better" (Sabin, 1995, p. 32). This practitioner resistance is not new or unique to behavioral health. When the first medical group practices emerged in Minnesota and California, they were viewed as a liberal social experiment or a form of socialized medicine by many solo practitioners (Starr, 1982). Some clinicians continue to express concerns about the potential adverse effects of managed care on the relationships between practitioners and patients (e.g., Emanuel and Dubler, 1995).

Proponents of managed care point to examples of managed care providing better coordination, better information systems and health education, and more standardization of best practices, and thus improved quality. In solo practice, it is extremely difficult to provide coordination and linkage with primary care and other practitioners. Quality management activities in managed care help to provide better matching of care with the needs of consumers and families and also reduce the number of unnecessary and ineffective procedures or visits. In addition, managed care information systems can support the collection and assessment of standardized encounter and other data to further understand what contributes to effective treatments and positive outcomes.

Medical ethicists Philip Boyle and Daniel Callahan frame the issues around managed care in the following way. Because even the vast amounts of money currently spent on health care are not sufficient to allow everyone to receive every potentially beneficial intervention, the resources must somehow be managed. Boyle and Callahan believe that a managed behavioral health care system offers more potential for quality, access, and equity than the current combination of fee-for-service and public systems of care. The argument then shifts from *whether* to manage care to *how* to manage care (Boyle and Callahan, 1993; Sabin, 1995).

PURCHASERS

Group purchasers of health care include employers, unions and associations, and federal, state, and local governments. Large private employers have been leaders in altering the buying practices in the health care market, based on their interest in increasing the value that they receive for health care spending (IOM, 1993) and in providing quality health care efficiently. Most large employers still continue the historical practice of offering substantial subsidies to their employees' health insurance premiums as part of a fringe benefits package that attracts qualified employees. Some large employers have developed their own standards for the purchase of behavioral health care (e.g., Digital Equipment Corporation), and increasingly, coalitions of employers such as the Pacific Business Group on Health are developing alliances to negotiate with health plans for standardized primary care benefits at lower prices (Brown, 1996).

Employers have always tried to evaluate the value of health care. To our employer groups, that is defined as a change in health status plus satisfaction, divided by cost.

Catherine Brown
Pacific Business Group on Health
Public Workshop, May 17, 1996, Irvine, CA

Traditionally, employers have been the main purchasers of managed care, but federal, state, and county governments have also looked to managed care to help control costs and increase the opportunity for accountability. As indicated in Table 1.2, approximately 224 million individuals are insured (as of 1995), and on behalf of these individuals, hundreds of private organizations and public agencies negotiate contracts with providers.

Expenditures for mental health and substance abuse treatment account for approximately 10 percent of all health care spending (Frank and McGuire, 1996). Although an estimated half of all individuals who have behavioral health problems do not receive care (see Table 1.3), the growth of spending for mental health and substance abuse treatment has been a matter of considerable concern to both private payers and state governments. In the late 1980s and early 1990s, the rates of growth in behavioral health care spending substantially exceeded the rise in general health care spending (England and Vaccaro, 1991).

State governments have moved to strengthen the bargaining power of health plan buyers by encouraging the creation of purchasing alliances that enable small group purchasers of health insurance to command more choice at better prices. Twenty states have adopted measures that encourage the formation of purchasing alliances (GAO, 1994). States also have an important consumer protection role by licensing and/or certifying practitioners and provider agencies, which will be discussed later in this report (see Chapter 4). In addition, states regulate insurance plans, such as HMOs, against standards of financial solvency, benefits, and health care practice.

Purchasers can set standards of quality for the health plans and practitioners from whom they purchase care or care management, generally as part of a contract. The standards used by purchasers are highly variable and idiosyncratic across

TABLE 1.2 U.S. Health Insurance Data (in millions), 1992–1995

Population Description	1992	1993	1994	1995
Total population	251.7	256.9	259.3	264.3
Insured population[a]	212.8	215.7	219.6	223.7
HMO enrollment	41.4	45.2	51.1	58.2[b]
Specialty MBHC enrollment[c]	78.1	86.3	102.5	110.9
Uninsured population	38.9	41.2	39.7	40.6

[a]HMO enrollment and Specialty managed behavioral health care (MBHC) enrollment are included in the category "Insured population" to illustrate their relative proportions. Due to potential double counting, they should not be added.

[b]1995 projection as of June 1996.

[c]Specialty MBHC has been defined as an entity managing fixed behavioral health, mental health and chemical dependency treatment benefit budgets on capitated, risk-based, or performance-based contracts (Open Minds, 1996). The term excludes public programs and most provider-sponsored integrated delivery systems (Stair, 1996).

SOURCES: EBRI (1996), GHAA (1996), HIAA (1996a), Open Minds (1996), and Stair (1996).

and within the public and private sectors, but the contract requirements are generally the arena in which the issues of outcomes and consumer satisfaction are addressed. In the committee's view, many new developments in these areas, such as the CMHS consumer-oriented report card, the American Managed Behavioral Healthcare Association's (AMBHA's) Performance Measures for Managed Behavioral Healthcare Programs, and state-level initiatives such as the Consumer Quality Review Teams used in Georgia, Pennsylvania, and Ohio, are likely to begin to be incorporated into contracts. For example, the Health Care Financing Administration (HCFA) is basing its contracts on the Healthplan Employer Data Information System developed by the National Committee for Quality Assurance (NCQA) (HCFA, 1996).

Public and private purchasers are concerned with the cost of health care. Indeed, in the public workshops conducted by the committee, several presenters referred to cost of care as the purchasers' primary consideration. The questions for this committee are how much purchasers weigh the importance of the quality of care in their search for good value and outcomes and how purchasers can be helped to maintain and improve the quality of care as they strive for greater value and efficiency.

THE MANAGED CARE INDUSTRY

Consumers, practitioners, and third-party payers (insurance) are traditionally viewed as the main partners that interact in the delivery of health care. Man-

TABLE 1.3 Utilization of Services for Behavioral Health Problems

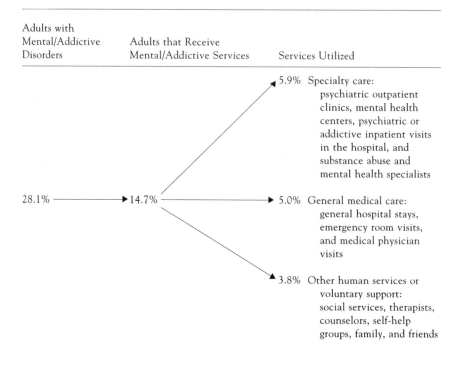

Adults with Mental/Addictive Disorders	Adults that Receive Mental/Addictive Services	Services Utilized
		5.9% Specialty care: psychiatric outpatient clinics, mental health centers, psychiatric or addictive inpatient visits in the hospital, and substance abuse and mental health specialists
28.1%	14.7%	5.0% General medical care: general hospital stays, emergency room visits, and medical physician visits
		3.8% Other human services or voluntary support: social services, therapists, counselors, self-help groups, family, and friends

NOTE: The prevalence of mental or addictive disorders in adults and their utilization of services was based on an Epidemiological Catchment Area (ECA) study sponsored by NIMH in 1990. Within the 14.7 percent of the adult population that utilize mental or addictive services, 6.6 percent did not have a diagnosable disorder. In addition, the percentages of the services utilized (i.e., specialty care, general medical care, and other human services or voluntary support) are estimated separately for each individual service. The same study reported that almost 9 percent of the patients used specialty services in combination with general medical care, while 7.5 percent utilized specialty services in combination with other human services. General medical services and other human services or voluntary support were used jointly by 3.4 percent of the population (Regier et al., 1993).

SOURCES: CMHS (1994) and Regier et al. (1993).

aged care alters the delivery of care by introducing a new control mechanism and method for formal negotiation of expected results among the stakeholders, with the expressed purpose of controlling costs through reducing unnecessary or inappropriate care. Managed care plans use a network of selected providers, which includes hospitals, residential programs, and practitioners. Managed care organizations also seek to influence the nature, quantity, and location of services that are delivered (IOM, 1996a). The contractual relationship between the purchaser and the managed care entity and between the managed care entity and its practitioners are critical in the specification of the incentives, controls, and goals for the plan (Frank et al., 1995).

We know that there is competition in the health care marketplace today. I don't think anybody doubts that. But it is very much a price-driven competition. And that, we think, is very dangerous to the quality of care that patients are receiving.

Margaret O'Kane
National Committee for Quality Assurance
Public Workshop, April 18, 1996, Washington, DC

From mid-1991 through mid-1995, there was a 46 percent increase in HMO enrollment (HIAA, 1996a) (see Figure 1.1). In 1995, of the 184 million Americans with private insurance, an estimated 161 million were enrolled in some form of managed care (HIAA, 1996b). In the public sector in 1995, approximately one third of Medicaid-eligible individuals and close to 10 percent of Medicare beneficiaries were enrolled in managed care plans (see Table 4.2 in Chapter 4). Growth in managed care is taking place primarily in large and medium-sized markets, and the penetration of managed care is greatest in the West, the upper Middle West, and the Northeast (IOM, 1996a).

Managed care has had a major impact on the traditional indemnity insurance industry, which was based on a system in which fees were paid for services provided. Some insurance companies, such as Prudential, Cigna, Aetna, Metropolitan Life, and Travelers, as well as the nonprofit Blue Cross and Blue Shield plans, have bought and developed their own managed care plans. During the mid- to late 1980s, the rate of growth in behavioral health care was greater than the growth in any other sector of health care. The mid-1980s also saw the emergence of a number of managed behavioral health care companies that offered to reduce the spiraling costs of behavioral health care (England and Vaccaro, 1991). A further discussion of these trends in the health care industry is presented in Chapter 2.

Another recent development in the health care industry is the increasing number of benefits consulting firms, such as Coopers and Lybrand, Ernst and Young, Hewitt Associates, KPMG Peat Marwick, McKinsey and Company, William R. Mercer, Towers Perrin, and The Wyatt Company. These companies are largely invisible to consumers and to many practitioners, but they have evolved from providing accounting and auditing services to becoming the main brokers of the managed care contracts negotiated by employers. In the past, benefits consultants worked primarily with purchasers in private industry, but with the expan-

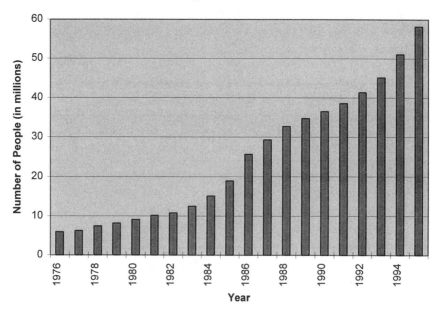

FIGURE 1.1   Number of HMO enrollees, 1976–1995. SOURCE: HIAA (1996a).

sion of managed care into the public sector, consultants are now providing technical assistance to state agencies that want to make informed purchases and hold managed care organizations accountable for the public dollars spent.

Key stakeholders in the industry also include the private national organizations that accredit both provider agencies and managed care entities. Technically, accreditation is voluntary, but many public and private payers encourage or require that their practitioners maintain accreditation. These accreditation entities address organizational capacity, internal management and quality improvement processes, and related issues. In general, accreditation standards are evolving, and the standards for individual practitioners are better developed than the relatively new standards for managed care plans. Chapter 6 of this report discusses five of the organizations involved in accreditation for managed behavioral health care: the Rehabilitation Accreditation Commission (CARF), the Council on Accreditation of Services for Families and Children (COA), the Joint Commission on Accreditation of Healthcare Organizations (JCAHO), NCQA, and the Utilization Review Accreditation Commission (URAC).

Managed care entities also carry out significant quality functions within their contracts and care networks. Examples of these functions include credentialing and recredentialing clinicians; practice guidelines; and profiles of practice patterns, outcomes, and consumer satisfaction for individual practitioners. These functions are sometimes labeled as the "black box" of managed care, because although they can be powerful and valuable forces, they are handled quite differently by individual managed care organizations and networks and are not always shared with practitioners or purchasers. One goal of this report is to address this variation by developing a framework for the evaluation of quality improvement activities. Figure 1.2 presents a summary of the committee's framework for quality improvement.

STATEMENT OF PRINCIPLES

The committee values the evidence-based approach to making health care decisions, and so made it a priority to review the available medical, psychosocial, and health services research on clinical outcomes. The committee also sought other empirical findings to inform the committee's deliberations, including current activities and surveys in the managed behavioral health care industry, such as those performed by AMBHA and the Institute for Behavioral Healthcare, as well as documents and reports from federal agencies such as the Center for Substance Abuse Treatment, and CMHS, NIMH, the National Institute on Drug Abuse, National Institute on Alcohol Abuse and Alcoholism, and HCFA.

The committee also reviewed descriptions of five accreditation organizations: CARF, COA, JCAHO, NCQA, and URAC. In addition, the committee reviewed the following previous reports by the IOM: *Controlling Costs and Changing Patient Care? The Role of Utilization Management* (1989), *Medicare: A Strategy for Quality Assurance* (1990a), *Clinical Practice Guidelines: Directions for a New Program* (1990b), *Broadening the Base of Treatment for Alcohol Problems* (1990c), *Treating Drug Problems* (1990d), *Employment and Health Benefits* (1993), *Primary Care: America's Health in a New Era* (1996a), and *Pathways of Addiction: Opportunities in Drug Abuse Research* (1996b).

However, the committee also recognized that many of the study's most important questions could not be answered solely by searching the available research and health care industry literature. To provide a context for this report, the committee developed a set of principles that is based on empirical evidence, but that also relies on a consideration of issues that may not have been examined empirically. These principles are reflections of a current understanding of strategies for improving the quality of care, as well as ethical concerns that have emerged through the individual committee members' professional and personal experiences in the delivery and study of health care.

1.   Helping to improve the quality of life for individuals, families, and those responsible for the legal and financial circumstances of those individuals and families should be the heart of all efforts to improve the quality of behavioral health care.

2.   Because treatment is effective for mental health and substance abuse problems, it is an essential part of health care and should be accessible to all.

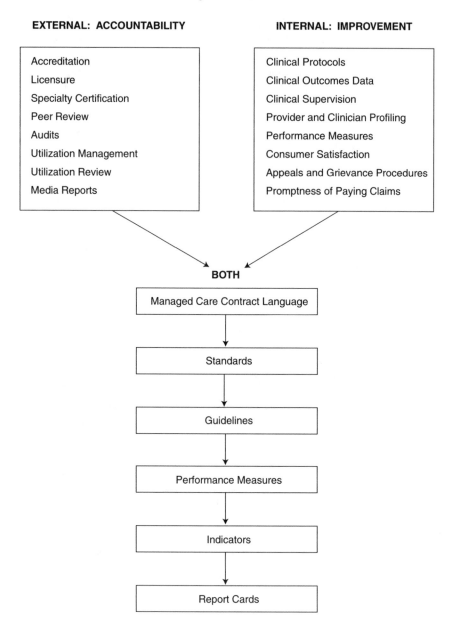

EXTERNAL: ACCOUNTABILITY

Accreditation
Licensure
Specialty Certification
Peer Review
Audits
Utilization Management
Utilization Review
Media Reports

INTERNAL: IMPROVEMENT

Clinical Protocols
Clinical Outcomes Data
Clinical Supervision
Provider and Clinician Profiling
Performance Measures
Consumer Satisfaction
Appeals and Grievance Procedures
Promptness of Paying Claims

BOTH

Managed Care Contract Language

Standards

Guidelines

Performance Measures

Indicators

Report Cards

FIGURE 1.2 Framework for quality assessment. The figure displays a wide array of activities that can have an impact on the quality of care. Impact may vary depending on the level of responsibility for quality of care within an organization, the regulatory mechanisms that apply, the nature and extent of the relevant outcomes research base, and other factors.

Behavioral conditions should be viewed as clinical conditions, both in the provision of (and access to) preventive interventions and treatment and in the requirements for quality and patient satisfaction.

3.   Activities to improve the quality of health care should be based on evidence of effectiveness whenever possible. Every group among the stakeholders—consumers, practitioners, purchasers, managed care companies, accreditation organizations, and other groups—must share responsibility for the quality of treatment. Commitment to improving quality should be inherent in any agreement to provide or receive care.

4.   The expense of successful and appropriate treatment for mental health and substance abuse problems can be a barrier and a burden, putting individuals and families at substantial financial risk. However, untreated behavioral health problems are also costly to individuals, families, businesses, and the rest of society. Thus, providing insurance coverage against the financial risks of behavioral health problems and guaranteeing access to treatment can be justified on grounds of fairness as well as efficiency.

5.   Managed care technologies offer an opportunity to increase access to preventive interventions and to control costs without imposing special limits and excessive cost-sharing. However, managed care can also bring risks of undertreatment and concerns about quality.

6.   Vulnerable and disabled populations are potentially most at risk from the failures in the managed behavioral health care market. Particular attention should be paid to the impact of managed care on such populations, which include children, seniors, people from diverse cultural backgrounds, people who live in rural and other medically underserved areas, people who live in poverty, people who have developmental and other disabilities, people with co-occurring disorders (e.g., depression and alcoholism), and people who have the most severe forms of mental illness and addiction.

7.   Quality improvement and accreditation are two important tools that can be used to protect and improve the quality of care. In general, quality mechanisms should be used to improve performance and reward best practices.

8.   This committee adopts the definition of quality of care developed by another IOM committee: "the degree to which health services for individuals and populations increase the likelihood of desired health outcomes and are consistent with current professional knowledge" (IOM, 1990a, p. 21).

9.   Quality of care includes several components. These include (1) a real opportunity for the person being treated to have a reasonable range of practitioners and treatment options from which to choose, and to provide informed consent (by the person being treated or by a designated representative, the approval of, and agreement with the decision or actions taken by the provider[s]); (2) the protection of confidentiality and privacy rights, balanced with the need to share clinical information to improve the coordination of care; (3) a demonstrated respect for the cultural context of the individual and community being served; and

(4) an emphasis on functional assessments, such as a return to work or school, as measures of success.

10.   Behavioral health problems require an array of preventive and treatment services that are coordinated into a continuum of care that integrates worksites and schools with all parts of the medical treatment system, as well as with community-based services.

ORGANIZATION OF THE REPORT

This report has been written for a broad audience, including the stakeholders who are concerned about quality: public and private purchasers, consumers and families, the managed care industry, professional organizations, accreditation organizations, practitioners in primary care and specialty sectors, and policymakers. Health care quality is complex, and it is addressed in numerous ways: accreditation; quality assurance programs; licensure, certification, and other credentialing activities; clinical practice guidelines; consumer satisfaction; report cards; and other means.

Donabedian (1966, 1980, 1982, 1984, 1988a, b, c) has described three interrelated ways to understand and measure quality: *structure*, *process*, and *outcomes*. *Structural measures* of quality include the types of services available, the qualifications of practitioners, staffing patterns, adherence to building and other codes, and other administrative information. *Process measures* of quality focus on procedures and courses of treatment, such as the numbers of individuals served; on the appropriateness of the care; and on ongoing efforts to maintain quality, such as practice guidelines and continuous quality improvement activities. *Outcome measures* of quality include health status changes after treatment and consumer satisfaction with the care that is provided, as well as short-term or intermediate outcomes.

To prepare this report, the committee adapted Donabedian's approach to address the past, present, and likely future of health care quality improvement. Chapter 1 is intended to provide a context for the report by describing the committee's consumer protection approach to quality measurement, including the statement of principles that it used in approaching this report. Chapter 2, Trends in Managed Care, describes current influences across the spectrum of health care delivery, including quality measurement activities and the changing roles of purchasers. Chapter 3, Challenges in Delivery of Behavioral Health Care, addresses quality measurement issues unique to managed behavioral health care, including the history of separate and distinct systems of care.

Chapter 4, Structure, describes the current delivery systems for behavioral health; these include substance abuse, mental health, and primary care in both the public and private sectors, as well as separate systems for children, seniors, the military, and Native Americans. Chapter 5, Access, discusses general concerns about access, measurement of access in the private sector, and specific concerns about vulnerable and high-risk populations in the public sector. (Access is viewed as a structural factor in the Donabedian framework, but the committee chose to consider access variables in a separate discussion.)

Chapter 6, Process, provides an overview of accreditation and quality improvement activities in their current forms. Chapter 7, Outcomes, reviews what is known from research about treatment outcomes. This chapter is supplemented by two papers in Appendixes B and C: Thomas McLellan and colleagues address questions of substance abuse outcomes research, and Donald Steinwachs discusses outcomes research in mental health.

In Chapter 8, Findings and Recommendations, the committee summarizes its concerns and presents specific recommendations for future steps that should be taken to address those concerns. In developing the recommendations, the committee was mindful of the rapid rate of change in the health care system and the need to anticipate new directions and trends. The report, then, is intended to provide a general, overarching framework that shows how all of the varied current and future quality improvement activities can relate and that also may support creative and collaborative initiatives to improve the quality of care.

REFERENCES

Boyle P, Callahan D. 1993. Minds and hearts: Priorities in mental health services. *Hastings Center Report Special Supplement* September/October:S3-23.

Brown C. 1996. *Purchasers' Perspectives on Quality*. Presentation to the IOM Committee on Quality Assurance and Accreditation Guidelines for Managed Behavioral Health Care. Irvine, CA. May 17.

CMHS (Center for Mental Health Services). 1994. *Mental Health, United States—1994*. Manderscheid RW, Sonnenschein MA, eds. DHHS Publication No. (SMA) 94-3000. Washington, DC: U.S. Government Printing Office.

CMHS. 1996. *Consumer-oriented Mental Health Report Card: The Final Report of the MHSIP Task Force on a Consumer-Oriented Mental Health Report Card*. Rockville, MD: Center for Mental Health Services.

Donabedian A. 1966. Evaluating the quality of medical care. *The Milbank Quarterly* 44:166-203.

Donabedian A. 1980. *Explorations in Quality Assessment and Monitoring: The Definition of Quality and Approaches to Its Assessment*. Vol. 1. Ann Arbor, MI: Health Administration Press.

Donabedian A. 1982. *Explorations in Quality Assessment and Monitoring: The Criteria and Standards of Quality*. Vol. 2. Ann Arbor, MI: Health Administration Press.

Donabedian A. 1984. *Explorations in Quality Assessment and Monitoring: The Methods and Findings of Quality Assessment and Monitoring, An Illustrated Analysis*. Vol. 3. Ann Arbor, MI: Health Administration Press.

Donabedian A. 1988a. Quality assessment and assurance: Unit of purpose, diversity of means. *Inquiry* 25:173-192.

Donabedian A. 1988b. The quality of care: How can it be assessed? *Journal of the American Medical Association* 260:1743-1748.

Donabedian A. 1988c. Monitoring: The eyes and ears of healthcare. *Health Progress* 69:38-43.

EBRI (Employee Benefit Research Institute). 1996. *EBRI Issue Brief*. February.

Emanuel EJ, Dubler NN. 1995. Preserving the physician-patient relationship in the era of managed care. *Journal of the American Medical Association* 273(4):323-329.

England MJ, Vaccaro VA. 1991. New systems to manage mental health care. *Health Affairs* 10(4):129-137.

Frank, RG, McGuire TG. 1996. Introduction to the economics of mental health payment systems. In: Levin BL, Petrila J, eds. *Mental Health Services: A Public Health Perspective*. New York: Oxford University Press.

Frank RG, McGuire TG, Newhouse JP. 1995. Risk contracts in managed mental health care. *Health Affairs* 14(3):50-64.

GAO (U.S. General Accounting Office). 1994. *Health Reform: Purchasing Cooperatives Have an Increasing Role in Providing Access to Insurance*. GAO/HEHS-94-142. Washington, DC: U.S. General Accounting Office.

Gerstein DR, Johnson RA, Harwood HJ, Fountain D, Suter N, Malloy K. 1994. *Evaluating Recovery Services: The California Drug and Alcohol Treatment Assessment (CALDATA)*. Fairfax, VA: Lewin-VHI and National Opinion Research Center at the University of Chicago.

GHAA (Group Health Association of America). 1996. *1995 National Directory of HMOs*. Washington, DC: Group Health Association of America.

HCFA (Health Care Financing Administration). 1996. *Growth in HCFA Programs and Health Expenditures*. Baltimore, MD: Health Care Financing Administration.

HIAA (Health Insurance Association of America). 1996a. *Sourcebook of Health Insurance Data, 1995*. Washington, DC: Health Insurance Association of America.

HIAA. 1996b. Personal communication to the Institute of Medicine. Washington, DC. September 3.

Iglehart JK. 1996. Health policy report: Managed care and mental health. *The New England Journal of Medicine* 334(2):131-135.

IOM (Institute of Medicine). 1989. *Controlling Costs and Changing Patient Care? The Role of Utilization Management*. Washington, DC: National Academy Press.

IOM. 1990a. *Medicare: A Strategy for Quality Assurance*. Washington, DC: National Academy Press.

IOM. 1990b. *Clinical Practice Guidelines: Directions for a New Program*. Washington, DC: National Academy Press.

IOM. 1990c. *Broadening the Base of Treatment for Alcohol Problems*. Washington, DC: National Academy Press.

IOM. 1990d. *Treating Drug Problems*. Vol. 1. Washington, DC: National Academy Press.

IOM. 1993. *Employment and Health Benefits: A Connection at Risk*. Washington, DC: National Academy Press.

IOM. 1996a. *Primary Care: America's Health in a New Era*. Washington, DC: National Academy Press.

IOM. 1996b. *Pathways of Addiction: Opportunities in Drug Abuse Research*. Washington, DC: National Academy Press.

Kessler RC, McGonagle KA, Zhao S, Nelson CB, Hughes M et al. 1994. Lifetime and 12-month prevalence of DSM-III-R psychiatric disorders in the United States. *Archives of General Psychiatry* 51:8-19.

Mechanic D, Schlesinger M, McAlpine DD. 1995. Management of mental health and substance abuse services: State of the art and early results. *The Milbank Quarterly* 73(1):19-55.

Miller RH, Luft HS. 1994. Managed care plan performance since 1980: A literature analysis. *Journal of the American Medical Association* 271(19):1512-1519.

NAADAC (National Association of Alcohol and Drug Abuse Counselors). 1996. *The Role of Alcohol and Drug Counselors in Behavioral Managed Care (Unpublished Manuscript.)* Arlington, VA: National Association of Alcohol and Drug Abuse Counselors.

Open Minds. 1996. *Managed Behavioral Health Market Share in the United States, 1996-1997*. Gettysburg, PA: Open Minds.

Regier DA, Narrow WE, Rae DS, Manderscheid RW, Locke BZ, Goodwin FK. 1993. The de facto U.S. mental and addictive disorders service system: Epidemiologic catchment area prospective 1-year prevalence rates of disorders and services. *Archives of General Psychiatry* 50:85-94.

Sabin JE. 1995. Organized psychiatry and managed care: Quality improvement or holy war? *Health Affairs* 14(3):32-33.

Shore MF, Beigel A. 1996. The challenges posed by managed behavioral health care. *The New England Journal of Medicine* 339(2):116-118.

Stair T. 1996. Personal communication to the Institute of Medicine. Open Minds. October.

Starr P. 1982. *The Social Transformation of American Medicine.* New York, NY: Basic Books.

SAMHSA (Substance Abuse and Mental Health Services Administration). 1995. *Substance Abuse and Mental Health Statistics Sourcebook.* Publication No. (SMA) 95-3064. Washington, DC: U.S. Government Printing Office.

2

Trends in Managed Care

Market forces are creating dramatic shifts in the structure and conduct of business in the health care delivery system. Employers, government agencies, and other purchasers of health care have become increasingly aggressive in demanding competitive prices from suppliers of health care services. The response to the new strategies in purchasing health care has been an acceleration in the growth of managed care organizations.

Managed care imposes organization, controls, quality measurement, and accountability on the delivery of health care to achieve the purchaser's goals for access to care, quality of care, effectiveness of care, and cost of care (Goldstein, 1989; Mechanic et al., 1995; Miller and Luft, 1994; Wells et al., 1995). The introduction and expansion of managed care strategies have altered the organization of general health care (e.g., Shortell et al., 1994) and have begun to influence the delivery of privately and publicly reimbursed mental health and substance abuse treatment. Because behavioral health care takes place in primary and specialty settings and because there is a distinct publicly paid and managed system for the delivery of behavioral health care, the introduction of managed care in one setting can change the relationship to health care in other settings.

Potential problems of the quality of and access to behavioral health care under the managed care system have long been concerns of policymakers. Demonstration projects in Medicaid within the private insurance industry provide some evidence of the impacts of managed care arrangements on utilization and quality (Mechanic et al., 1995). The evidence supports the ability of health maintenance organizations (HMOs) to control the costs of behavioral health care (Frank et al., 1995). There is also mounting evidence that specialty behavioral health companies and other approaches to managed care lower costs compared with the costs of indemnity insurance plans (e.g., Essock and Goldman, 1995; Frank et al., 1995).

This chapter discusses some of the major trends in managed care and their implications for behavioral health care: (1) the increasing rate of growth of managed care, (2) the rapid expansion in the use of managed care systems by public-sector populations, (3) the role of purchasers in managing costs, and (4) the recognition of quality assurance and quality improvement mechanisms as tools for purchasers in making informed decisions. The chapter provides an overview of different quality monitoring mechanisms, including accreditation, quality improvement, performance measurement, licensing, and other credentialing activities, and discusses consumer protections, including confidentiality. Although the responsibility for quality is diffuse, the committee believes that quality assurance and accreditation can be used as tools to help purchasers of care receive the most effective care at the lowest appropriate price.

THE CHANGING HEALTH CARE SYSTEM

Managed Care

Conventional insurance, also called indemnity or fee-for-service insurance, places few restrictions on the choice of practitioners whose services are covered. Practitioners are reimbursed on the basis of the numbers and types of services that they provide, which produces unintended consequences: an incentive for practitioners to provide more services and an incentive for patients to seek more services because they are paid for by a third party. Costs under indemnity coverage are typically controlled by higher copayments, strict limits on services, and lifetime limits on aggregate coverage.

In contrast, managed care imposes limitations on utilization by specifying which practitioners and which services are covered, and often also the number of allowable visits. Managed care comes in many forms and new structures continue to develop, making generalizations difficult. However, managed care plans have the following characteristics in common (HIAA, 1996):

•   they make arrangements with selected practitioners to furnish a specific set of health care services to enrollees;
•   they have explicit criteria and standards for the selection of practitioners;
•   they have formal programs for ongoing quality assurance, quality improvement, and utilization review; and
•   they have financial incentives for members to use the practitioners and procedures that are covered by the plan.

As discussed throughout this report, enrollment in managed care plans continues to increase in both the private and public sectors (see Table 1.2 and 1.4 in Chapter 1). Although many think of managed care as a recent phenomenon, it began in the 1930s with the first prepaid group practices, forerunners of what are now known as HMOs. Early practitioners of managed care believed that it was a way to improve quality and coordination of care, as well as to increase emphasis on prevention (Starr, 1982).

Since the mid-1980s, managed care has gone through three major phases (CSAT, 1994). The first phase focused on managing access to health care, primarily using utilization review and administrative barriers such as pre-admission certification. The second phase focused on managing benefits, and in addition to utilization review, added fee-for-service provider networks, selective contracting, and treatment planning. In the third phase, the focus is on managing care, with a shift from utilization review to utilization management and emphasis on appropriateness of care. The fourth phase, which has begun in the last few years, is outcomes management in an integrated services system with a full continuum of treatment services.

Many structures of managed care have evolved. As indicated in Table 2.1, the types of HMOs include staff model, group model, network model, independent practice association (IPA), and mixed model HMOs. HMOs rely on capitation (a prepaid, fixed amount, usually per enrolled member per month) and other incentives to control costs, including the use of nonphysician practitioners and lower-intensity treatments. The group practice structure of HMOs allows better coordination between primary care and specialty practitioners, because, for example, practitioners are co-located and medical records are more easily shared.

Another prominent type of managed care plan is the preferred provider organization (PPO), which offers more flexibility in choosing practitioners than HMOs but which still offers incentives for seeing selected practitioners. PPOs are networks of practitioners that are most often organized by insurers, managed care organizations, or groups of practitioners. The networks contract with groups of practitioners who agree to provide services for a negotiated fee schedule (HIAA, 1996). Individuals who want to see a practitioner who is outside of the network can do so, but there is a financial penalty.

Point-of-service plans (POS) combine features of HMOs and PPOs. They use a network of selected practitioners who are reimbursed by either capitation or fee-for-service. Individuals choose a primary care practitioner who controls access to specialists, and copayments for seeing practitioners within the plan are low. When individuals see practitioners outside the plan, they pay higher deductibles and copayments (HIAA, 1996).

Currently, the feature most associated with managed care is cost containment. Compared with indemnity plans, managed care plans have significantly lower rates of utilization of inpatient hospitalization, lower rates of utilization of more expensive and discretionary tests, increased utilization of preventive services, and mixed results on quality as measured through outcomes (Miller and

TABLE 2.1 Types of Managed Care Organizations

Type of Organization	Organization Description	Accreditation Bodies	Relevant Regulatory Bodies
Health Maintenance Organization (HMO) **Staff model** (*practitioners are salaried employees of the HMO*) **Group model** (*HMO pays a group of practitioners a negotiated, per capita rate, which is then distributed among the individuals*) **Network model** (*practitioners work out of their own offices under contract with the HMO*) **Individual Practice Association (IPA) model** (*practitioners continue individual or group practice with compensation by capitation and/or fee-for-service [FFS] plans*) **Mixed model** (*combination of two or more of the above*)	An organized system of health care that provides a comprehensive range of health care services to a voluntarily enrolled population in a geographic area on a primarily prepaid and fixed periodic basis	National Committee for Quality Assurance (NCQA) Accreditation Association for Ambulatory Health Care (AAAHC) Utilization Review Accreditation Commission (URAC) Joint Commission on Accreditation of Healthcare Organizations (JCAHO)	Federal licensing agencies, state insurance commissions, state departments of mental health, and state departments of public health
Preferred Provider Organization (PPO)	A network discount, FFS provider arrangement with incentives to stay inside the network; allows services outside of the PPO network at an increased copayment and/or deductible; has structured quality and utilization management	NCQA JCAHO URAC (after its purchase of the American Accreditation Program, Inc.)	State insurance departments

continues on next page

TABLE 2.1 Continued

Type of Organization	Organization Description	Accreditation Bodies	Relevant Regulatory Bodies
Point-of-Service (POS)	An organized system of health care provided by an HMO model with the option of the delivery of services outside of the network at a higher copayment or deductible	NCQA JCAHO URAC	State insurance departments
Management Services Organization (MSO)	An organization that provides practice management, administration, and support services to individual physicians or group practices	JCAHO	State insurance departments
Employee Assistance Programs (EAP)	Programs to assist employees, their family members, and employers in finding solutions for workplace and personal problems	The Employee Assistance Professional Association has a certification program (EAPA)	None
Managed Behavioral Health Care Organizations (MBHO)	An organized system of behavioral health care delivery usually to defined population or members of HMOs, PPOs, and other managed care structures; also known as a carve-out	Council on Accreditation of Services for Families and Children (COA) Rehabilitation Accreditation Commission (CARF) JCAHO NCQA URAC	State insurance departments State public health departments State mental health departments

SOURCES: EAPA (1995), JCAHO (1996), NCQA (1995), and United HealthCare Corporation (1994).

Luft, 1994). Because of the demonstrations of cost savings, managed care has become more attractive to public agencies; for example, in 1995, 32 percent of Medicaid recipients were enrolled in managed care plans (HCFA, 1996).

Another feature of managed care is the development of specialty networks or "carve-outs" for mental health and substance abuse, cancer, vision, dental, and other types of care. Managed behavioral health care companies have been among the fastest growing in the managed care sector. Currently, 88 percent of the individuals in managed care and a total of 125 million individuals are enrolled in a variety of managed behavioral health care products ranging from utilization review only to capitated carve-outs. Carve-out vendors may be specialized units within larger managed care organizations or they may be independent companies.

Staff model HMOs have traditionally provided mental health and substance abuse care by their own staffs, now called a "carved-in" arrangement. In the area of mental health, HMOs have typically been found to spend only 3 to 5 percent of their budgets on mental health, whereas spending for mental health care is 10 percent of the overall budget for the health care system in general (Schadle and Christianson, 1988). These findings have led to concerns among consumers and family members about undertreatment, especially for individuals with serious and persistent mental illness (Flynn et al., 1994; Gerson, 1994). Another concern relates to adverse or biased selection, referring to the tendency for managed care organizations to enroll "good risks" or healthy individuals (Frank et al., 1995).

Increasingly, advocates look to managed behavioral health care to improve the quality of care for individuals with behavioral health problems, and because increasing numbers of public-sector clients are being enrolled in carve-outs, quality improvement is a high priority. The American Managed Behavioral Healthcare Organization (AMBHA) has developed its report card with input from consumer groups, such as the National Alliance for the Mentally Ill (NAMI). The Mental Health Statistics Improvement Program (MHSIP) involved consumer groups (e.g., NAMI and the National Empowerment Center) in developing a report card to evaluate mental health services. Although it is intended for all mental health services and is not specific to managed behavioral health care, the report card involved industry groups in its development. Field testing of the report card began in the summer of 1996.

Employers as Purchasers

As discussed in Chapter 1, employers are interested in the value of their investments in health care. They control the nature of competition among the health plans that are allowed to compete for a firm's employees and dependents. Control of competition occurs via the prequalification of plans, the initial negotiation of premiums, and the definitions of benefits and performance standards. Employees are then permitted to choose among qualified health plans. In many cases the premium subsidy is structured so that the employee must pay for premium costs above the cost of the lowest-priced plan. This competition for enrollees is thought to exert pressure to reduce premiums and to offer the opportunity to compete in the area of quality as well. In addition, the increased use of capitated payment methods for reimbursing health plans creates strong financial incentives for plans to reduce health care spending. Capitation refers to the practice of having fixed rates of payment for the provision of a specified group of services to a defined group of recipients. Usually, payment is made on a per-member, per-month basis.

Although it is not the dominant payment method, the use of capitation to create incentives for providers and practitioners has expanded. It is estimated that in 1994 about 20 percent of the population was served by a physician who was reimbursed under a capitation arrangement (Business and Health Magazine, 1995). This passes the strong financial incentives of capitation along to individual providers of care. Report cards and public reporting of responses to patient satisfaction surveys provide opportunities for employers and employees to choose among competing health plans by comparing the relative value offered by various plans.

The result of the combination of aggressive buying by employers and the use of competition has been a dramatic shift in enrollment patterns across plan types. Recent surveys by several large benefits consulting firms indicate that the portion of individuals covered by employer-sponsored insurance and enrolled in traditional indemnity plans (with or without precertification) fell from 53 percent in 1991 to 35 percent in 1994. In particular, PPOs, POS plans, and HMOs accounted for 63 percent of enrollees in employer sponsored health insurance plans in 1994 (Foster Higgins, Inc., 1994).

In addition, some employers report that they have been successful in obtaining premium reductions from health plans seeking to participate in their employee health programs. The overall result has been for average employee health care costs to rise only modestly among larger employers, whereas the increases in costs for other purchasers have been larger (IOM, 1993).

Financial incentives, provider selection, and utilization management techniques are used alone and in combination within most managed care plans (Freeman and Trabin, 1994; Goplerud, 1995; IOM, 1989). Financial incentives can be applied to consumers (deductibles and copayments) and providers (capitation or some other form of risk-based contracting) to discourage the use of costly services. Mandating the use of specific provider networks limits consumers' ability to choose practitioners, reduces the number of providers that can be reimbursed for care, facilitates the negotiation of contracts with favorable rates, and permits more scrutiny of the quality of care than reimbursing individual practitioners on a fee-for-service basis. Finally, utilization management applies treatment guidelines, protocols, and professional judgment through prior review (are services appropriate and necessary?) and high-cost case management (a review of high-expenditure cases to facilitate less costly care) to reduce the expense of care and enhance the consistency and quality of care (IOM, 1989).

State Governments as Purchasers

States and counties have the responsibility for managing public systems of care, and their objectives with regard to health plans and services differ somewhat from the objectives of private employers. For example, a state may place priority on offering a minimum level of access to basic medical care to achieve the lowest "on-budget" cost. The configurations and structural relationships among the Medicaid agency, state mental health and substance abuse authorities, and child welfare systems are different in each state, as are the economic and political environments, so the routes to cost-effective care differ in each state (Essock and Goldman, 1995).

By August of 1996, 29 states had received federal waivers to restructure their Medicaid programs, often in response to state legislative mandates to expand coverage for poor people who would otherwise not qualify for Medicaid (GAO, 1995). Expansion of the numbers of people enrolled in the Medicaid program requires the realization of savings from care for currently covered enrollees to finance the expansion of coverage to new populations. One way to achieve the savings is through capitated health plans.

As of June 1995, about 32 percent of Medicaid program beneficiaries were enrolled in capitated managed health care plans (HCFA, 1996). This segment of the Medicaid market is growing rapidly. States are active buyers of managed care services for their Medicaid enrollees and make use of competition to enter the program to obtain favorable premiums. Because Medicaid enrollees do not pay premiums, competition for enrollees is used primarily as a quality control mechanism. That is, if a plan offers insufficient quality, enrollees may choose some alternative plan that might offer more satisfactory services.

CONCERNS WITH MANAGED CARE IN THE PUBLIC SECTOR

The introduction of managed care into already existing public-sector service systems represents a reorganization of service delivery and creates opportunities to address many limitations of the current systems of care for individuals with mental health and substance abuse problems. Purchasers with vision can use managed care arrangements to achieve specific goals: improve access to care, enhance the quality of care, better manage the cost of care, increase the effectiveness of care, and facilitate prevention initiatives. Indeed, increased use of managed care tools can be a key strategy to facilitate improved integration of the separate and distinct public and private systems of care that are a problematic aspect of mental health and substance abuse care.

However, debate on the use of managed care for behavioral health care (mental health and substance abuse treatment) can be intense because there is evidence that individuals with chronic conditions including mental illness and substance abuse may have more difficulty receiving adequate and effective services when they are enrolled in managed care plans (Christianson et al., 1989; Mechanic and Aiken, 1989). One study comparing psychiatric treatment within prepaid managed care plans and fee-for-service arrangements found that half of the individuals receiving care through a managed care plan developed new functional limitations over time, whereas those receiving care through a fee-for-service plan did not (Rogers et al., 1993).

Some believe that the techniques used by managed care plans can facilitate access to care and improve the quality of services because provider flexibility can be enhanced and care can be individualized; others are concerned that managed care models can inhibit access and interfere with appropriate and individualized care (e.g., Boyle and Callahan, 1995; Gold et al., 1995; Kassirer, 1995; Sabin, 1995; Schlesinger, 1995; Schlesinger and Mechanic, 1993; Surles, 1995). Moreover, the prepaid capitated financing characteristic of managed care plans is frequently distrusted because of the potential financial incentives to minimize care and maximize profits (e.g., Boyle and Callahan, 1995; Iglehart, 1996; Sharfstein and Stoline, 1992)

Financial Risk

Effective managed care programs manage expenditures. Purchasers can increase or decrease the amount of financial risk that a managed care organization assumes and can potentially reduce the incentives to limit access and utilization of expensive technologies, specialty services, and long-term care (Frank et al., 1995). One important component in managing costs is the analysis of the incentives and disincentives included in the contracts between the purchaser and the managed care organization and between the managed care organization and the provider. Frank and colleagues (1995) have examined public and private contracts for managed behavioral health care, and they suggest that purchasers may achieve a balance between cost control and access through the use of "soft" capitation, which shares risks between the purchaser and managed care organization, thereby reducing the potential profit and losses for the managed care organization. Soft capitation can promote reinvestment of "savings" into increased benefits or expanded eligibility by giving governments a share of the "profits."

Public providers of community-based services who are eager to share in the potential profits related to the use of capitation have negotiated subcapitation rates. They agree to provide necessary services to a specified population for a portion of the total capitation—a subcapitation. Subcapitated providers can profit from treating patients. Each subsequent layer of subcontracting draws an administrative fee, which reduces the funds ultimately available for direct services. Inexperience with managing populations of enrollees may also lead to setting rates that are too low, thereby threatening access and quality of care.

Integrated Services

Direct and insufficiently planned applications of private-sector managed care models to public-sector systems that serve men and women with serious mental illness and chronic substance abuse are unlikely to be successful. Many employer-purchased managed care plans explicitly exclude social and support services, and because they emphasize acute care, they tend to have little experience in the management of chronic and disabling conditions.

Changes in service systems may also threaten the continued viability of the agencies and providers that have served the more complex and vulnerable uninsured and publicly insured consumers with distinction. At the same time, many of the tools of private-sector managed care have relevance to public-sector systems. For example, integrated management information systems, decision-making algorithms, and methods of developing and improving provider networks have great applicability to public-sector systems. The ability of public systems to implement these strategies, however, may be limited by budgetary constraints, procurement policies, personnel capacity, and other factors.

Integration of service delivery across a broad range of services is a challenge to achieving effective and efficient services. Carve-in or integrated policies, most common in staff model HMOs, can increase the likelihood of coordination and communication among primary care and specialty providers. Carve-out vendors have the advantages of having better linkages with employee assistance programs, more specialized quality measurement tools, more specialized practitioners, and the ability to provide consistent benefits anywhere in the country (IOM, 1996).

Integration of services requires resource management that coordinates benefits from multiple entitlements and services from diverse and multiple providers. Case management to support transitions (transition management) can help individuals moving across settings and to care outside the system. Regular screening of populations and internal referral systems among key providers are needed to support aggressive case finding and early intervention. Multidimensional assessments need to include the medical, personal care, mental health, substance abuse, and social facets of need, but comprehensive approaches are very difficult to coordinate. One way to assist in coordination is to include in contracts requirements for linkages to support wraparound services such as transportation and child care (Institute for Health Policy, 1995).

BEHAVIORAL HEALTH IN THE NEW MARKETPLACE

As employers and states have moved in the direction of contracting with managed care organizations to care for at-risk individuals, providers, consumers, and policymakers have become concerned about the consequences of these developments with regard to access to care and the quality of treatment for individuals suffering from mental health and substance abuse problems. Individuals suffering from severe forms of mental and addictive disorders have been identified as being at risk for neglect under these new market arrangements (Boyle and Callahan, 1995). The question that stems from such concerns is, how can behavioral health care productively fit into the larger health care system?

This section focuses on one dimension of making markets more accommodating to behavioral health care. That dimension involves improving the information available on the quality of health plans in providing behavioral health care services. Information on quality is one aspect of the choices available to purchasers and policymakers in the behavioral health care arena. It is, however, an important choice and arises as an issue under all types of organizational and financial arrangements, albeit in different forms.

In many respects, the behavioral health care market is being transformed from transactions based on services to transactions based on people. Behavioral health care organizations are increasingly competing for the right to serve populations. In some cases, this competition comes in the forms described above, in which individuals choose from among competing health plans. In other cases, a purchaser (employers or a government) will carve out behavioral health care and will competitively select a single managed care vendor (Frank et al., 1995). Risk-sharing arrangements are increasingly common for both health plans and carve-out programs. These can involve establishing financial arrangements, utilization controls, and other mechanisms to share the financial risk of providing care among health plans or other providers, payers, and users of a health care plan. In a risk-sharing arrangement, health plans face at least some financial risk for the costs incurred on behalf of their enrollees.

Initial results from the transformation of behavioral health care markets are dramatic. Managed behavioral health care has shown that in many cases it can result in significant reductions in behavioral health care spending (Mechanic et al., 1995). Treatment patterns are changing, often in directions that have long been viewed as desirable. For example, in the mental health area, adoption of a managed behavioral health care program is often accompanied by a reduced reliance on hospital-based inpatient care and a greater emphasis on community-based alternatives (Callahan et al., 1994). In the substance abuse area, managed behavioral health care plans result in dramatic reductions in the use of 28-day inpatient programs and the expanded use of residential treatment programs.

Many of the criticisms of the new organizational and financial arrangements associated with managed behavioral health care stem from their efforts to respond to certain problems inherent in trying to insure health care. One of these problems involves the utilization effect of health insurance; the other is the problem of biased risk selection.

The utilization effect of health insurance (sometimes called moral hazard) refers to the tendency of those who are insured to use more health services—both appropriate and inappropriate—than those people would use if they were responsible for the full cost of care. Ideally, health plans could respond with strategies that selectively reduced inappropriate use of services. That this has proved very difficult in most areas of health care is indicated by research showing that most cost containment tools affect most needed and unneeded services. Behavioral health care may face particular challenges in calibrating strategies to minimize harm because measures of need, outcomes, appropriateness, and effectiveness—although improving—still lag behind efforts in other areas of health care.

Given the pressures on health plans to reduce costs, consumers who need behavioral health care may thus be especially vulnerable to cost control strategies that unselectively affect the quality and accessibility of appropriate services. Another problem for those who use behavioral health care in a competitive market is the challenge of functioning well in the consumer role. Particularly for individuals who are in crisis, it may be particularly difficult to negotiate the administrative requirements for obtaining care, or to challenge adverse administrative decisions.

Adverse (biased) selection creates market failure in several ways. Individuals typically know more than their health plans about their own health status. Hence, consumers will naturally choose plans that offer provisions that are best aligned with their anticipated health care needs. It is therefore possible that individuals with behavioral health problems and family members who act on their behalf will be more likely to foresee their use of health care services than other individuals. For this reason health plans that offer generous coverage and high-quality behavioral health care services or that allow relatively free access to services will disproportionately attract users of behavioral health services to their plans. Because mental and addictive disorders can be chronic and relapsing problems, people who experience these problems can incur additional medical expenses and thus can accumulate high overall costs for their care.

Under such circumstances, premiums based on population averages may be too low. Thus, there are strong incentives to compete for individuals who are "good risks" (McGuire, 1989). The implications will be that plans will compete to avoid attracting enrollees who are likely to use behavioral health care services. These competitive dynamics lead plans to limit coverage, access, and quality in the behavioral health care arena.

Another aspect of adverse selection occurs because purchasers of all types (individuals, employers, and governments) cannot obtain information on quality but do have access to information on price (Akerlof, 1970). When only this one aspect of information is measurable, purchasers may place excessive weight on price in the absence of reliable information on quality.

At the public workshops convened by the committee, a variety of parties from the managed behavioral health care industry and from the purchaser community suggested that price was most important to government and corporate purchasers. This is true both in the context of behavioral health carve-out purchases and for purchasers choosing plans that will be permitted to compete for a population of enrollees. The result is that plans will be rewarded by the market for achieving lower prices by reducing quality. Higher-quality, higher-cost providers will be disadvantaged in competition and possibly driven from the market. Again, because quality in the behavioral health care arena is more difficult to measure than in the general medical care behavioral health arena, services are particularly vulnerable to such quality reductions.

Whether we like it or not, behaviors are very financially driven. When I was in the managed care industry as director of provider networks, we moved a group from a fee-for-service group to a capitated group, and in the first month of the capitation, their inpatient rate dropped 50 percent. Now, the question is, did it drop from 100 percent too much to exactly the right amount, could it have dropped further, did it drop too much? I don't know that we were clear on that.

Michael Jeffrey
William R. Mercer
Public Workshop, May 17, 1996, Irvine, CA

The relative importance of biased risk selection and moral hazard will depend in part on the specific organizational and financial arrangements involved in choosing health care plans. For example, if a single behavioral health care vendor is chosen, the problems related to incentives created by risk selection are largely eliminated because the vendor would be the only source of care for a defined population. In contrast, if a purchaser allows individuals to select among competing health plans (either integrated or carved out), the plans' enrollees could present different levels of risk to the plans in terms of the likelihood of needing care. When a health plan attracts a more risky or more costly group than the average, or than the competition, it has experienced adverse selection (IOM, 1993).

In Medicaid programs and private insurance plans, choices about how to organize the purchase of behavioral health services are quite similar. In comparison, public mental health and substance abuse systems typically face more complexity with respect to moral hazard because these systems serve as the provider of last resort in the United States. Thus, these systems must serve all those who need treatment and who are unable to pay for care. However, there is no "denominator population" for which to construct a capitation rate (fixed rate of payment per enrollee per month) and thus no way to accurately estimate the possible costs of care. Thus, a managed care vendor serving the public system potentially may face more financial risk.

With the incentives to produce cost savings comes a risk of cost shifting, or a redistribution of payment sources, For example, when one payer obtains a discount on services from a particular provider group, the provider group might increase their costs to another payer to make up the difference. In the context of managed behavioral health care, the concern is that the costs of care for seriously mentally ill individuals might be shifted by private companies to the public sector.

Another way in which cost savings might be achieved is sometimes called "skimming," which refers to the practice of only enrolling the healthiest individuals in an insured population. Policies that might support this practice could include having very few behavioral health providers and practitioners in a network, or having them located in areas that are difficult to reach through public transportation. Another policy might be to define behavioral health problems, especially severe problems, as being outside of the responsibility of the health plan. Some of the ways to avoid these practices are discussed in a later section of this chapter on contracting and contract language.

HEALTH CARE QUALITY

Moving away from an exclusive interest in cost, purchasers are beginning to demand documentation that services are effective. Thus, the introduction of managed care can stimulate the development of treatment guidelines and standards of care, improve the delivery and monitoring of care, and encourage linkages between research and practice. Because plans are developed for the benefit of specific groups of eligible consumers, consumer report cards and measures of satisfaction can become important indicators of effectiveness.

Managed care and managed behavioral health care organizations are now competing on the basis of both quality of care and cost of care (England and Vaccaro, 1991). Digital Equipment Corporation's (1995) *HMO Performance Standards* reflect one purchaser's requirement for specific levels of quality in the health plans that it purchases for its employees and beneficiaries. Quality standards for behavioral health care are being promulgated and implemented by accreditation agencies (NCQA, 1996) and promoted by trade organizations (AMBHA, 1995).

Well-developed quality improvement initiatives use management information systems to monitor and manage clinical processes to enhance client outcomes. AMBHA's (1995) quality standards emphasize continuity of care, follow-up, and readmission rates. Digital Equipment Corporation's (1995) standards for behavioral health care require quality improvement plans, requirements for staffing levels and staff credentials, and access to case management to support the treatment interventions. These and other standards will be discussed further in Chapter 6, Process.

On a quarterly basis we feed back to all our providers how they've done compared to the rest of the plan in terms of their utilization statistics, their quality improvement statistics, their outcomes, the complaints and grievances, and their administrative compliance to the plan.

Peter Panzarino
Vista Behavioral Health
Public Workshop, May 17, 1996, Irvine, CA

Context for Accreditation and Outcome Measurement

Although accreditation approaches and measurement of outcomes are central issues in ensuring the quality of managed behavioral health care systems, a range of other factors and approaches critically shape, affect, and address the quality of care. The unique structure of behavioral health care itself creates fundamental quality issues. Since most commercial insurance coverage is limited, commercially paid care is fragmented between primary and specialty sectors and there is a substantial public sector that serves as a safety net. Cost shifting and other relationships between sectors of care are in themselves a crucial problem. Furthermore, the complex framework for quality is itself a challenge for ensuring and improving quality.

As Table 2.2 illustrates, responsibility for quality is divided, and fundamental issues of coverage, benefit adequacy, and system design exert a profound effect on quality. For example, the typically limited behavioral health care benefits in most commercial insurance plans—especially in an environment of cost control—lead to a shift of consumers with high levels of need to the public sector. In the public sector, state-to-state variability in funding patterns, organization, and service adequacy lead to idiosyncratic patterns of care.

The array of approaches to monitoring service processes and outcomes is also complex. Responsibility for addressing quality is diffuse. Providers use their own measures and approaches to improve the quality of the care that they provide (e.g., quality assurance and continuous quality improvement). Thus, the responsibility for quality starts at the level of the providers.

Accrediting organizations (historically, especially JCAHO) have required providers to develop and implement internal quality assurance systems. Pressure to develop *internal* quality improvement activities may paradoxically be a positive result of *external* accreditation approaches.

States regulate health care practice by licensing individual practitioners, for example, physicians, nurses, psychologists, and social workers (see Table 4.1). Different states have different approaches to licensure, for example, whether so-

TABLE 2.2 Ecology of Consumer Protection: Current Context

Inputs	Processes	Outcomes

Context/Environment of Coverage
Workplace
  Workplace to employee assistance program (EAP)
  EAP to Health Care
  Workforce improvement
Uninsured
Underinsured
Incarcerated
	Accreditation of Plans
	Tend to focus on commercial market
	Early in development
	Weak on disabled population and care other than medical care
		Consumer Satisfaction
		Internal, e.g., surveys
		External, e.g., Ohio Consumer Quality Review Team

	Quality Improvement In Plans	**Outcomes Measures** MHSIP Highly relevant to consumers in public sector

Benefits And Services
Commercial
  Broad populations
  Narrow, shallow benefits
Public sector
  Narrow population
  Deep, broad benefits
	State Certification Standards
	Standards for systems of care; certification or contract/plan specifications
		Covers wide range of issues, including quality of life and care other than medical care
		  Being field tested

	Standards for providers, not plans
	  Variable patterns
	  May duplicate accreditation
	  Cover care other than medical care
		NAMI roundtable
		  Pilot testing under way
		  Focuses on feasibility of collecting outcome data from individuals with depression and schizophrenia

	State Professional Licensure Standards
	Counselors
	Nurses
	Physicians
	Psychologists
	Social workers
		System Performance Standards
		AMBHA/PERMS[a]
		  Sums process measures
		  Wide database
		  Focuses on medical/ clinical issues

[a]PERMS, Performance-Based Measures For Managed Behavioral Healthcare Programs.

cial workers are licensed or whether nurses have prescription-writing privileges. However, the licensure standards within each profession are generally comparable from state to state. Licensure approaches require evidence of adequate training and credentials and of continuing education, and state licensure boards monitor problems of egregiously poor care, although instances of inadequate or inappropriate care are probably underreported.

States also license or certify provider agencies, for example, mental health centers, against minimum standards of staffing, facilities, and organization. This certification may be carried out by the funding agency or the state health department and is typically required if an agency is to receive state funding or to participate in the Medicaid program. State certification standards are somewhat variable in both coverage and intensity; they are a corporate analog of the licensure of individual professionals. State certification of agencies is usually not required for participation of the agency in commercially paid insurance plans. States also regulate insurance plans, such as HMOs, although the regulation of specialty managed care entities is in its infancy.

Prevention

In theory, the prepaid capitated health care system increases incentives for a plan to prevent health care problems and to identify emerging problems early. Investments in some prevention activities and early interventions may reduce the cost of treatment. Prevention services, however, often require years before their effects can be discerned, and managed care organizations may have relatively little incentive to prevent conditions they may never be required to treat because of enrollee mobility.

Among the most readily available quality standards for behavioral health care, only Digital Equipment Corporation's (1995) *HMO Performance Standards* address prevention and early intervention. Digital requires health promotion activities and health education and supports a strong employees assistance program (EAP), and thus does not require screening and early intervention for substance abuse and mental health problems (Digital Equipment Corporation, 1995).

In planning for this capitation, the managed care organizations were really convinced that they wanted to, they had the responsibility to, and to a great degree were motivated to keep these patients well and out of the hospital.

Don Austin
Oregon Health Department
Public Workshop, May 17, 1996, Irvine, CA

In public managed care programs there may be increased value for the inclusion of screening and the early identification of problems in the design of the benefits package. The Oregon plan for Medicaid recipients, for example, requires HMOs to screen Medicaid beneficiaries for the presence of substance abuse problems and to refer them for assessment and treatment if necessary. Similarly, some jurisdictions, such as Indian Health Service hospitals, require screenings for alcohol among trauma patients seen in emergency rooms.

Licensure and Certification

Before the federal government's adoption of the Hughes Act [the Comprehensive Alcohol Abuse and Alcoholism Prevention, Treatment and Rehabilitation Act of 1970 (P.L. 91-616)] and, at the state level, the decriminalization of public intoxication and the authorization of alternatives to incarceration for treatment, formal treatment for alcoholism was primarily provided in state mental hospitals and a small number of outpatient clinics and halfway houses (IOM, 1990a; NIAAA, 1971). Systems of care did not exist in most states. Both the Hughes Act and the Uniform Alcoholism and Intoxication Treatment Act (P.L. 94-371) included provisions for a state alcoholism authority that would plan, coordinate, fund, and regulate alcoholism treatment and prevention services in the state. Section 9 of the Uniform Act empowers the states with the authority to set standards for treatment facilities and to approve public and private facilities to deliver care (NIAAA, 1971).

Although the specific powers vary from state to state, third-party payers typically require state licensure or approval before they will provide reimbursement for care in a facility. State licensure or approval therefore became a key tool in the development of systems of care. Licensure and approval thus are required to legitimize programs, ensure quality, and protect consumers (Birch and Davis Associates, Inc., 1984; IOM, 1990b).

State regulations for treatment facilities usually establish requirements for space, staff, services, and record keeping. A review of state licensing practices completed in 1992 found that although all states specify requirements for treatment providers, compliance in some states is voluntary (Health Management Resources, Inc., and Birch and Davis Associates, Inc., 1992).

The introduction of managed care has challenged state licensing systems because some new models of care may not fit existing licensing categories (e.g., home detoxification services). Although the managed care plans may urge minimal state regulation to minimize their costs and maximize creative treatment planning, consumers may be less protected because standards of care have not been established for many emerging treatment techniques.

Thus, licensure has been developed for individual practitioners and facilities. The ability of licensure to control quality, however, is unclear. For example, licensure for mental health professionals emphasizes educational degrees, performance on written tests, familiarity with the statutes and regulations applicable in a given state, and specific courses of study. Actual effectiveness or skill during treatment is not tested directly, because it is assumed to have been attained during the accumulation of a required number of hours of supervised experience. Performance-based credentialing of the workforce, which bases certification on direct evidence of skills, has developed in some parts of the mental health workplace (e.g., biofeedback). In general, however, licensure as a consumer protection strategy has not been evaluated.

Counselor Certification

The workforce in behavioral health care is unusual in that it includes many counselors who have experience but not necessarily professional training. Counselor certification has been encouraged to legitimize the field of addictions counseling, demonstrate that individual counselors are qualified to provide counseling services, and promote the development of a professional identity (Birch and Davis Associates, Inc., 1984; Valle, 1979). Certification specifies counselor qualifications rather than educational degrees (Birch and Davis Associates, Inc., 1984; Valle, 1979).

Because the field of substance abuse counseling includes many men and women whose initial involvement with training is their personal experience of recovery, the need to demonstrate competence and skill has been especially acute. The development of credentialing standards was an early priority for the field and, with support from the National Institute on Alcohol Abuse and Alcoholism, trade groups collaborated and proposed 12 core competency areas and credentialing guidelines (Birch and Davis Associates, Inc., 1984). A review of state procedures for the certification of substance abuse counselors found that all states support certification, but in most states the certification is voluntary and coordinated through an independent nongovernmental entity, usually a trade group organization (Health Management Resources, Inc., and Birch and Davis Associates, Inc., 1992).

Debate about the role of individuals who are in recovery as counselors (experiential counselors) has persisted over the decades. Krystal and Moore (1963) debated the issue in the early 1960s; Krystal argued that alcoholism is a complex disease that requires professionally trained counselors, whereas Moore believed that psychotherapy is unnecessary in most cases and that physicians and psychologists should work closely with counselors who are themselves in recovery. In practice, experiential counselors became a major part of the workforce in the emerging alcoholism and drug abuse treatment programs. Counselors in recovery are more likely to be older and male and to work in residential treatment settings (McGovern and Armstrong, 1987; Mulligan et al., 1989).

Research on treatment effectiveness tends not to evaluate differences among types of practitioners. Within the managed care environment which emphasizes ambulatory care and lower-cost practitioners, it would seem to be desirable to employ counselors rather than psychiatrists or other mental health professionals. However, the role and status of experiential counselors appears to be limited. Although counselors with certification are more competitive, it appears that many managed care plans also require an individual to have graduate training and a master's degree to serve their members. The National Association of Alcoholism and Drug Abuse Counselors (a professional organization for certified addiction counselors) therefore advocates certification requirements for degreed and nondegreed counselors as evidence that counselors are not only professionally trained but are also skilled in the treatment of addictions (NAADAC, 1988, 1991, 1994).

Academic preparation does not make you a better clinician, to be honest. It may give you a better grounding in theory. It does not make you a better clinician.

Linda Kaplan
National Association of Alcohol and Drug Abuse Counselors
Public Workshop, April 18, 1996, Washington, DC

Loss of Current Providers

Public-sector service systems often appear to be a patchwork of service agencies that specialize in the unique and complex needs found among uninsured individuals and individuals with public insurance. The service providers may include state and county hospitals and clinics, as well as private nonprofit agencies such as community-based programs staffed with licensed, certified, and noncertified counselors. In contrast to the private sector, where individual practitioners must meet licensing and other standards, the public sector has a long tradition of accreditation at the program level. When managed care networks expand, they tend to recruit individual practitioners rather than programs. Consequently, networks may exclude the practitioners with the greatest understanding and experience working with publicly financed consumers of health care.

One strategy to limit the disruption of care is to require managed care organizations to include public-sector providers, such as halfway houses or therapeutic communities, in their service networks. Because they have operated under different types of accreditation, however, some publicly funded providers may have difficulty meeting the performance expectations and abiding with service and cost restrictions. For example, halfway houses are an important social support service when inpatient care is not available or not appropriate. Support for system development may be required for many providers to facilitate their change to a managed care environment.

Clinical Practice Guidelines

In an earlier report, the Institute of Medicine (IOM) (1990c) defined clinical practice guidelines as systematically developed statements that could be used to assist practitioner and patient decision-making about appropriate health care for specific clinical circumstances. They are intended to improve the quality, appropriateness, and effectiveness of care, and they have been used to help guide clinical decision-making, to assist organizations in developing their own clinical and risk management protocols, to guide payers in setting reimbursement policies, and to assist consumers in making informed choices regarding their health care (Edmunds, 1996).

Clinical practice guidelines are seen by federal policymakers as a key activity in rationalizing decision-making about the delivery of health care and in reducing variation for nonclinical reasons such as local patterns of practice (Edmunds, 1996). In its 1989 report to the U.S. Congress, the Physician Payment Review Commission recommended increases in funding for the development, implementation, and evaluation of practice guidelines and for outcomes research on which to base those guidelines (PPRC, 1989). In that same year, Congress passed legislation creating as a part of the U.S. Public Health Service the Agency for Health Care Policy and Research (AHCPR) to carry out those responsibilities (Gray, 1992).

National professional associations, such as the American Medical Association (AMA), the American Psychiatric Association, and federal agencies, particularly AHCPR, develop practice guidelines recommending treatment approaches for particular conditions such as depression in the primary care setting (DHHS, 1993). These guidelines are generally developed on the basis of a review of the literature regarding treatment effectiveness and use a professional consensus development process.

Approximately 1,600 guidelines from 45 national medical groups and several other organizations are listed in the directory of guidelines published by the AMA (1993). Hundreds of proprietary guidelines have been developed in the managed care sector. Consequently, it is not unusual to find conflicting recommendations, various degrees of involvement by clinicians in their development, and various amounts of research cited as evidence. Some guidelines are intended to reduce costs by eliminating unnecessary and ineffective procedures and improving the coordination of care, but others can increase costs by recommending additional services and procedures.

Guidelines developed by a consulting firm, Milliman and Robertson, Inc., are used by health plans at Prudential, Cigna, U.S. Healthcare, Kaiser Permanente, and many Blue Cross and Blue Shield affiliates, affecting a combined total of 50 million members, subscribers, or covered lives. The Harvard Pilgrim Health Plan has undertaken an evaluation of the impact of the guidelines of Milliman and Robertson, Inc., on cost and quality of care, with implications for future practice (Myerson, 1995).

Guidelines have the potential to allow for the coordination of the delivery of care, improve the quality of care, and standardize the collection of clinical data for use in outcomes research. The development of guidelines can help to bring about consensus and agreement among a variety of practitioners and purchasers about best practices. The use of practice guidelines by providers is increasingly required by accreditation bodies. However, much remains to be learned about the effective implementation of guidelines to produce changes in provider behavior and influence practice patterns.

QUALITY IMPROVEMENT AND QUALITY ASSURANCE

Donabedian's (1980, 1982, 1985) pioneering efforts to define and measure the quality of health care recognized that consumer sentiments and desires were essential components of quality measurement and that analysis of cost could not be divorced from the assessment of quality. In many ways, his discussions anticipated contemporary debate about the need to balance quality and cost within managed care environments. Donabedian's categorization of variables into "structure" (staff and facility resources and standard procedures), "process" (the delivery of care), and "outcome" (the results of care) continues to provide a useful conceptual framework for analysis of the variables that can affect the quality of medical products and health care services.

Concepts of total quality management and continuous improvement evolved from efforts of Japanese manufacturers to improve products, increase productivity, and reduce costs (e.g., Deming, 1986; Imai, 1986; Juran, 1988). During the 1980s, however, improvements in the quality of care occurred slowly, in part because the tools used to measure health care quality and monitor health care processes had not been developed and it was unclear how health care practitioners and systems could adapt the quality improvement tools developed for industrial environments (Berwick et al., 1991).

Quality improvement represents an evolution and enhancement of the technology developed for quality control and assurance. Quality was originally managed through inspection—finished products were examined to detect flaws, and if they were not satisfactory, they were returned for additional work or discarded. The approach was therefore inherently reactive: errors were corrected after they occurred. Short-term goals were emphasized and production quotas were used to monitor productivity. There was also an adversarial element, in that an inspector or supervisor would review the product and judge the quality of the product and, implicitly, the quality of the worker responsible for the product. Systems based on this model (results-oriented management) do not encourage innovation, do not empower workers to assume greater responsibility, and encourage games that inhibit the identification and correction of problems (Imai, 1986; Scholtes, 1988).

Quality improvement strategies, on the other hand, attempt to prevent problems from occurring so that corrective efforts are not required. Management and supervision become proactive and emphasize processes (process-oriented management); individuals are not blamed, processes are reviewed and critiqued, barriers that inhibit quality are eliminated, workers are encouraged and empowered to participate and assume responsibility, and products are designed to meet the needs and desires of both internal and external customers (Imai, 1986; Scholtes, 1988).

An IOM committee that examined quality review and assurance for Medicare (1990b) compared quality assurance and quality improvement models. They found that although both emphasize outcomes and stress the linkages between processes, the models differed on five dimensions (IOM, 1990b):

• First, quality improvement models require continuous efforts at improvement even when high levels of quality have been achieved; quality assurance efforts, in contrast, would be directed at other issues once specific problems were resolved.

• Second, a consumer perspective is essential to quality improvement efforts and identifies communication and interorganizational relationships that may be overlooked in quality assurance reviews.

• The third difference between the two approaches is a quality improvement interest in patient needs, experiences, and satisfaction that is usually not part of quality assurance.

• Fourth, quality improvement efforts attempt to improve mean performance levels, whereas quality assurance reviews focus on the identification and removal of outliers.

• The last difference is the role of leadership; quality improvement programs require the organizational leadership to assume overall responsibility for persistent improvements in quality and to empower individual workers to participate in and contribute to the transformation of the organization.

The IOM (1990b) review also cautioned that there were few demonstrations of the application of quality improvement techniques to clinical care issues, and the usefulness of these tools to health care was unknown. Nonetheless, by 1992 an IOM committee that examined clinical guidelines found growing interest in quality improvement models within health care settings (IOM, 1992). The National Demonstration Project was an early effort to begin a transformation of health care and increase the use of quality improvement techniques (see Box 2.1).

The key to quality improvement is a change in perspective. Instead of assessing quality through inspection of people and products, processes and systems are created and monitored to prevent flaws and problems, and because quality is determined by the customer, products and services are designed to meet consumer needs and expectations (Berwick et al., 1991; Imai, 1986). Quality improvement also requires the application of scientific methods to the analysis and monitoring

BOX 2.1
National Demonstration Project on Quality Improvement
in Health Care: Applications and Implementation

In 1987 and 1988, the National Demonstration Project on Quality Improvement in Health Care worked with 21 U.S. health care organizations and examined the application of the quality management technology developed for manufacturing processes to the delivery of health care. Ten management principles guided efforts in the National Demonstration Project (Berwick et al., 1991):

1. work requires processes—individuals and departments are both consumers and suppliers, and medical care relies on increasingly complex and interdependent processes;
2. relationships and communication between consumers and suppliers must be sound—organizations that meet customer needs better will be more effective and more successful;
3. defects in quality are usually related to problems in process—systems are more influential than individuals, and changing or berating individuals will not improve processes;
4. poor quality is costly—defective processes and products are a significant expense, and prevention of defects and problems reduces expenses;
5. quality improvement requires an understanding of the causes of variability—failure to control variation leads to quality problems, and variation must be controlled to enhance quality;
6. select the most critical processes for attention—it is impossible to control and measure everything, so clearly define goals and identify the most important sources of problems;
7. use scientific and statistical thinking—measurement helps workers understand processes, facilitates hypothesis testing about the causes of problems, and provides prompt feedback on results;
8. all employees must be involved—senior management provides leadership and eliminates barriers, whereas line staff provide ideas and expertise;
9. new organizational structures are often required to achieve improvements—quality teams and councils cross organizational levels and facilitate integration of efforts; and
10. management must plan for quality, control for quality, and improve quality.

of processes, that is, statistical thinking. Decisions are based on data rather than intuition, so information systems are built and graphical tools are used to monitor critical processes and track the effects of alterations in the delivery of a service or the production of a product

Using these tools, workers are empowered to continually adjust the process and make consistent and persistent improvements in both process and outcomes. Gradual improvement in all aspects of life, but particularly the quality of the environment, process, and products of work, is embodied in the Japanese word *kaizen* (ky'zen) (Imai, 1986). A commitment to *kaizen* requires a careful understanding of processes, systems, and consumers and the application of strategies and tools to the production and delivery of high-quality products and services. The focus on long-term gradual improvement by using scientific methods and by paying attention to consumer needs characterizes true quality improvement orientations.

Quality Improvement in Health Care

Application of quality improvement methods has expanded substantially in health care settings. An annual review of the U.S. health care system reported that 94 percent of hospital chief executives believed that quality improvement programs would enhance efficiencies and reduce costs; 61 percent anticipated increased market share because of quality improvement initiatives (Business and Health Magazine, 1993). Increasingly, accreditation agencies and purchasers expect organizations to have formal quality improvement programs and assess the quality improvement processes as part of their review of a health care organizations (e.g., AMBHA, 1995; CARF, 1996; Digital Equipment Corporation, 1995; NCQA, 1996; URAC, 1996). Similarly, the federal Health Care Financing Administration is responsible for monitoring the quality of services for Medicare recipients and is supporting a quality improvement initiative that emphasizes continuous quality improvement methods, makes information available to the public, is consistent with state and private certification and accreditation programs, and employs multiple measures of quality and performance (GAO, 1996).

Improvements in patient care and outcomes are the ultimate result of quality improvement technology within health care settings. Applications are inhibited, however, because of the variable presentation of illnesses, variations in practice patterns, the hierarchical structure of patient care, and the complexity of hospitals and managed care programs. The "gold standard" for effectiveness continues to be randomized clinical trials, which are prohibitively expensive.

It is therefore noteworthy, for example, that the Northern New England Cardiovascular Disease Study Group applied quality improvement techniques and documented a significant reduction in hospital mortality associated with coronary artery bypass graft surgery in a multi-institutional regional environment (O'Connor et al., 1996). Clinicians, administrators, and researchers from the five hospitals in Vermont, New Hampshire, and Maine where coronary artery bypass graft surgery is performed created a patient registry in 1987 and began a quality improvement initiative in 1990. The initiative involved three kinds of intervention: feedback of outcome data to practitioners, training in continuous quality improvement techniques, and site visits to other medical centers.

Data from 1993 suggested a cumulative reduction of 74 deaths from the mortality levels expected before the quality improvement intervention—a 24 percent reduction. The five institutions made multiple changes in procedures and techniques, so there was no single cause for the decline in mortality; rather, the observed improvements were due to the net effect of their efforts to learn and improve (Berwick, 1996).

Berwick (1996), in commenting on the study group's report, suggests that this type of discovery may be more valuable than randomized clinical trials for cumulative improvement and for the identification of techniques that enhance health care and reduce costs. It is also critical, he argues, that such information be reported to and published in peer-reviewed journals and not be guarded as proprietary information. The techniques and outcomes will be most useful if they are incorporated into clinical guidelines and protocols

Quality Improvement in Behavioral Health Care

Comparable demonstrations of the successful application of quality improvement methods to improved patient outcomes do not appear to exist for mental health and substance abuse treatment services. Both public- and private-sector treatment systems, however, have begun to adapt and apply quality improvement technologies.

In Massachusetts, for example, the Quality Improvement Collaborative is a peer-reviewed total quality management initiative designed to foster the introduction and use of continuous improvement protocols within all of the substance abuse treatment programs under contract with the Massachusetts Department of Public Health's Bureau of Substance Abuse Services (Fishbein and McCarty, in press). Detoxification centers adopted and implemented a model clinical record, and methadone services standardized evaluations of their clients' progress and linked a client's progress to the phases of care; evidence of improvements in patient care, however, are not yet available.

The Massachusetts Medicaid program has also applied quality improvement methods to the management of relationships with its suppliers (managed care organizations and health care providers) and reports improved responsiveness among the suppliers of health care (Friedman et al., 1995). As a result of this initiative, the managed behavioral health care organization responsible for the management of mental health and substance abuse services for the Massachusetts Medicaid program developed its own quality improvement program (Nelson et al., 1995).

Report Cards and Performance Standards

Consumer ratings of service industries have been available for many years but have only recently become available for health care. With the emergence of managed care and consideration of competing health plans, purchasers need to make decisions about what benefits they need, the amount of out-of-pocket expenses or copayments that are desired, and the choice of providers and practitioners within a plan or network. In the public sector, purchasers need to make policy decisions on behalf of publicly insured individuals in the context of the local and regional political and economic environments.

A majority of the health care quality information has been geared toward employers and other purchasers, but there is a growing emphasis on providing information that will help consumers select managed care plans that provide quality and an array of services. Quality in these terms is usually measured as patient satisfaction with the services that have been received. Common dimensions include access to care, perceived quality of the contact with the provider, and outcomes of the contact, such as improvements in health status.

One area of controversy has to do with the quality of the data that are used to prepare report cards. Many health plans produce their own report cards as part of a marketing strategy, and without some kind of independent verification of the data, there may be an incentive to misrepresent information. Another major concern has to do with the comparability of data from different plans, because they may have had different benefit structures, different member populations with different levels of risk, and other differences. One approach has been taken by the Pacific Business Group on Health (PBGH), a nonprofit coalition of public and private purchasers. PBGH has developed a model plan design that all members must adopt, information systems are comparable so that performance can be measured in the same ways across plans, and the data are collected and analyzed in a format that can be audited (Brown, 1996).

Contracts for Purchasing Care

The structure of the contract between a payer and a managed care organization and the means for monitoring and enforcing the contract are among the most important ways to influence the quality of care (Essock and Goldman, 1995). Contracts and contract language in the purchasing agreement should specify expectations about benefits and covered services, standards of care, ways of ensuring that the standards and other quality measures are met, and incentives and disincentives associated with the vendor's performance. For example, if a state agency is concerned about the possibility of a managed care organization "dumping" patients with serious mental illness into the public system, the contract could specify that the organization will have to pay a financial penalty for every day that a person covered by the contract spends in a state hospital (Essock and Goldman,

1995). As a positive financial incentive, a contract might include a bonus based on the number or proportion of individuals who experience reduction in symptoms and other positive outcomes.

Some large purchasers, such as the Digital Equipment Corporation and Pacific Business Group on Health, have developed their own set of standards and monitoring guidelines and requirements and include those in their contracts with managed care organizations. Some other purchasers have adopted these standards, but others may in the future require use of the standards developed by the National Committee for Quality Assurance, which are based in part on the American Managed Behavioral Healthcare Association's performance measure set, or the report card developed by the Center for Mental Health Services. These behavioral health performance measurement systems will be discussed further in Chapter 6.

In an effort to control costs and improve efficiency and quality, many states are contracting with managed behavioral health companies. The development of contracts that protect and enhance care for publicly insured individuals is a new responsibility for state agencies, and technical assistance manuals for public purchasers of managed care have been developed by the Center for Substance Abuse Treatment (1994, 1995) and by the Bazelon Center for Mental Health Law (1995).

ETHICAL ISSUES IN MANAGED BEHAVIORAL HEALTH CARE

Quality of care necessarily raises ethical issues. Most ethical issues related to managed behavioral health care are not new or unique to managed care, either medical or behavioral health managed care. Many of these concerns also existed under fee-for-service systems, but public awareness of these concerns has been increasing as managed care has expanded. The intent of this section of the report is to review the most salient ethical concerns in relation to the quality of care. Generally, these issues revolve around confidentiality, patient autonomy, the practitioner-patient relationship, and the patient's right of appeal.

Confidentiality

Designating the primary care physician as the coordinator of care and requiring prior authorization for treatment and other case management activities inherent in managed care increase the necessity for sharing medical information. The primary concern about confidentiality under managed care focuses on the claim that there is a greater demand to release confidential patient information in managed care systems than under fee-for-service systems. Information is disclosed when authorization for treatment is sought and when patients are referred from one service provider or practitioner to another. These risks for breach of confidentiality are not new under the managed care system, although they are perhaps more accelerated in this system because of increased efforts to centrally manage the care.

Patients have increased concerns about confidentiality related to mental health or substance abuse treatment because of their fear of being stigmatized. Who is bound in the confidential relationship and thus obligated to protect the use of or prevent further disclosure of the information? The most relevant element is therefore the obligation of managed care plans to designate explicitly who can release and receive information and the limits to which it can be used. Ethicists agree that insurers, providers, and practitioners have a duty to safeguard the release of sensitive information through policy directives, information system protections, and quality assurance mechanisms (IOM, 1993).

Confidentiality Regulations in Substance Abuse Treatment

A unique aspect of treatment for alcoholism and drug abuse is the presence of federal regulations (42 CFR Part 2) that require that the confidentiality of information about individuals in substance abuse treatment be maintained. The regulations prohibit unauthorized disclosure of patient-specific information and limit the ways in which disclosure can occur legally. The Hughes Act (P.L. 91-616), its reauthorization (P.L. 93-282), and the Drug Abuse Prevention, Treatment, and Rehabilitation Act of 1972 (P.L. 92-255), as amended by P.L. 93-282, stipulate that treatment records are confidential and required the development of federal regulations to govern the disclosure of information from patient records (Legal Action Center, 1988, 1991; Lopez, 1994; NIDA, 1980).

The regulations protect the privacy of individuals entering care and help assure men and women seeking care that their participation in treatment cannot be disclosed without their consent. The requirements are more restrictive than those related to doctor-patient or attorney-client privilege (Legal Action Center, 1991). All substance abuse treatment services that receive federal assistance, tax exemptions, or authorization to conduct business are covered by the regulations. Most treatment programs follow the guidelines developed by the Legal Action Center (1991) to facilitate the disclosure of patient information and maintain compliance with the regulations.

Without special safeguards, the computerized information systems used to record diagnostic and billing information and to share clinical records within a health plan could violate the federal regulations. The confidentiality of patient records and any information about participation in treatment for alcoholism and drug abuse therefore becomes an especially complex issue within the context of managed behavioral health care.

Patient Autonomy

Patient autonomy can be defined as the right of an individual to exercise free will, have choice among options, and be the decision maker in managing his or her health care. Therefore, from this perspective patient autonomy has always had certain limitations. When one seeks care from another, there is an implicit understanding that the practitioner assumes some role in managing the person's health. To the degree that an individual allows payment for his or her health care by a third party, that party becomes a stakeholder in the process and the patient's autonomy begins to be restricted.

Managed care limits the choices that patients have regarding what services are available and who will provide them. This is part of the rationale under which managed care systems were created. The ethical concern is whether the restriction of choice results in limitations that affect the outcome of care. Even to the degree that managed care may mean less care, one cannot presume that this means worse or less effective care, although exposures in the media and litigated cases have occasionally provided evidence that this can occur (e.g., Goleman, 1996).

Individuals have a responsibility to learn as much as they can about their health plans, including the nature of their benefits (Council on Ethical and Judicial Affairs, 1995). Respect for autonomy assumes that a patient is capable of self-determination, but the capacity of an individual patient to make sound decisions that are in his or her best interest is influenced by the nature and course of the illness, as well as by individual personality and preferences. This is true for all illnesses (Povar, 1991).

Thus, the choices made by a patient may not be those recommended by the patient's clinician or family. Disregarding patient preferences by not offering options can have measurable effects on the patient's compliance as well as the patient's outcome (Povar, 1991). This further complicates the issue of patient autonomy. However, in spite of these factors, patient autonomy and the right to make choices need to be ensured, even though reasonable limitations may exist.

Practitioner-Patient Relationship

The discussion of patient autonomy leads directly to the issue of the practitioner-patient relationship. In medicine, this relationship has always been considered to be based on trust (Council on Ethical and Judicial Affairs, 1995). Critics on both sides argue about the impact that managed care has on this relationship. Advocates say that a primary care physician maintains, by definition, a principal and ongoing association with the patient, serving as the coordinator of his or her medical care. Opponents of managed care believe that the structure of the system distances a patient from the physician. Large group practices, provider panels, prior authorization requirements, and arbitrary assignment of a patient to a practitioner or a series of practitioners can erode the practitioner-patient relationship.

There is general agreement that disrupting an established relationship is usually disadvantageous. The ethical question seems to be to what degree is this allowable without having an effect on the effectiveness of care? Do insurers and providers have an obligation to minimize the likelihood of this happening? Are such mechanisms as policy directives, service delivery structures, and quality reviews adequate safeguards and guarantees for preserving the practitioner-patient relationship?

Society's expectations are the ultimate test of the fit of our measures of quality. We believe that creative dialogue about quality with consumers and persons experiencing recovery from mental illness is a professional and ethical requirement that will change and increase with society's expectations.

Sarah Stanley
American Nurses Association
Public Workshop, April 18, 1996, Washington, DC

The role that patients play in managing their health is a theme common to the ethical concerns of confidentiality, patient autonomy, and the practitioner-patient relationship. Several factors influence what this role can or should be. These include the patient's individual personality, life situation, health history, and functional capacity and cultural background; the nature and course of the illness(es); the effectiveness of health services; and the availability of community support. The manner in which all of these dynamics converge significantly affects the effectiveness of care provided. In the course of events, the decisions made and the outcomes of these decisions can be misunderstood, or can be confusing or disturbing for patients. Patients can feel victimized by the very systems that are supposed to care for them.

To empower patients, they need to receive adequate information regarding choices of treatment and to be able to provide informed consent. Social change and public policy have increased the need to involve patients in their treatment decisions. Health care providers and practitioners, ethicists would agree, have a moral duty to provide systems that empower patients, allow them to be responsible for making treatment decisions, and give them opportunities to appeal decisions made by others on their behalf.

Summary of Ethical Concerns

Addressing the ethical issues in mental health care and addiction treatment is especially complex. This is because of the unique impact that mental illness and addiction have on the reasoning and behavior of individuals and the continuing stigma associated with mental illness and addiction. Much more than physical illness, mental illness and addiction are viewed as social as well as medical problems. The question is not whether managed care should continue in light of these ethical concerns. Rather, it is how managed care must best address and respond to these critical issues.

SUMMARY

This chapter has discussed some of the major trends affecting health care delivery. One major trend is the increasing numbers of individuals enrolled in managed care plans, which take a variety of forms with different delivery and financing structures. A second trend is the increasing numbers of individuals in the public sector who are being enrolled in managed care plans, including a large number of individuals with chronic and severe health problems. A third trend is the shift from exclusive concern with the cost of care to increasing interest in the quality of care, which can be described as the overall value derived from expenditures on health care on the basis of evidence of effectiveness and positive outcomes from care.

John Ruskin, a nineteenth century businessman, said something I think helps us to determine where we have gotten in this field. He said: it is unwise to pay too much, but it is worse to pay too little. When you pay too much, you lose a little money. That is all. But when you pay too little, you sometimes will lose everything, because the thing you bought was incapable of doing the thing it was bought to do.

William Dennis Derr
Employee Assistance Professionals Association
Public Workshop, April 18, 1996, Washington, DC

Quality assurance in health care takes many forms, including licensure and certification of providers and practitioners, practice guidelines, report cards, performance measures, and regulatory approaches such as accreditation. Evidence of the effectiveness of different approaches is still preliminary because of the variety of quality improvement strategies and the complexity of health care. However, the committee believes that there is increasing support and consensus about the importance of quality improvement throughout the health care system.

REFERENCES

Akerlof G. 1970. The market for lemons: Qualitative uncertainity and the market mechanism. *Quarterly Journal of Economics* 84:488-500.
AMBHA (American Managed Behavioral Healthcare Association). 1995. *Performance Measures for Managed Behavioral Healthcare Programs.* Washington, DC: The AMBHA Quality Improvement and Clinical Services Committee.
AMA (American Medical Association). 1993. *Directory of Practice Parameters, 1993 Edition.* Chicago: American Medical Association.
Bazelon Center for Mental Health Law. 1995. *Managing Managed Care for Publicly Financed Mental Health Services.* Washington, DC: Bazelon Center for Mental Health Law.
Berwick DM. 1996. Harvesting knowledge from improvement. *Journal of the American Medical Association* 275:877-878.
Berwick DM, Godfrey AB, Roessner J. 1991. *Curing Health Care: New Strategies for Quality Improvement.* San Francisco: Jossey-Bass Publishers.
Birch and Davis Associates, Inc. 1984. *Development of Model Professional Standards for Counselor Credentialing.* Rockville, MD: National Institute on Alcohol Abuse and Alcoholism.
Boyle PJ, Callahan D. 1995. Managed care in mental health: The ethical issues. *Health Affairs* 14(3):7-22.
Brown C. 1996. *Purchasers' Perspectives on Quality.* Presentation to the IOM Committee on Quality Assurance and Accreditation Guidelines for Managed Behavioral Health Care. Irvine, CA. May 17.
Business and Health Magazine. 1993. *The State of Health Care in America: 1993.* Montvale, NJ: Medical Economics Publishing.
Business and Health Magazine. 1995. *The State of Health Care in America: 1995.* Montvale, NJ: Medical Economics Publishing.
Callahan JJ, Shepard DS, Beinecke RH, Larson M, Cavanaugh D. 1994. *Evaluation of the Massachusetts Medicaid Mental Health/Substance Abuse Program.* Submitted to the Massachusetts Division of Medical Assistance, Mental Health Substance Abuse Program. Waltham, MA: Institute for Health Policy, Brandeis University.
CARF (The Rehabilitation Accreditation Commission). 1996. *1996 Standards Manual and Interpretive Guidelines for Behavioral Health.* Tucson, AZ: The Rehabilitation Accreditation Commission.
Christianson JB, Lurie N, Finch M, Moscovice I. 1989. Mainstreaming the mentally ill in HMOs. *New Directions for Mental Health Services* 43:19-28, Fall.
Council on Ethical and Judicial Affairs, American Medical Association. 1995. Ethical issues in managed care. *Journal of the American Medical Association* 273(4):330-335.
CSAT (Center for Substance Abuse Treatment). 1994. *Managed Healthcare Organizational Readiness Guide and Checklist.* Rockville, MD: Center for Substance Abuse Treatment.
CSAT. 1995. *Purchasing Managed Care Services for Alcohol and Other Drug Treatment: Essential Elements and Policy Issues.* Rockvillle, MD: Center for Substance Abuse Treatment.
Deming WE. 1986. *Out of the Crisis.* Cambridge, MA: MIT-CAES.
DHHS (U.S. Department of Health and Human Services). 1993. *Depression in Primary Care: Clinical Practice Guideline No. 5.* Rockville, MD: Agency for Health Care Policy and Research.
Digital Equipment Corporation. 1995. *HMO Performance Standards.* Maynard, MA: Digital Equipment Corporation.

Donabedian A. 1980. *Explorations in Quality Assessment and Monitoring: The Definition of Quality and Approaches to Its Assessment.* Vol. 1. Ann Arbor, MI: Health Administration Press.

Donabedian A. 1982. *Explorations in Quality Assessment and Monitoring: The Criteria and Standards of Quality.* Vol. 2. Ann Arbor, MI: Health Administration Press.

Donabedian A. 1985. *Explorations in Quality Assessment and Monitoring,: The Methods and Findings of Quality Assessment and Monitoring, An Illustrated Analysis.* Vol. 3. Ann Arbor, MI: Health Administration Press.

EAPA (Employee Assistance Professionals Association, Inc.). 1995. *Glossary of Employee Assistance Terminology.* Arlington, VA: Employee Assistance Professionals Association, Inc.

Edmunds M. 1996. Clinical practice guidelines: Opportunities and implications. *Annals of Behavioral Medicine* 18(2):126-132.

England MJ, Vaccaro VA. 1991. New systems to manage mental health care. *Health Affairs* 10(4): 129-137.

Essock S, Goldman HH. 1995. States embrace of managed mental health care. *Health Affairs* 14(3):34-44.

Fishbein R, McCarty D. In press. Quality improvement for publicly-funded substance abuse treatment services. In: Gibelman M, Demone HW, Jr., eds. *Private Solutions to Public Problems.* New York: Springer Publishing.

Flynn LM, Panzetta, AF, Shumway, DL. 1994. Can managed behavioral healthcare plans serve the severely mentally ill? *Behavioral Healthcare Tomorrow* March:40-48.

Foster Higgins, Inc. 1994. *Managed Behavioral Healthcare: Quality and Access Survey Report.* Washington, DC: American Managed Behavioral Healthcare Association.

Frank RG, McGuire TG, Newhouse JP. 1995. Risk contracts in managed mental health care. *Health Affairs* 14(3):50-64.

Freeman MA, Trabin T. 1994. *Managed Behavioral Healthcare: History, Models, Key Issues, and Future Course.* Rockville, MD: Center for Mental Health Services.

Friedman MD, Bailit MH, Michel JO. 1995. Vendor management: A model for collaboration and quality improvement. *Journal of Quality Improvement* 21:635-645.

GAO (U.S. General Accounting Office). 1995. *Block Grants: Characteristics, Experience, and Lessons Learned.* GAO/HEHS-95-74. Washington, DC: U.S. General Accounting Office.

GAO. 1996. *Medicare: Federal Efforts to Enhance Patient Quality of Care.* GAO/HEHS-96-20. Washington, DC: U.S. General Accounting Office.

Gerson SN. 1994. When should managed care firms terminate private benefits for chronically mentally ill patients? *Behavioral Healthcare Tomorrow* March/April:31-35.

Gold MR, Hurley R, Lake T, Ensor T, Berenson R. 1995. A national survey of the arrangements managed-care plans make with physicians. *The New England Journal of Medicine* 333:1678-1683.

Goleman D. 1996. Critics say managed-care savings are eroding mental care. *The New York Times,* 24 January, C9.

Goldstein L. 1989. Genuine managed care in psychiatry: A proposed practice model. *General Hospital Psychiatry* 2:271-277.

Goplerud E. 1995. *Managed Care for Mental and Substance Abuse Services.* Rockville, MD: Substance Abuse and Mental Health Services Administration.

Gray BH. 1992. The legislative battle over health services research. *Health Affairs* 11(4):38-66.

Health Management Resources, Inc., and Birch and Davis Associates, Inc. 1992. *Final Report: State Standards and Licensing, Certification, Accreditation, and Reimbursement Requirements for Drug Abuse Treatment Programs.* Vol. 1. Technical report submitted to the National Institute on Drug Abuse.

HCFA (Health Care Financing Administration). 1996. *Medicaid Managed Care Enrollment Report.* Baltimore, MD: Health Care Financing Administration.

HIAA (Health Insurance Association of America). 1996. *Source Book of Health Insurance Data, 1995.* Washington DC: Health Insurance Association of America

IOM (Institute of Medicine). 1989. *Controlling Costs and Changing Patient Care? The Role of Utilization Management.* Washington, DC: National Academy Press.

IOM. 1990a. *Broadening the Base of Treatment for Alcohol Problems.* Washington, DC: National Academy Press.

IOM. 1990b. *Medicare: A Strategy for Quality Assurance.* Vol. 1. Washington, DC: National Academy Press.

IOM. 1990c. *Clinical Practice Guidelines: Directions for a New Program.* Washington, DC: National Academy Press.

IOM. 1992. *Guidelines for Clinical Practice: From Development to Use.* Washington, DC: National Academy Press.

IOM. 1993. *Employment and Health Benefits: A Connection at Risk.* Washington, DC: National Academy Press.

IOM. 1996. *Primary Care: America's Health in the New Era.* Washington, DC: National Academy Press.

Iglehart JK. 1996. Managed care and mental health. *The New England Journal of Medicine* 334(2):131-135.

Imai M. 1986. *Kaizen: The Key to Japan's Competitive Success.* New York: McGraw-Hill Publishing Company.

Institute for Health Policy. 1995. *Enabling Support Services Within Mental Health and Substance Abuse Services.* Paper submitted to the Substance Abuse and Mental Health Services Administration.

JCAHO (Joint Commission on Accreditation of Healthcare Organizations). 1996. *Comprehensive Accreditation Manual for Health Care Networks.* Chicago, IL: Joint Commission on Accreditation of Healthcare Organizations.

Juran JM, ed. 1988. *Juran's Quality Control Handbook.* New York: McGraw-Hill.

Kassirer JP. 1995. Managed care and the morality of the marketplace. *The New England Journal of Medicine* 333:50-52.

Krystal H, Moore RA. 1963. Who is qualified to treat the alcoholic? A discussion. *Quarterly Journal of Studies on Alcohol* 24:705-718.

Legal Action Center. 1988. *A Guide to the New Federal Regulations.* New York: Legal Action Center.

Legal Action Center. 1991. *A Guide to the Federal Regulations: Updated and Revised.* New York: Legal Action Center.

Lopez F. 1994. *Confidentiality of Patient Records for Alcohol and Other Drug Treatment: Technical Assistance Publication Series 13.* DHHS Publication No. (SMA) 95-3018. Rockville, MD: Center for Substance Abuse Treatment.

McGovern TF, Armstrong D. 1987. Comparison of recovering and non-alcoholic alcoholism counselors: A survey. *Alcoholism Treatment Quarterly* 4(1):43-60.

McGuire TG. 1989. Financing and demand for mental health services. In: Taube C, Mechanic D, Hohmann A, eds. *The Future of Mental Health Services Research.* DHHS Publication No. ADM 89-1600. Rockville, MD: National Institute on Mental Health.

Mechanic D, Aiken LH. 1989. Capitation in mental health: Potentials and cautions. *New Directions in Mental Health* 43:5-181.

Mechanic D, Schlesinger M, McAlpine DD. 1995. Management of mental health and substance abuse services: State of the art and early results. *The Milbank Quarterly* 73:19-55.

Miller RH, Luft HS. 1994. Managed care plan performance since 1980. *Journal of the American Medical Association* 272 (19):1512-1519.

Mulligan D, McCarty D, Potter D, Krakow M. 1989. Counselors in public and private alcoholism and drug abuse treatment programs. *Alcoholism Treatment Quarterly* 6(3/4):75-89.

Myerson AR. 1995. Helping insurers say no. *The New York Times,* 20 March, C1, C8.

NAADAC (National Association of Alcoholism and Drug Abuse Counselors). 1988. *Position Statement: Accessibility of Treatment by Certified Alcohol and Drug Abuse Counselors.* Washington, DC: National Association of Alcoholism and Drug Abuse Counselors.

NAADAC. 1991. *Position Statement: Quality Treatment from Qualified Professionals.* Washington, DC: National Association of Alcoholism and Drug Abuse Counselors.

NAADAC. 1994. *Position Statement: Health Care Reform and Addiction Treatment Providers.* Washington, DC: National Association of Alcoholism and Drug Abuse Counselors.

NCQA (National Committee for Quality Assurance). 1995. *Standards for Accreditation, 1995 Edition.* Washington, DC: National Committee for Quality Assurance.

NCQA. 1996. *Accreditation Standards for Managed Behavioral Healthcare Organizations.* Washington, DC: National Committee for Quality Assurance.

Nelson DC et al. 1995. Outcomes measurement and management with a large Medicaid population: A public/private collaboration. *Behavioral Healthcare Tomorrow* 4(3):31-37.

NIAAA (National Institute on Alcohol Abuse and Alcoholism). 1971. *First Special Report to the U.S. Congress on Alcohol and Health.* DHEW Publication No. (HSM) 73-9031. Rockville, MD: National Institute on Alcohol Abuse and Alcoholism.

NIDA (National Institute on Drug Abuse). 1980. *Legal Opinions on the Confidentiality of Alcohol and Drug Abuse Patient Records: 1975-1978.* DHHS Publication No. (ADM) 81-1013. Rockville, MD: National Institute on Drug Abuse.

O'Connor GT, Plume SK, Olmstead EM, Morton JR, Maloney CT, Nugent WC, et al. 1996. A regional intervention to improve the hospital mortality associated with coronary artery bypass graft surgery. *Journal of the American Medical Association* 275:841-846.

Povar GJ. 1991. What does quality mean? Critical ethical issues for quality assurance. In: Palmer RH, Donabedian A, Povar GJ, eds. *Striving for Quality in Health Care: An Inquiry into Policy and Practice.* Ann Arbor, MI: Health Administration Press.

PPRC (Physician Payment Review Commission). 1989. *Annual Report to Congress.* Washington, DC: Physician Payment Review Commission.

Rogers WH, Wells KB, Meredith LS, Sturm R, Burnam MA. 1993. Outcomes for adult outpatients with depression under prepaid or fee-for-service financing. *Archives of General Psychiatry* 50(7): 517-525.

Sabin JE. 1995. Organized psychiatry and managed care: Quality improvement or holy war? *Health Affairs* 14(3):32-33.

Schadle M, Christianson JB. 1988. *The Organization of Mental Health Care, Alcohol, and Other Drug Abuse Services Within Health Maintenance Organizations.* Vol. 1. Excelsior, MI: InterStudy.

Schlesinger M. 1995. Ethical issues in policy advocacy. *Health Affairs* 14(3):23-29.

Schlesinger M, Mechanic D. 1993. Challenges for managed competition from chronic illness. *Health Affairs* 12(suppl):123-137.

Scholtes PR. 1988. *The Team Handbook: How to Use Teams to Improve Quality.* Madison, WI: Joiner Associates, Inc.

Sharfstein SS, Stoline AM. 1992. Reform issues for insuring mental health care. *Health Affairs* 11(3):84-97.

Shortell SM, Gillies RR, Anderson DA. 1994. New world of managed care: Creating organized delivery systems. *Health Affairs* 13:46-64.

Starr P. 1982. *The Social Transformation of American Medicine.* New York: Basic Books, Inc.

Surles RC. 1995. Broadening the ethical analysis of managed care. *Health Affairs* 14(3):29-31.

United HealthCare Corporation. 1994. *The Managed Care Resource: The Language of Managed Health Care and Organized Health Care Systems.* Minnetonka, MN: United HealthCare Corporation.

URAC (Utilization Review Accreditation Commission). 1996. *National Network Accreditation Standards.* Washington, DC: Utilization Review Accreditation Commission.

Valle S. 1979. *Alcoholism Counseling.* Springfield, IL: Charles C Thomas.

Wells KB, Astrachan BM, Tischler GL, Unutzer J. 1995. Issues and approaches in evaluating managed mental health care. *The Milbank Quarterly* 73(1):57-75.

3

Challenges in Delivery of
Behavioral Health Care

The most unusual aspect of the care and financing system for mental health and substance abuse is the presence of a distinct and substantial publicly managed care system that serves as a safety net. Thus, public services are available for those with public insurance, as well as for those who have private insurance, under circumstances that will be described in this chapter. Public services are funded through a large number of categorical programs administered by different agencies, creating both duplication and gaps in service, and these programs almost always have different eligibility requirements. In addition, funding is fragmented, which leads to fragmented service delivery.

Another challenge is that much mental health and substance abuse care, for perhaps as many as half of all episodes, is provided in primary care settings, not in specialty programs (IOM, 1996). Despite clinical practice guidelines, continuing education courses, and other training programs, however, primary care practitioners tend to underdiagnose depression, substance abuse, and other behavioral health problems (IOM, 1996). This is changing, but there is a great need to improve the quality of mental health and substance abuse care delivered in primary care settings and also to better coordinate the care delivered in primary care and specialty sectors (IOM, 1996).

In addition, a significant portion of the public care system for individuals with the most disabling conditions extends beyond health care services to rehabilitative and support services, including housing, job counseling, literacy, and other programs. The coordination of these services requires collaborative and cooperative relationships among many agencies, including public health, mental health, social services, housing, education, criminal justice, and others. Most of these services are not covered by private insurance and have not been developed by most private behavioral health care companies.

Any approach to reform of mental health and substance abuse care services or to the problem of accountability must reckon with these factors, which are not simultaneously present in any other substantial sector of health care services. The dynamics of the three interrelated sectors—privately funded primary and specialty health care and public health care systems—are complex and also highly idiosyncratic from state to state, community to community, and plan to plan. An additional layer of complexity comes from the historical separation of treatment systems for mental health, drug abuse, alcohol abuse, and the primary care system in both the public and private sectors.

This chapter will set out the committee's views about the unique challenges in the delivery of behavioral health care. The chapter includes a description of the prevalence and costs of mental health and substance abuse problems, the difficulties and fragmentation of the current system for the delivery of care, the role of primary care, and a description of some of the support services that are needed for the long-term management of mental health and substance abuse problems. Historical perspectives on separate systems are also provided.

EXTENT AND IMPACT OF BEHAVIORAL HEALTH PROBLEMS

Prevalence

The social consequences of mental health and substance abuse problems are much greater than generally appreciated. The prevalence of these conditions in society is quite large, and the economic burdens are substantial.

The most recent estimates of the prevalence of behavioral health disorders suggest that almost a third of the adult population experiences some impairment due to a behavioral health problem in any one year (Kessler et al., 1994). The most common problems experienced by the adult population annually are anxiety disorders (17 percent), alcohol dependence (7 percent), and affective disorders (11 percent) (Kessler et al., 1994) (see Table 3.1).

Many of the most serious and often disabling mental disorders (e.g., schizophrenia, major depression, bipolar illness, or manic depression) affect a total of 1 to 2 percent of the adult population annually. The incidence and prevalence of child and adolescent problems is not as well established, but levels of emotional disturbance that affect functioning are noted in about one of every eight children and adolescents (SAMHSA, 1996) (see Table 3.2a). Estimated annual prevalence of drug use among children and adolescents is presented in Table 3.2b.

Estimates of the impact of mental health and substance abuse problems reveal the substantial effects of these conditions. The direct and indirect costs to society have been estimated at $257 billion for substance abuse (Rice, 1995) (see Table 3.3) and $148 billion for mental illness in 1990 (Rice, 1995; Rice and

TABLE 3.1   Estimated Annual Prevalence of Behavioral Health Problems in the United States (Ages 15–54)

Behavioral Health Problems	Prevalence (percent)
All behavioral health problems	29.5
Any mental disorder	22.9
Any affective disorder	11.3
Major depressive episode	10.3
Manic episode	1.3
Dysthymia	2.5
Any anxiety disorder	17.2
Panic disorder	2.3
Agoraphobia without panic disorder	2.8
Social phobia	7.9
Simple phobia	8.8
Generalized anxiety disorder	3.1
Other disorders	
Antisocial psychosis	N/A[a]
Nonaffective psychosis[b]	0.5
Substance abuse or dependence	11.3
Alcohol abuse without dependence	2.5
Alcohol dependence	7.2
Drug abuse without dependence	0.8
Drug dependence	2.8

[a]N/A, not available.
[b]Nonaffective psychosis includes schizophrenia, schizo-phreniform disorder, schizoaffective disorder, and atypical psychosis.
SOURCE: Kessler et al. (1994).

Miller, 1996; Varmus, 1995) (see Table 3.4). Mental health and substance abuse factors are associated with a majority of suicides, whereas alcohol abuse alone is implicated in 50 percent of all homicides and 30 percent of all accidental deaths (NIAAA, 1990). One third of all criminal justice costs relate to mental health and substance abuse problems (Rice et al., 1990), and general health care costs are significantly increased by the presence of these disorders (NAMHC, 1993). Perhaps the simplest summary of the scope of these conditions is that mental health and substance abuse problems are comparable in magnitude to cancer and heart disease (see Table 3.5).

Underestimating the Scope of the Problem

Although the stigma associated with seeking treatment for mental or addictive disorders is a significant factor in masking the scope of these problems by keeping them "in the closet," the unusual fragmentation of these sectors of care is

TABLE 3.2a Sample of Estimated Annual Prevalence of Behavioral Health Problems in Children and Adolescents

	Lavigne et al., 1996	Bird et al., 1988	Offord et al., 1989	Costello et al., 1988	Anderson et al., 1987	Velez et al., 1989
Methods	Child (Play observation and developmental evaluation) Parent (Checklist and Interview)	Child (Interview) Parent (interview)	Child (Checklist) Parent (Interview) Teacher (Checklist)	Child Interview Parent (Interview)	Child (Interview) Parent (Checklist) Teacher (checklist)	Child (Interview) Parent (Interview)
Sample size	N = 510	N = 777	N = 2,679	N = 789	N = 782	N = 776
Age	2–5 years (percent)	4–16 years (percent)	4–16 years (percent)	7–11 years (percent)	11 years (percent)	11–20 years (percent)
All mental disorders	21.4	18	18.1	22.0	17.6	17.7
Attention deficit disorder (w/wo hyperactivity)	2.0	9.9	6.2	2.2	6.7	4.3
Oppositional disorder	16.8	9.5	—	6.6	5.7	6.6
Conduct disorder	—	1.5	5.5	2.6	3.4	5.4
Separation anxiety	—	4.7	—	4.1	3.5	5.4
Overanxious disorder	—	—	9.9	4.6	2.9	2.7
Simple phobia	—	2.3	—	9.2	2.4	—
Depression (dysthymia)	—	5.9	—	2.0	1.8	1.7
Functional enuresis	—	4.7	—	4.4	—	—

NOTE: The prevalence rates listed above reveal the range of rates estimated for specific disorders among different age groups. Studies are under way at NIMH and CMHS to update these estimates.

SOURCES: Anderson et al. (1987), Bird et al. (1988), Costello (1989), Costello et al. (1988), Lavigne et al. (1996), Offord et al. (1989), and Velez et al. (1989).

TABLE 3.2b   Estimated Annual Prevalence of Drug Use Among Children and Adolescents, 1995

Age	National Household Survey on Drug Abuse, 1995 Findings (SAMHSA, 1996) 12–17 years (percent)	Monitoring the Future Study, 1995 Findings (Johnston et al., 1996)		
		8th graders (percent)	10th graders (percent)	12th graders (percent)
Any illicit drug use	18.0	21.4	33.3	39.0
Marijuana use	14.2	15.8	28.7	34.7
Cocaine use	1.7	2.6	3.5	4.0
Alcohol use	21.1*	45.3	63.5	73.7
Cigarette use	26.6	19.1*	27.9*	33.5*

*Indicates past month prevalence.

SOURCES: Johnston et al. (1996) and SAMHSA (1996).

also part of the problem. A first factor is that, unlike most other health conditions, separate publicly managed health care systems are maintained for mental illness and substance abuse treatment. The publicly managed systems, with responsibility divided between federal, state, and local governments, and also divided for mental illness and substance abuse care, permit a de facto catastrophic insurance function that allows private purchasers to strictly limit behavioral health care coverage because they know that they will not be leaving their employees without an alternative. The magnitude of the public-sector role is substantial, especially in caring for individuals with histories of chronic mental illness, alcoholism, and drug dependence.

The public-sector commitment is not just in the form of public insurance programs like Medicare and Medicaid but is also through state and local funding of systems of care. Estimated 1994 mental health care costs were about $81 billion, of which state and local funding was about $22 billion (Oss, 1994). In several states, Medicaid supports about one third of the community mental health center program and may be the sole funding source for community support and rehabilitation services funded through state mental health agency appropriations and reimbursed by Medicaid (AMBHA and NASMHPD, 1995). Thus, the public role is much larger than that in the rest of the health care system, and there is a fragmented division of labor between the public and private sectors. This makes estimating total treatment costs more difficult.

High Indirect Costs

Some costs incurred in the care of behavioral health disorders—especially for

TABLE 3.3 Estimated Annual Economic Costs of Substance Abuse, 1990 (millions)

Type of Cost	Illicit Drugs	Alcohol	Nicotine	Total
Total	$66,873	$98,623	$91,269	$256,765
Core Costs	14,602	80,763	91,269	186,634
Direct	3,197	10,512	39,130	52,839
Mental health/specialty organizations	867	3,469	–	4,336
Short-stay hospitals	1,889	4,589	21,072	27,550
Office-based physicians	88	240	12,251	12,579
Other professional services	32	329	a	361
Prescription drugs	–	–	1,469	1,469
Nursing homes	–	1,095	3,858	4,953
Home health services	–	–	480	480
Support costs	321	790	–	1,111
Indirect	11,405	70,251	52,139	133,795
Morbidity[b]	7,997	36,627	6,603	51,227
Mortality[c]	3,408	33,624	45,536	82,568
Other Related Costs	45,989	15,771	–	61,760
Direct	18,043	10,436	–	28,479
Crime	18,035	5,807	–	23,842
Motor vehicle crashes	–	3,876	–	3,876
Fire destruction	–	633	–	633
Social welfare administration	8	120	–	128
Indirect	27,946	5,335	–	33,281
Victims of crime	1,042	576	–	1,618
Incarceration[d]	7,813	4,759	–	12,572
Crime careers[e]	19,091	–	–	19,091
	6,282	–	–	6,282
Fetal Alcohol Syndrome	–	2,089	–	2,089

NOTE: The costs in 1990 for illicit drugs and alcohol abuse are based on socioeconomic indexes applied to 1985 estimates (Rice et al., 1990); direct costs for cigarette smoking are deflated from 1993 direct cost estimates (MMWR, 1994); indirect costs for cigarette smoking are from Rice et al. (1992).

[a]Amounts spent (nicotine) for other professional services are included in office-based physicians.

[b]Value of goods and services lost by individuals unable to perform their usual activities because of drug abuse or unable to perform them at a level of full effectiveness.

[c]Present value of future earnings lost; illicit drugs and alcohol are discounted at 6 percent and nicotine is discounted at 4 percent.

[d]Value of lost productivity of incarcerated individuals.

[e]Value of lost productivity of people who engage in criminal activity as a result of drug abuse.

SOURCE: Rice (1995).

TABLE 3.4   Estimated Annual Economic Costs of Mental Disorders by Disorder, 1990 (millions)

Type of cost	Total Mental Disorders	Anxiety Disorders	Schizo-phrenia	Affective Disorders	Other Disorders
Total	$147,847	$46,551	$32,538	$30,373	$38,385
Core Costs	141,887	46,184	29,292	29,073	37,338
Direct	67,000	10,748	17,296	19,215	19,741
Mental health organizations	19,516	1,985	6,520	4,873	6,138
Short-stay hospitals	13,392	388	2,595	4,695	5,714
Office-based physicians	3,655	356	406	1,171	1,722
Other professional services	6,599	645	710	2,047	3,197
Nursing homes	16,478	5,460	5,316	4,543	1,159
Drugs	2,191	1,167	397	406	221
Support costs	5,169	747	1,352	1,480	1,590
Indirect	74,887	35,436	11,996	9,858	17,597
Morbidity[a]	63,083	34,161	10,694	2,195	16,033
Noninstitutionalized population	58,988	33,105	8,837	1,556	15,490
Institutionalized population	4,095	1,056	1,857	639	543
Mortality[b]	11,804	1,275	1,302	7,663	1,564
Other Related Costs	5,960	367	3,246	1,300	1,047
Direct	2,292	229	599	656	808
Crime	1,777	178	464	508	627
Social welfare administration	515	51	135	148	181
Indirect	3,668	138	2,647	644	239
Incarceration	573	58	150	164	201
Family caregiving	3,095	80	2,497	480	38

NOTE: 1990 costs are based on socioeconomic indexes applied to 1985 cost estimates.

[a]Value of goods and services lost by individuals unable to perform their usual activities or unable to perform them at a level of full effectiveness.
[b]Present value of future earnings lost discounted at 6 percent.

SOURCE: Rice and Miller (1996).

TABLE 3.5 Estimated Annual Costs of Illness for Selected Diseases and Conditions (billions of dollars)

Disease	Year	Total	Direct	Indirect	Other Related[a]
Drug addiction, total[b,c]	1990	$256.8	$52.8	$133.8	$61.8
Alcohol[b]	1990	98.6	10.5	70.3	15.8
Illicit drugs[b]	1990	66.9	3.2	11.4	46.0
Nicotine[b]	1990	91.3	39.1	52.1	[d]
Mental disorders, total	1990	147.8	67.0	74.8	6.0
Anxiety disorders	1990	46.5	10.7	35.4	0.4
Schizophrenia	1990	32.5	17.3	12.0	3.2
Affective disorders	1990	30.4	19.2	9.9	1.3
Other disorders	1990	38.4	19.7	17.6	1.1
Diabetes	1992	137.1	91.1	46.6	[d]
Heart disease[e]	1991	125.8	70.9	54.9	[d]
Cancer (all sites)[e]	1990	96.1	27.5	68.7	[d]
Alzheimer's disease	1992	87.9	13.3	74.6	[d]
Arthritis	1992	54.6	12.7	41.8	[d]
Stroke	1993	30.0	17.0	13.0	[d]
AIDS	1992	N/A[f]	10.3	N/A	[d]

NOTE: Data in table may not sum to totals due to rounding.

[a]Other related costs of drug addiction include direct and indirect costs of crime, motor vehicle crashes, fire destruction, and social welfare administration.

[b]Total includes costs of AIDS and fetal alcohol syndrome.

[c]The year 1990 is used as the base year because it is the most recent date for which the total costs of drug addition to society has been estimated. More recent figures were not available at the time of the study.

[d]Not calculated.

[e]Includes costs of adverse health effects of prescription drugs.

[f]N/A, not available.

SOURCES: NHLBI (1994), Rice (1995), Rice and Miller (1996), and Varmus (1995).

patients with the greatest disabilities cared for in public-sector programs—are not health care-related costs. The services needed by these individuals may include housing supports, job training and rehabilitation, and a wide variety of other forms of assistance not considered and rarely funded by health insurance. Partly because of the disability associated with serious mental health and substance abuse problems and partly because of poor private insurance coverage for treatment of these conditions, many people with serious conditions permanently lose employment and require income maintenance benefits for extended periods. Because they are transfers rather than social costs, these expenses often are not included in estimates of total costs.

Some of the problems attributed to behavioral health disorders have already been mentioned, including higher mortality, disability, and lost employment. In general, levels of impairment are comparable for mental disorders and common medical disorders. Because of this pattern and poor access to treatment, a significant proportion of societal costs due to behavioral health problems are not a result of treatment costs but are due to lost productivity and related costs.

The Potential of Treatment

In broad terms, research on treatment outcomes seeks to answer questions such as whether an intervention has been successful, whether it is more effective than other treatments, whether its effectiveness is better with some groups than with others, whether the setting of care makes a difference, and so on. Outcomes research has many subfields, including quality of care, consumer satisfaction, quality of life, provider-patient relationships, patterns of practice, technology assessment, cost-effectiveness, and bioethics (e.g., Brook and Lohr, 1985; Bunker, 1988; Eddy, 1990; Greenfield et al., 1992; Guadagnoli and McNeil, 1994; Lohr, 1988). Surprisingly little is known about the comparative effectiveness of different practitioners, because most outcomes research focuses on the treatment setting or approach rather than the practitioners who deliver care.

It is exceedingly difficult if not impossible to generalize about the findings from treatment research in behavioral health, which includes drug abuse, alcohol abuse and alcoholism, and mental illness. Research histories stretch back decades in some cases, such as methadone maintenance, whereas other areas are relatively recent. Studies tend to be published in dozens of specialty journals, and relatively few studies have been published in mainstream medical journals. Moreover, the quality of the evidence is generally viewed outside the fields as unconvincing, and this is given as one reason for justifying a lack of insurance coverage for behavioral health.

For at least 20 years, drug abuse researchers have been studying treatment effectiveness, including work with cocaine abuse, methadone maintenance, and marijuana abuse (e.g., Hubbard et al.,1989; IOM, 1990a, 1996; McLellan et al., 1980, 1982). Research on drug abuse treatment has shown consistently that effectiveness depends on the length of time in treatment, the intensity of treatment, and the availability of aftercare to maintain recovery (CSAT, 1995). Alcoholism treatment research is generally a research "culture" separate from drug treatment research, but the two areas of research have come to many of the same conclusions: no single treatment approach works for everyone, but most people benefit from a combination of modalities (e.g., IOM 1990b; McLellan et al., 1996).

Drug and alcohol treatment research thus focuses on the use of a particular substance. In contrast, much more clinical uncertainty is associated with the diagnoses in mental health. Still, mental health outcomes research studies tend to be concentrated according to diagnosis; the majority of research has been conducted on depression, anxiety disorders, schizophrenia, and attention deficit and hyperactivity disorder in children (Burnam, in press). Randomized controlled clinical trials have been conducted to test the effectiveness of medications, whereas other studies have compared the differential effects of therapeutic strategies, such as cognitive therapy or psychosocial support for depression (McLellan et al., 1996). Thus, generalizations are difficult to make with the existing data, but it would be appropriate to say that individuals can benefit from a variety of treatment strategies, including medication and psychotherapy or counseling, and that most practitioners seek to find an effective combination for each individual whom they treat.

In the committee's view, then, the available evidence suggests that most forms of mental health and substance abuse treatment are effective for some of the many people affected by behavioral health problems (see Box 3.1), but much remains to be learned about which treatments work best for which individuals to improve their functioning and reduce their symptoms. The lack of systematic studies of treatment outcomes, however, is not unique to behavioral health. From an outcomes research perspective, relatively little has been done to substantiate the majority of medical practice. In other words, the accuracy and reliability of diagnosis and the effectiveness of behavioral health treatment are viewed as comparable to equivalent measures for medical care in general (NAMHC, 1993).

In the mental health field, there is justified optimism about improving the effectiveness of treatment. In the case of schizophrenia alone, for example, improved medications including clozapine and risperidone have become available in recent years, other antipsychotic medications will soon be made available, and the effectiveness of relatively new psychosocial treatments including assertive community treatment and multiple family group treatment has been validated (AHCPR, 1995). There is more evidence that the long-term prognosis of recovery is better than was previously thought, even for the most serious disorders (Harding et al., 1992). Thus, the mental health field shares considerable optimism that was neither present nor justified in past generations.

In the drug treatment field, there is confidence about the effectiveness of treatment when it is delivered appropriately. Some of the most recent data have been developed in the National Treatment Improvement Evaluation Study (NTIES) sponsored by the Center for Substance Abuse Treatment (CSAT) (1995). CSAT is supporting pilot studies to develop and test outcomes monitoring measurement systems in a number of states. Preliminary data indicate that treatment is effective in reducing drug use and associated crime and that the reductions are more likely to be maintained with case management and ongoing aftercare (CSAT, 1995). In essence, the challenge for the drug treatment field is not so much developing more evidence of treatment effectiveness as it is convincing decision makers that investments in treatment are worthwhile and cost-effective.

Treatment effectiveness is discussed further in Chapter 7, Outcomes, and in the papers by McLellan et al. and Steinwachs, in Appendixes B and C, respectively.

BOX 3.1
The Case for Treatment of Mental Disorders and Addiction

Mental Disorders

- In the United States, more than 50 million Americans are faced with a mental disorder or addiction each year. Of these Americans, fewer than half receive treatment (Regier et al., 1993).

- Anxiety disorders affect more than 23 million Americans in a given year. On average, anxiety disorders cost $625 per patient for inpatient treatment. Outpatient treatment for anxiety disorders commonly costs as little as $500 a year, with the same results (NIMH, 1995).

- Affective or mood disorders affect nearly 18 million Americans annually, exacting an enormous human toll and cost to the U.S. economy—$43.7 billion a year in treatment, disability, and lost productivity, a figure comparable to that for heart disease. Nearly 85 percent of people with unipolar depression or dysthymia also respond positively to antidepressant medication or psychotherapy, either alone or in combination (NIMH, 1995).

- Schizophrenia, one of the most chronic and disabling mental disorders, affects about 1 percent of the U.S. population, with economic costs from treatment and lost income totaling more than $30 billion annually. However, new antipsychotic medications are helping to reduce the symptoms of schizophrenia, as well as the adverse side effects of past medications (NIMH, 1995).

Addiction

- In the United States, more than 18 million people who use alcohol and 5 million who use illicit drugs are in need of substance abuse treatment. Of that number, fewer than one in four receive treatment (Institute for Health Policy, Brandeis University, 1993).

- A 1994 California study of the cost-effectiveness of alcohol and other drug treatment programs found an average return to taxpayers of $7 for every $1 invested (Gerstein et al., 1994).

- The same study found that the level of criminal activity declined by two-thirds, from 73.6 percent before treatment to 20.3 percent after treatment (Gerstein et al., 1994).

- In California, hospitalizations were reduced by approximately one-third after treatment, including a reduction of 58 percent in drug overdose admissions and a reduction of 44 percent in mental health admissions (Gerstein et al., 1994).

- In Minnesota, an evaluation of Consolidated Chemical Dependency Treatment Fund activity found that almost 80 percent of treatment costs were offset in the first year alone. The savings were achieved through reductions in medical and psychiatric hospitalizations, detoxification admissions, and arrests (Minnesota Department of Human Services, Chemical Dependency Division, 1995).

- The Health Insurance Association of America estimates savings of from $48,000 to $150,000 in costs for maternity care, physicians' fees, and hospital charges for each delivery that is uncomplicated by substance abuse (CSAT, 1995).

THE ROLE OF PRIMARY CARE

Primary care has been defined by the Institute of Medicine (IOM) as follows:

Primary care is the provision of integrated, accessible health care services by clinicians who are accountable for addressing a large majority of personal health care needs, developing a sustained partnership with patients, and practicing in the context of family and community (IOM, 1996, p. 32).

In this definition, integrated care refers to comprehensive, coordinated, and continuous services whose processes are seamless across different levels of care. Accountability refers to the responsibility for quality of care, patient satisfaction, efficient use of resources, and ethical behavior. The context of family and community refers to an understanding of the importance of living conditions, cultural background, and the impact of family dynamics on health status and also recognizes the caregiving role of families. The committee agrees with this definition and endorses it.

In a given year, an estimated 10 to 20 percent of the general population consult with a primary care physician about a mental health problem (Hankin and Otkay, 1979; IOM, 1996; Schulberg and Burns, 1988). More than a dozen studies have looked at the rate of recognition of mental health and substance abuse problems in primary care settings (IOM, 1996). Most often a person will present with a physical complaint, and about half the time the primary care clinician will recognize the underlying behavioral health issues (Bridges and Goldberg, 1985; Kirmayer et al., 1993). In the small number of cases in which the presenting problem is emotional or psychological, the mental health or substance abuse diagnosis is correctly determined about 90 percent of the time (Bridges and Goldberg, 1985).

Depression is the best known and most widely studied behavioral health problem in primary care, and the only guidelines for behavioral health treatment in primary care settings are for depression (AHCPR, 1993). The Medical Outcomes Study (Sturm and Wells, 1995) followed individuals with severe depression and compared the treatment effectiveness of treatment by primary care physicians, psychiatrists, and other mental health professionals. The quality of care provided by psychiatrists was found in that study to be significantly better than the quality of care given by primary care practitioners, but the cost of care was significantly less in the general medical sector.

Some studies have demonstrated that the integration of mental health and substance abuse professionals into primary care settings can improve patient outcomes with minimal changes in costs (Katon et al., 1995; Schulberg et al., 1995). For this integration to work, clear clinical protocols and standards of care are needed, the mental health professionals should be on-site, and the relationship between the patient and the primary care provider should continue (IOM, 1996). In summary, there is evidence that treatment in primary care settings given by behavioral health professionals can be effective and cost-effective.

We encourage physicians to have enough skill to be able to know when there is a problem and something needs to be done, and then enough self-awareness to know whether they are the ones to do it or somebody else should.

Linda Bresolin
American Medical Association
Public Workshop, April 18, 1996, Washington, DC

The alternative to integration is carve-outs, in which patients are referred to completely separate systems for behavioral health care. These systems sometimes consist of contracts with private mental health professionals who work on a capitated or fee-for-service basis. More often, they include plans with teams of psychiatrists, psychologists, family therapists, social workers, substance abuse counselors, or various combinations of these professionals. The rapid growth in carve-outs has been attributed to the failures of primary care clinicians to adequately diagnose and treat individuals who have mental health and substance abuse problems (England and Vaccaro, 1991; Iglehart, 1996).

One advantage of carve-outs is that they operate separately from primary care and thus reserve resources that might be displaced in an integrated system. They also protect a patient's confidentiality through the use of separate clinical records and billing systems. Conversely, the separation of systems can make the coordination of care more difficult. At this time, there is no clear evidence that carve-outs provide care that is any more or less effective than the care provided in integrated systems. In both systems, however, there are disincentives for primary care practitioners to identify and treat mental health and substance abuse problems (IOM, 1996). The provision of care depends almost entirely on the fee structure and on the time needed to conduct the procedures that are reimbursed. When primary care clinicians are not paid for the time that they spend interviewing primary care patients about mental health and substance abuse problems, the incentive structure works against the identification and treatment of mental health and substance abuse problems. These issues are discussed in detail in the IOM (1996) report *Primary Care: America's Health in a New Era*, and interested readers are referred to that report.

We're working with our primary care docs to use a screening instrument. The patients can fill this out in the office, and it can be faxed directly to us and optically scanned. We can get the information back to the primary care doc while the patient is still in the office. We can help the doc make a decision as to whether or not this is a patient that can be managed in their own setting, or needs to be referred out, based on the depression guidelines that we helped create with them.

Peter Panzarino
Vista Behavioral Health
Public Workshop, May 17, 1996, Irvine, CA

A challenge for quality assurance is to assess, monitor, and regulate mental health and substance abuse care in primary care settings. This is a pervasive problem, given the high percentage of mental health and substance abuse care provided in these settings, but the breadth of the issue is tempered by the fact that there may be less risk of serious problems in this arena, in that many patients whose mental health and substance abuse problems are treated in primary care settings are less ill or disabled (IOM, 1996). On the other hand, failure to recognize or appropriately treat a mild depression or dysthymia, for example, may have modest short-term consequences but may also fail to prevent an otherwise unnecessary escalation of the illness into severe depression.

The challenges in monitoring behavioral health care in primary care settings are magnified by the increased scope and complexity of the health conditions that are expected to be treated in the primary care settings, the wide variability in the extent of psychiatric training received by family physicians and other primary care practitioners, and the rapid development of new treatments that makes it increasingly difficult for practitioners to stay current. However, as a matter of policy, the committee agrees with the IOM Committee on the Future of Primary Care and its recommendation to develop and evaluate collaborative care models with primary care clinicians and behavioral health professionals (IOM, 1996).

SPECIAL ISSUES FOR QUALITY IN BEHAVIORAL HEALTH CARE

Many challenges are related to measuring, ensuring, and improving the quality of care in specialty settings and, especially, in managed behavioral health care settings. The field of managed behavioral health care is new, diverse, and highly competitive. Therefore, it is not regulated as intensively as more traditional forms of managed care. For example, both the federal government and the states regulate health maintenance organizations (HMOs) as insurance entities and in terms of the practice of health care (See Table 2.1 in Chapter 2). There is little regulation, however, of insurance or medical care issues in managed behavioral health care companies. This issue will be discussed further in Chapter 6, Process, which includes a description of the accreditation process.

General Dynamics of Care and Coverage

Changing Coverage

Coverage for behavioral health care continues to change. The history of coverage for alcoholism is a good example. Until relatively recently, most health insurance did not include coverage for alcoholism. In 1968, alcoholics were excluded from 60 percent of the general hospitals, and 40 percent of the Blue Cross and Blue Shield plans explicitly excluded coverage for alcoholism treatment (NIAAA, 1974). NIAAA advocated for the inclusion of alcoholism treatment as a benefit under health insurance and encouraged employers to support treatment for alcoholic employees (IOM, 1990a). The agency also contracted with the Joint Commission on Accreditation of Hospitals to develop accreditation standards for hospitals and specialty treatment services, supported counselor credentialing standards, and had Blue Cross and Blue Shield develop a model benefit package (Regan, 1981). Resistance to the inclusion of alcoholism treatment benefits in employer-sponsored health plans, however, was still strong.

Because a voluntary expansion of benefits appeared unlikely, states changed insurance regulations and laws to mandate coverage for alcoholism treatment in group health insurance plans (NIAAA, 1974; Scott et al., 1992). The first states to require coverage for inpatient alcoholism treatment were Wisconsin (in 1972), Illinois, Massachusetts, Minnesota, and Washington State (NIAAA, 1974; Scott et al., 1992). Massachusetts also required coverage for outpatient care. The National Association of Insurance Commissioners in 1981 adopted a model of benefits for alcoholism treatment —30 days of inpatient care and 30 outpatient visits per year (Scott et al., 1992). A 1991 review found that 41 states either require coverage (23 states) or require that coverage be offered (18 states); most of the states, however, have never altered the original benefit, so the value of the benefits may have eroded (Scott et al., 1992).

Although insurance mandates were an important policy strategy and stimulated the development of many private-sector alcoholism treatment services, health care financing and reimbursement systems evolved to better control the costs associated with alcoholism treatment. The Employee Retirement Income Security Act of 1974 (ERISA) exempts self-insured employers from state insurance mandates; thus, state insurance mandates have decreasing influence on the structure of health care. Employer-purchased managed care plans therefore may not need to be responsive to insurance mandates. As a result, managed care strategies are altering the organization and delivery of private- and public-sector services.

Current Coverage for Behavioral Health

Currently, the vast majority of individuals who have health insurance also have some coverage for behavioral health treatment (see Chapter 1). As has already been discussed, a substantial number of people with behavioral health disorders—especially those with less acute or disabling conditions—receive some care from their primary care practitioners.

Although most private health plans provide some coverage for care of behavioral health problems, most of these plans and Medicare have coverage limits that tend to be more restrictive than the coverage limits for treatment of physical illnesses. Annual limits on the number of outpatient visits and inpatient hospital days are common (IOM, 1993). Other limits in insurance coverage (low lifetime coverage caps, restricted benefits, higher coinsurance) mean that most private health care coverage does not offer protection against catastrophic mental or addictive disorders.

Service-Sector Boundaries

In thinking about health care in general, the special problems faced by uninsured individuals are usually recognized. Behavioral health care faces a distinct problem: in addition to the substantial population of uninsured individuals, who by definition have no coverage for specialty care, the limits described above create gaps in coverage for the privately insured. This is where the public sector comes in. Since the establishment of asylums for the treatment of mental illness in the 19th century, the public system has specialized in the care and support of indigent individuals with the most serious and protracted conditions. In fact, it can be argued that the existence of this public safety net has mitigated against improvements in private coverage.

Individuals who have severe mental illness thus are a group with special needs under managed care, and advocates have identified specific concerns about how well those needs will be met. Less frequently identified as having special needs are those individuals who do not have severe mental illness but who have severe personality disorders or post-traumatic stress disorder. These patients often use extensive treatment resources with little clear improvement. If private coverage for these patients is limited, they may leave the prepaid system or pay out of pocket for their treatment. They do not usually qualify for public-sector services, but they may need more than private coverage may provide.

The result of this counterproductive division of labor is that private coverage tends to be available for the time-limited and traditional treatments for behavioral health problems (e.g., benefits for limited inpatient treatment and limited

TABLE 3.6   Uses of Funds for Mental Health and Substance Abuse: United States, 1990

Population Group	No of Subjects (millions)	Amount per Capita	Total Amount (billions of dollars)
Privately insured	160.4	$138	$22.2
Medicaid	22.1	430	9.5
Medicare	31.2	71	2.2
Uninsured	35.0	575	20.1
SMI[a]	5.6	3,205	17.9
Non-SMI	29.4	75	2.2
Total	248.7	217	54.0

[a]SMI, severe mental impairment.

SOURCE: Frank and McGuire (1996).

counseling or psychotherapy). However, individuals with serious or prolonged disorders or the parents of children with serious or prolonged disorders can easily use up their private insurance coverage benefits, creating economic hardships for them and their families. The end result is that the public system will pay for their care. Table 3.6 provides the relative contributions of the private and public sectors.

> In a number of states we are seeing what we refer to as a divided benefit. Managed care organizations are responsible for the acute care benefit for children, while the public sector retains responsibility for extended care for those with serious emotional disorders.
>
> *Sybil Goldman*
> *National Technical Assistance Center*
> *Georgetown University*
> *Public Workshop, April 18,1996, Washington, DC*

Therefore, advocates have strong concerns that reforms could threaten this system. On the other hand, the current divisions of labor between the public and private sectors contribute to many consumers being stuck in a lifetime of public care and unemployment. They find it necessary to remain poor to maintain their Medicaid eligibility, which is needed to cover the costs of medication and other treatments. The problem is compounded because they typically have not been able to obtain private coverage because of their "preexisting condition." Reforming a system with these interrelated problems is extremely difficult, although the Kassebaum-Kennedy bill of 1996 was aimed to ensure job-to-job coverage.

Drug and alcohol problems are pervasive in our society, whether we address them or not. And I could sum it up this way: they don't just fade away. They go to another funding stream.

Gwen Rubinstein
Legal Action Center
Public Workshop, April 18, 1996, Washington, DC

Cost Shifting

In both public- and private-sector service systems, financial arrangements may promote cost-shifting—the cost of caring for untreated problems is shifted to another service system. Untreated alcohol and drug dependency, for example, leads to increased utilization of emergency rooms and acute care hospitals. Similarly, men and women with serious mental illnesses may be more likely to be incarcerated for public order offenses if community services and supports are not provided. For individuals in need of long-term care, costs and responsibilities may be shifted to the family and other support systems, and family members increasingly provide relatively complicated medical care because patients with managed care plans are discharged rapidly from acute care hospitals.

Although the fundamental dynamics associated with separate public and privately paid systems have been remarkably stable in recent years, the evolution of financing and care in each sector has been remarkable. Understanding these dynamics is central to designing relevant accountability and consumer protection systems, as the following section will show.

DEVELOPMENTS IN THE PRIVATE SECTOR

Since World War II there have been dramatic expansions of privately paid behavioral health care. National data on patterns of care in the past 50 years reveal that powerful trends have been at work. The expansion of employer-financed group health insurance during and after World War II set the stage for more accessible behavioral health care. The number of members in such plans grew from 12 million in 1940 to more than 100 million by 1955, fueled by substitution of benefits for wages under wage and price controls and then by the preferential tax treatment of benefits (Bodenheimer and Grumbach, 1994).

Following this expansion of basic health care coverage, dramatic increases in the use of behavioral health care occurred. In response to reduced stigma, better evidence of treatment effectiveness, and consumer demand, many companies added behavioral health benefits for their employees' health plans during the 1980s.

Not surprisingly, the costs of these benefits increased rapidly and, in fact, increased faster than the costs in the rest of the health care system. As a direct result of these increased costs of employee benefits, companies and insurance plans turned to specialty managed care firms to rein in the costs of care. By 1995, more than 125 million Americans were enrolled in some form of managed behavioral health care plan, running the gamut from utilization review plans to fully capitated managed care plans, and the rate of increase in the penetration of managed care versus indemnity plans in behavioral health care exceeded that of health care in general (Oss, 1994).

Although there is variability in the performance of managed behavioral health care plans and companies, several trends in this field are evident. First, specialty behavioral managed care approaches have clearly demonstrated their ability to contain costs, reducing the rate of growth in costs of behavioral health care in all known instances and, in fact, actually reducing costs in the majority of instances. Second, the primary strategy used by this sector has not been to limit benefits per se but rather to limit or manage access to high-cost services, primarily hospitalization. Generally, these plans have maintained and sometimes increased access to outpatient treatment, whereas they have limited outpatient costs by using selective provider contracting, fee discounts, and various utilization management activities. Third, the field is becoming more competitive, and competition is having several effects: price increases are small, larger companies are increasingly dominating the market, and the use of a variety of sophisticated methods are being introduced to manage access.

The strengths of the private-sector managed behavioral health care industry include demonstrated competence at managing care for a privately insured population and the development of management tools relevant to this task, for example, information systems and provider credentialing approaches. The weaknesses of this sector include a lack of experience with managing comprehensive treatment and providing support to the more disabled population served in the public sector. More states are contracting with managed care firms to manage Medicaid behavioral health care services, but this is a new trend: currently, Medicaid covers only a portion of the costs of mental health and substance abuse care and support for individuals in the public sector.

QUALITY AND CONSUMER PROTECTION CHALLENGES

The high degree of competition for behavioral health care contracts is itself a factor regarding quality. Competition can drive prices down or quality up. There is much evidence of intense price competition, but there is not much evidence that contract decisions tend to be made primarily on the basis of quality. On the other hand, it is clear that competition is encouraging adaptation and innovation in the field and that the rapid development of new products and approaches is occurring. This is a positive sign for the quality of care, but it is one that raises challenges for accreditation and quality assurance approaches. These issues will be discussed further in Chapter 6, Process.

The variability in the structure, funding, focus, and competency of public mental health and substance abuse systems and the fact that they are primarily directed by the 50 state governments creates challenges for behavioral health care and for consumer protection, quality assurance, and accreditation. Solutions that rely on the action of the federal government must recognize the limited, if pervasive, role of federal funding (e.g., Medicaid). Other approaches that are national in scope, for example, recommendations on accreditation, must recognize that it is not clear whether these approaches will be adopted at the state and local levels and that their implementation may be variable from state to state.

VARIABILITY AT THE STATE LEVEL

Although there is much variability from state to state, public behavioral health care services are coordinated and funded through state authorities for mental health and substance abuse. Those authorities revolve around organized systems of care, are managed by designated not-for-profit agencies or units of county governments, and provide broad and diverse services. Public behavioral health care systems usually employ many elements of managed care, such as alternatives to hospitalization, case management to coordinate services for needy individuals, and crisis intervention services.

We have a public mental health system that helps us, that delivers both care and services and helps us to be stable in our own communities, despite having disabling mental illnesses.

Ray Bridge
Northern Virginia Consumers Association
Public Workshop, April 18, 1996, Washington, DC

Many who provide and receive care in the public mental health and substance abuse service systems believe that these systems generally have done well in managing coordinated, long-term treatment and providing support for individuals who have chronic conditions.

The weaknesses of public mental health and substance abuse care systems relate to their broad missions, limited resources, and governmental auspices. They typically include poorly developed administrative infrastructures, including the information systems needed to manage large amounts of clinical and outcomes data, and a lack of experience with the managed care tools relevant to the needs of a privately insured population (CSAT, 1994). In addition, the state-to-state variability in public mental health and substance abuse care is a significant challenge, underlined by the lack of a broad federal commitment to financing care and magnified by devolution, in which many responsibilities are shifting from the federal government to the states.

Solutions to improving mental health and substance abuse care must build on the recognition that these are complex clinical and social problems involving medical, social, and disability factors manifested variably over time. Yet the service systems that have evolved to deal with them are fragmented between private and public responsibilities and among various levels of government. The juxtaposition of these factors led Marmor and Gill (1989) to conclude that basic aspects of U.S. political character and governance (e.g., suspicion of governmental solutions, the separation of powers, and federalism) mitigate against adequate solutions in the area of serious mental illness.

HISTORICAL PERSPECTIVE ON SYSTEMS

The historical development of services for the treatment of alcoholism, drug abuse, and mental illness reflects prevailing political currents and a persistent ambivalence toward full recognition of these illnesses as medical rather than moral or criminal justice problems. Although alcoholics and drug addicts were frequently admitted to mental health institutions and sought care from psychiatrists and psychologists, poor-quality and ineffective services were the consequences of little understanding of addiction, and after completing withdrawal, chemically dependent patients were difficult to treat in the mental health system (IOM, 1990a, b). Similarly, individuals with serious mental illnesses received poor care in alcoholism and drug abuse treatment programs (IOM, 1990a, b).

As a result, the service systems evolved and matured relatively independently. The history of tension between the service systems continues to inhibit full integration of the service systems. It is therefore important to understand how autonomous service systems developed, the needs that they addressed, and the unique role of public funding in the creation and delivery of services for individuals struggling with mental illness, alcoholism, or drug abuse. Box 3.2 provides a timeline with highlights of the discussions presented in the following sections.

BOX 3.2
Historical Perspective on the Development of Behavioral Health Systems

1784   Dr. Benjamin Rush, a signer of the Declaration of Independence and surgeon general of the Continental Army, publishes a pamphlet entitled "An Inquiry into the Effects of Ardent Spirits on the Mind and Body" and pioneers the view of alcoholism as a medical rather than moral problem.

1820s   Studies of public welfare and mental illness recommend a general shift from home care by families to institutional care in asylums, and in the next decade asylums come under state authority.

1840s   Washingtonian Societies promote the potential for self-reform and foster the first residential treatment programs for inebriation.

1845   New York City establishes a police force, in part to deal with chronic inebriates causing public disorder problems in the Bowery.

1852   President Franklin Pierce vetoes legislation to establish a federal land-grant program to aid in the construction of asylums, thus moving the responsibility for mental health care to the states.

1890s   Rescue missions and shelters provide outreach to homeless inebriates and offer programs based on prayer, food, shelter, and work.

        Commercial insurance companies begin to offer policies for specific diseases, disability, accidents, and death. Most sickness benefits are provided by small immigrant benefit societies and local chapters of fraternal orders and unions, and only about a third of industrial workers have them.

1906   The American Association for Labor Legislation is formed and begins to advocate for health insurance.

1908   Nobel Prize winner Elie Metchnikoff's work helps to develop the theory of "autointoxication" related to narcotic dependence.

1913   The Rockefeller Institute creates the Bureau of Social Hygiene to study substance abuse and its impact and role in society and on criminality.

1914   The Harrison Narcotic Act leads to U.S. Treasury Department regulations that the maintenance of addicts on narcotics to prevent withdrawal would not be legitimate medical practice. Physicians who issue prescriptions for that purpose are prosecuted.

1919   Congress ratifies the 18th Amendment to the Constitution, also known as Prohibition.

1926   An independent body, the Committee on the Costs of Medical Care (CCMC), is formed by prominent economists, physicians, and public health specialists. Over 5 years, CCMC conducts research and publishes 27 studies on the costs and utilization of medical care.

continues on next page

BOX 3.2 Continued

1930	President Herbert Hoover creates the Federal Bureau of Narcotics within the U.S. Treasury Department, under the leadership of Harry Anslinger. Until his retirement in 1962 at age 70, Anslinger supports prosecution and incarceration and opposes community-based services for addiction treatment.
1932	CCMC releases its final report, which calls for reductions in economic barriers to medical care and endorses the promotion of group practice and group payment for care. Not all CCMC members agree; an editorial in the *Journal of the American Medical Association* and an article in *The New York Times* denounce the proposals as socialized medicine.
1933	Congress passes the 21st Amendment to the Constitution, repealing Prohibition.
1935	Alcoholics Anonymous begins in Dr. Bob's kitchen in Akron, Ohio.
	The first formal drug treatment program opens at a U.S. Public Health Service Narcotic Hospital in Lexington, Kentucky, and becomes a major research and teaching center for the treatment of opiate addiction.
1942	Yale Center for Alcohol Studies is established.
1945	The Knickerbocker Hospital in New York becomes the first hospital to open an Alcoholics Anonymous (AA) ward for the treatment of alcoholics.
1949	The National Institute of Mental Health (NIMH) is established as the successor to the U.S. Public Health Service's Division of Mental Hygiene, and alcohol and narcotics become part of its responsibilities.
1956	The American Medical Association (AMA) issues a statement declaring that alcoholism is a disease.
1958	Synanon is founded in California and becomes the first therapeutic community to provide residential treatment for heroin addicts.
1961	The Joint Committee on Narcotic Drugs of the American Bar Association (ABA) and the AMA releases a report criticizing prosecution and enforcement strategies and recommending more research on drug treatment.
1962	The U.S. Supreme Court decision in *Robinson v. California* holds that a state can establish a compulsory treatment program for narcotics addicts and that such treatment can involve periods of involuntary confinement with penal sanctions for failure to comply.
1963	The Community Mental Health Centers Act provides the first federal assistance for local treatment of addiction under the rubric of mental illness. Prevention services were declared essential and made mandatory for such centers to qualify for federal funds. The Act also lead to the deinstitutionalization of patients in state hospitals.
	Daytop Village, a second-generation therapeutic community, opens in New York City.

1964 The U.S. Congress creates the Military Medicare Program, later called the Civilian Health and Medical Program of the Uniformed Services.

1965 In his Great Society speech to U.S. Congress, President Lyndon Johnson announces "unconditional war on poverty in America." Seven months later, he signs Medicare and Medicaid into law.

1966 Decisions in two U.S. Circuit Courts (*Easter* v. *District of Columbia* and *Driver* v. *Hinnant*) rule that public intoxication is an involuntary consequence of the illness of alcoholism and that incarceration for an involuntary behavior is not permissible.

The Narcotic Addict Rehabilitation Act is passed, allowing judges and prison officials to refer narcotics-addicted probationers and prisoners to the Lexington and Ft. Worth treatment facilities as part of their sentence.

1967 Reports from the U.S. and District of Columbia Crime Commissions and the Cooperative Commission of the Study of Alcoholism conclude that criminal law is an "ineffective, inhumane, and costly device" for the prevention and control of alcoholism, including public drunkenness.

1968 The U.S. Supreme Court decision in *Powell* v. *Texas* upholds a conviction for public intoxication, but a majority of justices hold that alcoholism is a disease and that involuntary drinking is a symptom of the disease.

Alcoholics are excluded from 60 percent of general hospitals, and 40 percent of Blue Cross plans explicitly exclude coverage for alcoholism treatment.

Hospital chains and multihospital systems begin to appear.

1969 Senator Harold Hughes, a freshman senator and former governor of Iowa who is in recovery, chairs public hearings on the extent and effects of alcoholism.

The ABA and the AMA issue a joint statement, "Principles Concerning Alcoholism," that urges state governments to stop handling alcoholism as a criminal offense.

1970 Congress adopts the Comprehensive Alcohol Abuse and Alcoholism Prevention, Treatment and Rehabilitation Act (Hughes Act) authorizing federal funding for the treatment and prevention of alcoholism and creating the National Institute on Alcohol Abuse and Alcoholism within NIMH.

The Comprehensive Drug Abuse Prevention and Control Act of 1970 (Controlled Substances Act) authorizes the diversion of drug-involved offenders from the criminal justice system into drug abuse treatment and becomes the first legislation to specify a role for physicians in drug treatment.

1971 President Richard M. Nixon declares "war on drugs" as a response

continues on next page

BOX 3.2 Continued

to public concern about drug-related crime in urban areas and growing drug use among adolescents and young adults.

President Nixon announces "a new national health strategy" and calls on the Congress to establish planning grants and loan guarantees that would help increase the number of health maintenance organizations (HMOs). At the time 30 HMOs were in operation, and the administration's goals were to create 1,700 HMOs by 1976 and to see 90 percent of the population in HMOs by the end of the decade.

The RAND Corporation begins the Health Insurance Experiment, which studies different ways of financing medical care until 1988.

1972 Wisconsin becomes the first state to require insurance coverage for inpatient treatment of alcoholism. Illinois, Massachusetts, Minnesota, and Washington State follow in 1974.

The Drug Abuse Office and Treatment Act of 1972 establishes the Special Action Office for Drug Abuse Prevention (SAODAP) in the Executive Office of the President. Headed by Jerome Jaffe, M.D., SAODAP coordinates the first federal funding for drug abuse treatment through the TASC (Treatment Alternatives to Street Crime) model with programs in Wilmington, Delaware, and Philadelphia, Pennsylvania.

1973 The Drug Enforcement Administration is established to control supply and enforce the regulation of controlled substances.

The U.S. Congress passes the HMO Act, requiring businesses with more than 25 employees to offer at least one qualifying HMO as an alternative to traditional insurance. Uncertainty about which plans would qualify leads to delays by employers in offering them, whereas hospitals and physicians largely view HMOs as competitors and oppose them.

1974 Reauthorization of the Hughes Act supports a reorganization and the development of separate and independent federal institutes for alcoholism, drug abuse, and mental health within the Alcohol, Drug Abuse and Mental Health Administration.

Model legislation known as the Uniform Alcoholism and Intoxication Treatment Act (Uniform Act) calls for a coordinated network of services to ensure that service boundaries do not prevent access to needed care. By 1981, 34 states have passed a version of the legislation.

The Employee Retirement Income Security Act is enacted, exempting self-insured employers from state mandates.

The National Health Planning and Resource Development Act establishes about 200 Health Systems Agencies to be run by boards with consumer representatives.

1978 The U.S. Congress authorizes law enforcement agencies to seize the assets of drug dealers, including money, real estate, and vehicles.

Congress amends the HMO legislation to increase federal aid for HMO development after it is found that hospital expenses for federal employees in Kaiser HMO plans are one-third the national average. By mid-1979 there are 217 HMOs with a total enrollment of 7.9 million people, about 4 percent of the U.S. population.

The President's Commission on Mental Health, chaired by Rosalynn Carter, releases a report calling for a broader view of mental health that would include social and community supports, attention to underserved groups, change in the insurance structure to increase access to care, and better measures of the prevalence of behavioral health disorders in the United States.

1980 The U.S. Public Health Service releases measurable objectives for improving national health status, risk reduction, and health services. Now known as *Healthy People 2000*, this initiative helps to form a national consortium of public agencies and professional organizations.

1981 The Omnibus Budget Reconciliation Act creates the Block Grant Program, which combines federal funding streams in an attempt to improve efficiency, reduce redundancy, and eliminate burdensome reporting requirements. The Alcohol, Drug Abuse, and Mental Health Services Block Grant represents a cut of 26 percent, compared with a 12 percent cut overall.

The National Association of Insurance Commissioners adopts a model benefit for alcoholism treatment with 30 days of inpatient care and 30 outpatient visits per year.

After several large mergers, three-quarters of the beds in for-profit hospital chains are operated by three companies (HCA, Humana, and American Medical International).

1984 The Crime Control Act increases federal mandatory minimum sentencing provisions for drug-related crimes.

The Justice Assistance Act of 1984 is passed, authorizing a criminal justice block grant program to encourage local and state governments to address problems of drug-related crime and substance-abusing offenders.

Studies by John Wennberg at Dartmouth University and Robert Brook and colleagues at the RAND Corporation begin to show regional variations in medical care practice patterns, revealing the lack of scientific evidence for much of the practice of medicine.

Mid-1980s Spending by employers on behavioral health services begins increasing at a rate of 50 percent a year, primarily because of inpatient care of adolescents and substance abusers in private psychiatric hospitals. Managed behavioral health companies begin to emerge as cost-saving alternatives to fee-for-service plans.

1986 The RAND Corporation undertakes the Medical Outcomes Study, a landmark 4-year longitudinal observational study that compares the use of services, quality of care, and health outcomes of adult outpatients in different practice settings, including a staff model HMO and fee-for-service office-based practices.

continues on next page

BOX 3.2 Continued

1988   The Anti-Drug Abuse Act mandates the creation of the Office of National Drug Control Policy and stiffens penalties for drug possession.

Surgeon General C. Everett Koop issues a report stating that cigarettes and other forms of tobacco are addictive.

1989   President George Bush appoints William J. Bennett as the first "drug czar" of the new Office of National Drug Control Policy.

The first Drug Court is established in Miami. Also known as "Treatment Court," this is a program run by criminal justice programs to treat addicted nonviolent offenders before trial. By 1996, more than 100 drug courts exist nationwide.

The Agency for Health Care Policy and Research is created by the U.S. Congress as part of the U.S. Public Health Service, with a mandate to conduct and fund research on the effectiveness of care and treatment outcomes, to develop clinical practice guidelines, and to disseminate research findings.

1992   The Alcohol, Drug Abuse, and Mental Health Administration (ADAMHA) Reorganization Act organizes its three research institutes (The National Institute on Drug Abuse, the National Institute on Alcohol Abuse and Alcoholism, and NIMH) under the National Institutes of Health. The service components of ADAMHA are reorganized into the Substance Abuse and Mental Health Services Administration, as the Center for Substance Abuse Treatment, Center for Substance Abuse Prevention, and Center for Mental Health Services.

1993   President Bill Clinton proposes The Health Security Act, which is comprehensive health care reform with an emphasis on consumer choice, report cards, outcomes research, and expanded coverage of behavioral health. After a year of congressional hearings and other legislative proposals, no legislation is passed.

1996   Congress debates legislative proposals for incremental health care reform, and the Senate passes the Kassebaum-Kennedy bill on job-to-job coverage with a provision advocating parity of mental health coverage with medical coverage. The provision is dropped from the final version of the bill passed by Congress and signed by President Bill Clinton. House and Senate negotiators agree to a compromise that requires parity for existing lifetime or annual limits, does not mandate mental health services, does not include substance abuse or chemical dependency, and exempts small businesses with 2 to 50 employees. The compromise version is passed as part of the annual appropriations bill for the Departments of Housing and Urban Development and Veterans Affairs.

SOURCE: Aaron and Musto (1981), Baumohl (1986, 1990), GAO (1995), Hewitt (1995), Hutt (1967), Iglehart (1996), IOM (1990a), Kurtz and Regier (1975), Lewis (1988), McCarty et al. (1991), Morrison and Luft (1990), Musto (1996), NIAAA (1971, 1974); Pike (1988), President's Commission on Mental Health (1978), Room (1976), Scott et al., (1992), Smithers (1988), Starr (1982), and W. Bill (1957).

Mental Health Services

Historical Overview

In 1996, when national legislation began to address parity of mental health care coverage, the origins of mental health care in the United States seemed even more distant. During the colonial era, however, individuals who had mental disorders were jailed or placed in poorhouses (Hamilton, 1944). Dr. Benjamin Rush began a study of mental illness at Pennsylvania Hospital in 1800, and by the 1840s, 18 hospitals were exclusively devoted to caring for the mentally ill (Hamilton, 1944).

In 1834, at the urging of Dorothea Dix, the Massachusetts legislature voted to make all indigent mentally ill individuals wards of the state. In 1890, the state of New York passed a law requiring that all mentally ill individuals be moved out of jails and poorhouses and into state hospitals, and other states passed similar legislation (Bromet and Parkinson, 1992). By the turn of the century, most states had established state-supported mental hospitals, and by the 1930s, nearly all state mental hospitals had established outpatient clinics, partly to eliminate overcrowding and partly because of the growth in outpatient psychiatric services in those years (Caton, 1984).

In 1946, Congress passed the National Mental Health Act, which created the National Institute of Mental Health (NIMH), thus establishing the first federal responsibility for prevention, diagnosis, and treatment. In 1963, President John Kennedy proposed the development of comprehensive community mental health centers, which led to the passage of the Community Mental Health Centers (CMHC) Act of 1963. By 1980, there were more than 700 community mental health centers across the country, reflecting a federal investment of more than $1.5 billion (Bromet and Parkinson, 1992).

In 1977, President Jimmy Carter signed an executive order establishing the President's Commission on Mental Health. The commission made a total of 100 recommendations addressing community linkages, expanding services to underserved populations, phasing down large state mental hospitals, and developing of a case management system (Bromet and Parkinson, 1992). One of the great unintended consequences of the shift from state hospitals to community mental health centers, given the lack of adequate resources, was an increase in the number of homeless mentally ill individuals.

Discredited and demoralized during the era of deinstitutionalization (dating roughly from the 1963 CMHC Act and the 1965 enactment of Medicaid until 1980), public mental health and substance abuse systems have improved dramatically in the past 15 years. Several forces and developments have contributed to this change.

The Community Support Model and the Reagan Legacy

It is ironic that federal agency (NIMH) leadership during a time of presidential initiatives to limit the federal government was so crucial in improving public-sector mental health care. Yet this was clearly the case. The Community Support Program (CSP) was a small demonstration effort in NIMH that had a significant impact on improving public mental health care. CSP promoted guidelines that urged a coordinated, community-based, long-term, and practical approach to caring for serious mental illness and provided a new and relevant conceptual model at a time when the field was searching for new solutions. Through a mix of national meetings and targeted demonstration grants aimed at implementing the new model, CSP leveraged change in all the states.

President Ronald Reagan's "new federalism" approach, emphasizing a diminished federal role in favor of state responsibility, was also a boon to the improvement of public-sector programs. Mental health had fundamentally been a state responsibility since the founding of asylums in the 19th century. Indeed, President Franklin Pierce's veto of 1852 legislation to establish a land-grant program aiding construction of asylums—as an unwarranted assumption of federal responsibility—set the tone for the federal government's role in mental health, and the states picked up the slack.

Medicaid

An aggressive federal role had developed in the 1960s with CMHC and Medicaid legislation. Although both pieces of legislation would play a positive role in improving public care in the long run, in the short term each undercut state responsibility. CMHC funding was channeled directly from the federal government to local programs, bypassing state government and thus creating obstacles in the way of states seeking to ensure community-based care for patients being discharged from state hospitals. Sometimes, however, the CMHC was a state entity.

Medicaid was designed to be administered by the state welfare agency, since at the time of its enactment this was the only relevant agency existing in every state. This strategy also undercut the role of state mental health agencies, although at first Medicaid had only a limited mental health benefit. But changes around 1980 made both programs more relevant to the state mental health agencies. President Reagan's block grant approach gave the states control of the federal mental health block grant, albeit with a 26 percent cut in funding, and this helped states better coordinate programs. At the same time, changes in Medicaid to make it more relevant to the community-based care of seriously mentally ill individuals—resulting from recommendations of the President's Commission on Mental Health in 1978—provided a viable source of funding for CSP programs. As a result of the improved (CSP) service approach, better state coordination, and targeted funding, public-sector care has steadily improved since 1980.

Alcoholism Services

In the United States, efforts to treat alcoholism began with the observations of Dr. Benjamin Rush in 1785 (IOM, 1990a). The temperance movement grew in strength during the 19th century (Aaron and Musto, 1981; Rorabaugh, 1979), and concern about inebriates led to informal and formal treatment systems. Washingtonian Societies, formed during the 1840s, promoted the potential for self-reform and fostered the first residential treatment programs for inebriation (Baumhol, 1986, 1990). In the 1850s and 1860s, formal publicly sponsored asylums for the treatment of inebriation were proposed, but the few that opened were frequently converted to institutions for the mentally ill (Baumhol, 1990). The Massachusetts State Hospital for Dipsomaniacs and Inebriates, for example, opened in 1893, but it was treating shell-shocked veterans of World War I by 1918 (Baumhol and Room, 1987). At the end of the 19th century, rescue missions and shelters provided outreach to homeless inebriates and offered programs based on prayer, food, shelter, and work (Glaser et al., 1978; Stoil, 1987).

The most pervasive strategy for the treatment and control of inebriates, however, was arrest and jail (McCarty et al., 1991). New York City established a police force in 1845, in part to deal with chronic inebriates causing public disorder problems in the Bowery (Murtagh, 1956). With the passage of the Volstead Act in 1919 and the imposition of Prohibition between 1920 and 1933, the control of alcohol and alcohol abuse was fully relegated to the criminal justice system and the need for formal treatment institutions dissipated (Aaron and Musto, 1981; IOM, 1990a). Resources dedicated to alcoholism treatment were directed elsewhere.

Contemporary treatment systems for alcoholism and drug abuse therefore began shortly after the repeal of Prohibition. In retrospect, the first programs were more likely to be based on personal experience than scientific research. The women and men who helped one another initiate and sustain a stable recovery were guided primarily by trial and error. Born in June of 1935 in Dr. Bob's kitchen in Akron, Ohio, and gradually replicated in homes and meeting rooms all over the United States (W., Bill, 1957), Alcoholics Anonymous (AA) meetings provided peer support for individuals seeking sobriety. The demonstrations of stable recovery from alcohol dependence among individuals involved in AA encouraged a reevaluation of the social and medical processes used to intervene with alcoholics and inebriates. Moreover, men and women in recovery began to advocate for more humane treatment for alcoholics.

The scientific and medical basis for understanding and treating alcoholism began with Jellinek's work in the 1940s and the 1942 establishment of the Yale Center for Alcohol Studies (IOM, 1990a). Formal treatment programs began to develop in the 1940s and 1950s. Yale Plan Clinics tested outpatient strategies for the treatment of alcoholism. AA meetings were held in mental health institutions and prisons (W., Bill, 1957). The first hospital-based treatment services were also developed. Bill W. (a co-founder of AA) recalled that in 1945 the Knickerbocker Hospital in New York City became the first hospital to open an AA ward for the treatment of alcoholics (W., Bill, 1957). In 1951, Boston established a 300-bed rehabilitation program at Long Island Hospital for the treatment of alcoholics; a 3-year follow-up study of 101 men found 12 of them to be sober and living independently (Myerson, 1956). Most hospitals were reluctant to admit alcoholics. Although the American Medical Association (AMA) recognized in a 1956 policy statement that alcoholism was an illness that physicians and hospitals could address (Committee on Alcoholism, 1956), an NIMH review during the 1960s found that many hospitals actively discriminated against alcoholics in admissions for health and psychiatric services (Plaut, 1967). Most chronic alcoholics therefore were still cared for in the criminal justice system. The dominant treatment intervention was arrest for public inebriation, detoxification in the drunk tank, and a drying out period on the state farm.

Courts in major metropolitan areas were overwhelmed in processing arrests for public intoxication (The President's Commission, 1967). Advocates challenged state laws that permitted the arrest and incarceration of individuals for chronic inebriation and appealed convictions for public intoxication. Decisions in two U.S. circuit courts in 1966 (*Easter* v. *District of Columbia* and *Driver* v. *Hinnant*) ruled that public intoxication was an involuntary consequence of the illness of alcoholism and that incarceration for an involuntary behavior was not permissible (Hutt, 1967; Kurtz and Regier, 1975; NIAAA, 1971; Room, 1976).

The stage was set for a U.S. Supreme Court decision in 1968 (*Powell* v. *Texas*). Although the Court's 5 to 4 decision upheld a conviction for public intoxication, a reading of the majority and minority opinions indicated that a majority of justices held that because alcoholism is a disease, inebriation is an involuntary consequence of the illness and, because homeless individuals cannot drink in private, homeless alcoholics cannot be convicted of public intoxication (NIAAA, 1971). The three court rulings drew attention to the lack of formal treatment systems for alcoholism, encouraged the decriminalization of public intoxication, and stimulated state and federal legislation that promoted the development of publicly funded continuums of care for the treatment of alcoholism (McCarty, 1995).

At the federal level, Senator Harold Hughes, a freshman senator and former governor of Iowa who was in recovery, chaired public hearings across the nation during 1969 on the extent and effects of alcoholism; publicly recognized men and women acknowledged their recoveries and testified to advocate for a national program to address alcoholism and to develop more humane systems of care (Hewitt, 1995). The Comprehensive Alcohol Abuse and Alcoholism Prevention, Treatment, and Rehabilitation Act of 1970 (Hughes Act) was introduced and sponsored by Senator Hughes and was signed into law by President Richard M. Nixon as P.L. 91-616 after campaign supporters dissuaded his veto of the legislation (Hewitt, 1995; Lewis, 1988; Pike, 1988; Smithers, 1988).

The Comprehensive Act is generally known as the Hughes Act and authorized a federal infrastructure and federal funding for the treatment and prevention of alcoholism. The act authorized the creation of the National Institute on Alcohol Abuse and Alcoholism (NIAAA) within NIMH, created a National Advisory Council on Alcohol Abuse and Alcoholism to foster policy development, required states to designate state alcoholism authorities, established federal formula grants for states to facilitate the creation of comprehensive state plans for the treatment and prevention of alcoholism, mandated treatment and prevention services for federal employees, encouraged hospitals to admit and treat alcoholics, protected the confidentiality of patient records, and funded research.

Many credit the Hughes Act for the development of contemporary public and private treatment systems for alcoholism and alcohol abuse (Hewitt, 1995; IOM, 1990a; Lewis, 1988). The 1974 (P.L. 93-282) and 1976 (P.L. 94-371) reauthorizations of the Hughes Act supported the development of independent institutes for alcoholism, drug abuse, and mental health within the Alcohol, Drug Abuse, and Mental Health Administration (ADAMHA) and authorized incentive grants to encourage states to adopt the Uniform Act (Hewitt, 1995; Lewis, 1988).

The Uniform Alcoholism and Intoxication Treatment Act (Uniform Act) was model legislation drafted to guide state reforms. The model act prohibited prosecution of alcoholics solely because of alcohol consumption (i.e., it decriminalized public intoxication) and supported the development of a comprehensive continuum of care to promote recovery from alcoholism; the initiative also created a state authority to fund, regulate, and coordinate treatment and prevention services and established a citizens' advisory council (NIAAA, 1971). More than two-thirds of the states (i.e., 34 states) fully implemented the provisions of the Uniform Act (Finn, 1985). A review of the act's implementation concluded that the burden of public intoxication on the criminal justice system was dramatically reduced and that a change in the health care delivery system occurred (Scrimgeour and Palmer, 1976).

At the state level, the Uniform Act fostered the development of treatment services and empowered a public authority to develop and regulate services (McCarty, 1995). The legislation encouraged the development of community-based treatment services and typically specified the creation of emergency detoxification services, short-term inpatient care, residential care in halfway houses, and outpatient services. Voluntary treatment was emphasized. Implementation differed in each state, and consequently, state systems for the treatment of alcoholism vary substantially in structure, organization, and size.

In many states, men and women in recovery formed private, nonprofit, community-based organizations to operate the continuum of care specified in the Uniform Act. State authorities used the grassroots activism to lobby for additional resources and build continuums of care that often relied on individuals with personal histories of addiction and recovery to deliver care. Service systems in many areas continue to reflect this history and highlight a persistent tension between professional practitioners and experiential practitioners.

Drug Abuse Treatment

Passage of the Harrison Narcotic Act of 1914 marked a policy evolution from reliance on informal social influences to the vigorous use of enforcement, prosecution, and incarceration to control the distribution, sale, and use of heroin and cocaine in the United States (Courtwright et al., 1989; Musto, 1973). The act requires legitimate manufacturers and distributors of narcotics to register, pay a tax on transactions, and record all transactions. Federal enforcement agencies interpreted the legislation as prohibiting the use of prescribed narcotics to maintain individuals dependent on opiates, and U.S. Supreme Court rulings in 1919 upheld the constitutionality of the legislation (King, 1953; Musto, 1973).

The unintended consequences were to inhibit the treatment of opiate and cocaine abuse and dependence in medical settings, stifle development of treatment services, and enhance the segregation of addiction treatment from medical care (Jaffe, 1979; Schur, 1962). As a result, for much of the 20th century there was little systematic effort to develop effective treatment options.

The only formal treatment programs for most individuals dependent on opiates, cocaine, or marijuana were two U.S. Public Health Service Narcotic Hospitals. Federal funding for programs for the isolation and rehabilitation of narcotic addicts was authorized in 1929; the first hospital opened in Lexington, Kentucky, in 1935, and a second, smaller program began in Fort Worth, Texas, in 1938 (Courtwright et al., 1989; Walsh, 1973). Most of the hospitalized individuals were sentenced to the facilities for drug crimes, but individuals could also voluntarily commit themselves. Lexington was the major research and training center for the treatment of opiate addiction

Many individuals (perhaps 90 percent or more), however, relapsed quickly after release (Courtwright et al., 1989; Schur, 1962). The poor outcomes were due in part to a lack of community-based aftercare and follow-up services (Walsh, 1973). The institutions were maintained, despite high relapse rates, because the hospitals were effective at removing and isolating addicts from their communities. Harry J. Anslinger, the director of the Federal Bureau of Narcotics from the time of its creation in 1930 until his retirement at age 70 in 1962, strongly supported prosecution and incarceration for individuals with addictions and opposed community-based services (Courtwright et al., 1989). Control of the two narcotic hospitals was transferred to the Bureau of Prisons (Fort Worth in 1971 and Lexington in 1974); elimination of the hospital function was consistent with increased reliance on community-based services (Walsh, 1973).

Support for more humane policies and effective treatments emerged in the late 1950s and early 1960s. The Joint Committee of the American Bar Association and the American Medical Association on Narcotic Drugs (1961) released an interim review of drug policies in 1958. The report critiqued prosecution and enforcement strategies and recommended increased research, including establishment of an experimental outpatient clinic that could potentially provide drugs to addicts. A final report was released in 1961. In June 1962, the U.S. Supreme Court ruled in *Robinson v. California* that prosecution of individuals simply because they were addicted to illegal drugs was cruel and unusual punishment; medical treatment, not incarceration, was appropriate (Courtwright et al., 1989). New treatment strategies also appeared during this embryonic period.

In 1958, Chuck Dederich, a recovering alcoholic, opened a residential treatment program for heroin addicts known as Synanon (Courtwright et al., 1989; Jaffe, 1979). Synanon did not accept public funds and was based to some extent on the treatment strategies used by Maxwell Jones (1953), a British psychiatrist, and on the AA model, using recovering addicts and group encounters to confront residents to take responsibility and live without using drugs (Courtwright et al., 1989; IOM, 1990b). Synanon demonstrated that recovery from heroin abuse was possible and became the prototype for therapeutic communities.

Daytop Village, the first second-generation therapeutic community, began in 1963 with support from the city of New York and was designed to correct the deficits that the founders identified in the Synanon model. Reentry to the home community was planned, research on effectiveness was encouraged, staff included professionally trained individuals, and many unorthodox practices were avoided (interview with William B. O'Brien in Courtwright et al., 1989).

About the same time that Daytop Village opened, Vincent Dole and Marie Nyswander began a program of research with heroin addicts at Rockefeller University. Dole and Nyswander administered various narcotics to addicts to assess their effects. They found that individuals given methadone stabilized and that their social and interpersonal functioning improved (interview with Vincent Dole in Courtwright et al., 1989). Despite opposition from the Federal Bureau of Narcotics, they continued their work and published their first research report in the *Journal of the American Medical Association* (Dole and Nyswander, 1965). Methadone maintenance research programs began in 1965 with support from New York City (Courtwright et al., 1989).

Replication and expansion of these early treatment initiatives were inhibited until an infrastructure to support state and federal treatment systems developed during the late 1960s and early 1970s. The Narcotic Addict Rehabilitation Act of 1966 (P.L. 89-793) created a federal program for the civil commitment to and treatment of individuals dependent on narcotics and provided a framework for the evolution of a federally funded drug treatment system during the early 1970s (Besteman, 1992). NIMH consolidated the administration of research, training, and treatment related to drug abuse in the Division of Narcotic Addiction and Drug Abuse and funded community-based outpatient programs to provide assessments and aftercare (Besteman, 1992). A 1968 census of drug treatment programs identified 183 facilities (private and public) located primarily in urban areas of the Northeast (Connecticut, Massachusetts, New Jersey, and New York), Midwest (Illinois), and the West Coast (California); most (77 percent) had opened within the previous 5 years and reflected the influence of the Narcotic Addict Rehabilitation Act (Jaffe, 1979).

The most important federal initiative was President Nixon's declaration of a "war on drugs" (IOM, 1990b). Responding to concern about drug-related crime in urban areas and to growing drug use among adolescents and young adults, President Nixon's 1969 message to the U.S. Congress emphasized reduced access to illegal drugs while supporting the need for treatment and prevention services (IOM, 1995). The Comprehensive Drug Abuse Prevention and Control Act of 1970 (P.L. 91-513) legislatively clarified, for the first time since the passage of the Harrison Act in 1914, the roles of physicians in the treatment of narcotic addiction and authorized the secretary of the U.S. Department of Health, Education, and Welfare to determine methods for treating addiction (IOM, 1995).

In June 1971, President Nixon issued an executive order creating the Special Action Office for Drug Abuse Prevention (SAODAP) within the Executive Office of the President and appointed Jerome Jaffe, M.D., as the director (Besteman, 1992; IOM, 1990b; Jaffe, 1979). The Drug Abuse Office and Treatment Act of 1972 (P.L. 92-255) provided legislative authority for SAODAP; the legislation also authorized direct funding for community-based treatment and formula grants for state treatment systems if a state drug abuse treatment authority was designated and a state plan was submitted (Besteman, 1992). The legislation promoted a coordinated federal strategy to reduce the incidence of drug abuse (IOM, 1995).

SAODAP implemented services quickly: the use of inpatient facilities was limited, unused inpatient capacity was converted to outpatient services, treatment guidelines were issued, administrative costs were limited to 8 percent, and waiting lists were purchased to dramatically improve access to community-based outpatient and residential services (Besteman, 1992).

Under Dr. Jaffe's leadership, the office participated in the development of the 1972 federal methadone regulations and promoted the expansion of methadone treatment capacity (IOM, 1995). SAODAP purchased outpatient and residential services based on a "treatment slot" (i.e., "the projected utilization of capacity to deliver a given mix of services. . . to a population of clients" [Jaffe, 1979, p.11]) rather than a more traditional fee-for-service model. Jaffe (1979) felt that this approach encouraged flexible care for the clients based on their individual needs and discouraged incentives to maximize revenues from each client through the provision of more services. From the beginning, therefore, publicly funded drug abuse treatment programs were organized and financed by using reimbursement and administrative structures that differed from those used by the rest of medical services.

The federal infrastructure evolved rapidly. In 1971, the creation of NIAAA within NIMH and advocacy from the alcoholism treatment field for an identity separate and distinct from that of mental health fostered interest in reorganization of the federal authorities for mental health, alcoholism, and drug abuse. ADAMHA was formed (P.L. 93-282) in 1974, and three separate institutes were created: NIMH, NIAAA, and the National Institute on Drug Abuse (NIDA) (Besteman, 1992; Lewis, 1988). The director of SAODAP, Robert DuPont, M.D., became the first director of NIDA (Besteman, 1992; IOM, 1990b).

NIDA consolidated federal funding for services into grants to states rather than direct funding for service providers, and the states were encouraged to develop treatment systems (Besteman, 1992; IOM, 1990b). New federal awards required a transition of support to state funding and stimulated increased state appropriations for the treatment of drug abuse (Besteman, 1992). Federal funding and oversight declined throughout the 1970s, and NIDA increasingly emphasized biomedical research (IOM, 1990b).

Federal funding and oversight for the treatment of alcoholism, drug abuse, and mental illness declined most dramatically in 1981 when the Omnibus Budget Reconciliation Act (P.L. 97-35) combined funds from direct project grants and state formula grants into the Alcohol, Drug Abuse, and Mental Health Services Block Grant (Lewis, 1988; McCarty, 1995). Total funding was reduced 26 percent, but reporting requirements that were perceived as burdensome to the states were eliminated (IOM, 1990a; GAO, 1995). Treatment advocates perceived the reduction of federal support for the treatment and prevention of alcoholism, drug abuse, and mental illness as a major retreat, and the administrator of ADAMHA stated publicly that the federal government was unlikely to resume its role in the treatment of alcohol and drug abuse (Lewis, 1982).

In a period of less than 20 years (1964 through 1981), alcohol and drug abuse treatment services incubated in NIMH and community-based mental health centers. After brief developmental periods in separate federal institutes, they were transitioned to states to grow into treatment systems that reflected the unique needs and personalities of the states, and these services varied substantially among the states. Three separate treatment systems evolved with federal support and incentives, because (1) alcoholism and drug abuse treatment were not integrated with medical or psychiatric care, (2) drug abuse and crime policies frequently overlapped, and (3) there was strong advocacy for autonomy in the alcoholism treatment field.

Ultimately, the funding reductions associated with the implementation of the Alcohol, Drug Abuse, and Mental Health Services Block Grant may have facilitated integration of alcoholism and drug abuse treatment systems in many states. The cutbacks required program consolidations and, even if it was not immediate, created pressures that weakened many services and encouraged the eventual combination of treatment systems. At the same time, the men and women seeking treatment were increasingly likely to report abuse of both alcohol and other drugs.

Block grant requirements emphasized an increased capacity for the treatment of drug abuse and priority access to treatment for pregnant women abusing drugs and injection drug users (GAO, 1995). In many states, the best source of additional capacity was a strong alcoholism treatment system. Consequently, during the 1980s, state authorities for alcoholism and drug abuse were combined, and treatment services for alcoholism and drug abuse began to be fully integrated.

Criminal Justice System

Background

As just described, a unique relationship has developed between the criminal justice system and the public addiction treatment system. During the 1960s and 1970s the numbers of crimes related to illegal drug use increased dramatically. The drug of abuse of most concern to politicians and policymakers was heroin, which had been shown to be related to highly recidivistic criminal behavior, particularly income-generating property crimes. Thus, programs were born to interrupt the drug-crime cycle.

During the 1980s the drug of abuse among offenders shifted from heroin to cocaine, and by the late 1980s crack cocaine had become a major concern. Research such as the National Institute of Justice's Drug Use Forecasting (DUF) project, begun in the 1980s, showed alarmingly high rates of substance abuse among offenders nationwide (IOM, 1990b, 1996). With the simultaneous increase in the human immunodeficiency virus infection rate among intravenous drug abusers, efforts to direct treatment resources to the criminal justice population intensified. At the same time, criminal penalties related to drug abuse increased nationwide, mandatory minimum prison sentences were imposed and increased for drug-related crimes, and many drug misdemeanors were upgraded to felonies (IOM 1990b, 1996). By the end of the decade, the criminal justice system was flooded with substance-abusing offenders.

Another factor that has added to the pressure on the treatment system is the increasing interest of public policymakers in addressing the toll of drunk driving on society. This has led to the development of specialized intervention and referral programs that mandate drivers convicted for driving under the influence to involuntarily participate in treatment programs. Jurisdictions vary in the degree to which courts use referrals for evaluation and treatment and in the use of treatment as a sentencing option (IOM, 1990a).

Extent of the Problem

The National Institute of Justice's DUF report on adult and juvenile arrestees provides drug use information for those arrested or detained for committing crimes. DUF data indicate that nationally in 1994, 69 percent of males and 72 percent of females tested positive for an illicit drug at the time of arrest (NIJ, 1995). These rates are significantly higher than the current use data reported in the National Household Survey on Drug Abuse, which report 7.9 percent for males and 4.3 percent for females (SAMHSA, 1996).

The Center for Substance Abuse and Treatment (CSAT) has also provided funding for technical assistance to individual states for studies of drug use by their incarcerated populations. Recent studies conducted by the Criminal Justice Policy

Council, State of Texas, and the Illinois Department of Alcoholism and Substance Abuse and Illinois Department of Corrections have found similar high rates of illicit drug use among inmates entering state correctional systems. In Texas, 34.7 percent of male inmates and 43.8 percent of female inmates reported that they had used illicit substances in the month before being incarcerated. In Illinois, 65.6 percent of male inmates and 62.4 percent of female inmates indicated that they had used illicit drugs in the month before being incarcerated.

Treatment

The Bureau of Justice Statistics has reported that inmates sentenced for drug offenses accounted for 54 percent of the federal prison population in 1990 and over 20 percent of the total state prison population in 1991 (BJS, 1992). Treatment programs based in prisons are most often therapeutic communities, which operate in varying degrees of separation from the general prison population, and 12-step approaches are also found (IOM, 1996).

Because of the numbers of persons addicted to drugs who are arrested for drug-related crimes, the public sector has developed a variety of treatment programs designed to serve addicted nonviolent offenders. These programs may be operated as pretrial drug courts, the programs may be alternatives to incarceration, or they may be treatment programs operated within correctional institutions. Funding for some of these programs is available through the Substance Abuse Prevention and Treatment Block Grant, and for others through CSAT's discretionary funds. CSAT has also provided technical assistance to support the development of state correctional treatment plans. The goal of these programs, in addition to the treatment of addiction, is to remove a substantial number of people from jails and prisons to relieve overcrowding, although an unintended consequence is to increase the pressure on community-based programs.

Most of the treatment of drug-involved offenders takes place in community-based settings as an alternative to incarceration or as a condition of parole or probation (IOM, 1996). The best-known example is Treatment Alternatives for Special Clients (formerly known as Treatment Alternatives to Street Crimes), which is found in more than 25 states. In general, programs that link treatment to parole and probation produce favorable results (Chavaria, 1992; IOM, 1996; Van Stelle et al., 1994).

Researchers have found that drug treatment is less expensive than the alternatives, including incarceration, probation, and drug control strategies and costs less than the costs of crime and lost productivity associated with untreated addiction (Gerstein et al., 1994; IOM, 1996). A RAND Corporation study analyzed the costs required to achieve a 1 percent reduction in cocaine usage by comparing treatment (demand control) with three strategies for controlling the supply: domestic enforcement, interdiction, and source country control. At a cost of $34 million, treatment was the least expensive, with the costs of the other strategies ranging from $250 million to $800 million (Rydell and Everingham, 1994).

Implications for Managed Care

The result of criminal justice system involvement with treatment for addictions is that a number of people are mandated to attend treatment programs for a specified amount of time. These models are consistent with a sentencing rather than a medical or a clinical necessity approach. This situation places requirements on programs to serve clients for a minimum period of time, which is often unrelated to the client's medical need or clinical progress. Nonetheless, the requirement exists, and compliance is necessary for the offender to complete his or her obligation to the court.

Consistent with national trends, some health care in prisons is provided under contract with independent managed care organizations. Although specialty behavioral health companies are not yet contracting with prisons, the committee believes that it should be possible to provide appropriate substance abuse treatment within the criminal justice framework. Planning should involve the criminal justice and the addiction treatment experts and must address the lack of fit of the managed care principles with the current structure of the criminal justic system.

Employee Assistance Programs

The field of employee assistance programming began in the mid-1930s, coinciding with the founding of AA. Major corporations such as the New England Telephone Company, Western Electric Company, E. I. DuPont de Nemours & Company, Eastman Kodak Company, and Illinois Bell Telephone Company recognized the negative impact that alcoholism had on employee productivity (Presnall, 1981). These companies chose to develop programs that encouraged the use of AA, which was at that time referred to as occupational alcoholism programming or occupational programming. In the beginning of the field of employee assistance programming, the primary focus was on dealing with the employed alcoholic; however, employers such as Caterpillar Tractor Company and DuPont also addressed mental health problems (Presnall, 1981).

Several events over the next 20 years began to establish a foundation for the field. The Yale (later Rutgers) Center for Alcohol Studies was founded in 1942, and in the 1950s, along with the National Council on Alcoholism, collected and disseminated information on effective programs in different companies (IOM, 1990a). The passage of the Hughes Act in 1970 created the single most important influence on the growth of the field of employee assistance programming. The Hughes Act established NIAAA, which included the Occupational Programs Branch. In 1972, the Occupational Programs Branch provided funding for each state in the country to hire two professionals known as occupational program consultants.

The occupational program consultants received extensive training and were charged with influencing the growth of employee assistance programs (EAPs) within the states that they represented. As a result, hundreds of EAPs were formed, typically with public agencies providing services to employers. The first professional association for those working within the field was founded during this period of growth. The Association of Labor-Management Administrators and Consultants on Alcoholism later became the Employee Assistance Professionals Association (EAPA), as it is known today (EAPA, 1996).

The 1980s brought about the evolution of the private-sector side of the EAP field. Individuals who had been trained in the public sector began moving to the private sector and established private companies to serve employers. The number of employers contracting for EAP services grew at a rapid pace during this decade as employers realized that they had to deal effectively with mental health and substance abuse problems to be competitive in the marketplace. During the 1980s, EAPA led an effort to establish the principal credential for professionals within the field, called the certified employee assistance professional. By 1996, the number of certified employee assistance professionals had grown to more than 4,000 (EAPA, 1996).

In the 1990s, the EAP field experienced the same kinds of transitions as other sectors in the health care industry. The public-sector EAP effort began to diminish as public funding decreased, and employers began to debate whether to have internal programs or to contract those services out to external vendors. The acquisition of local and regional companies offering EAPs began to take place as delivery systems began consolidating. Employers began to ask for "integrated services," referring to the linkage of EAPs with managed care services. This integration creates system efficiencies and avoids the potential for overlap of services. Employers also began seeking the consultation of employee assistance professionals on a multitude of issues such as stress, violence, change, child and elder care, disability management, regulatory compliance, financial and legal matters, and critical incidents (EAPA, 1996).

For more than 60 years, the EAP field has grown from a simple approach of assisting major employers in dealing with their employees with alcohol problems to a sophisticated approach of servicing the employer as a consultant in the workplace on a wide array of behavioral issues. EAPs maintain a set of core technologies, and on this foundation, it has become recognized as a critical component in the effective management of difficulties of employees and reducing the impact of these problems on workplace productivity.

SUMMARY: SYSTEM INTEGRATION

Currently, state and federal budget reductions are again creating pressures and incentives to integrate services. By now, many states have initiated integration of the state authorities for mental health and substance abuse. Although state agency integration is primarily an issue of merging staff and reducing duplication, in most states, the mental health and substance abuse treatment systems are still distinct and separate. Thus, differences in patient populations, organizational cultures, programmatic philosophies, and funding mechanisms will continue to inhibit full integration for some time.

> We are in the process of moving ultimately toward integrated delivery systems. We have a long way to go to get there. It may take seven to ten years for that to occur.
>
> *Robert Valdez*
> *Deputy Assistant Secretary for Health, Department of Health and Human Services*
> *Public Workshop, April 18, 1996, Washington, DC*

The IOM (1996) report on the future of primary care has called for the development of models of coordinated, integrated care, including better integration among mental health and primary health care professionals. Studies of existing models would help to identify the best practices in the coordination of all care, particularly primary and behavioral health care. Carved-out behavioral health services do not necessarily lead to poor coordination of care or to coordination poorer than that in a fee-for-service system. However, the separation of primary care and behavioral health care systems brings risks to coordination and integration that may not be in the best interest of patients and consumers.

REFERENCES

Aaron P, Musto D. 1981. Temperance and prohibition in America: A historical overview. In: Moore MH, Gerstein DR, eds. *Alcohol and Public Policy: Beyond the Shadow of Prohibition.* Washington, DC: National Academy Press.

AHCPR (Agency for Health Care Policy and Research). 1993. *Depression in Primary Care.* Publication No. 93-0551. Rockville, MD: Agency for Health Care Policy and Research.

AHCPR. 1995. *PORT and PORT-II Abstracts.* AHCPR Publication No. 95-0070. Rockville, MD: Agency for Health Care Policy and Research.

AMBHA (American Managed Behavioral Healthcare Association) and NASMHPD (National Association of State Mental Health Program Directors). 1995. Public mental health systems, Medicaid re-structuring, and managed behavioral healthcare. *Behavioral Healthcare Tomorrow* September/October:63-69.

Anderson J, Williams S, McGee R, Silva P. 1987. DSM-III disorders in preadolescent children. *Archives of General Psychiatry* 44:69-76.

Baumohl J. 1986. On asylums, homes, and moral treatment: The case of the San Francisco Home for the Care of the Inebriate, 1859-1870. *Contemporary Drug Problems* 13:395-445.

Baumohl J. 1990. Inebriate institutions in North America: 1840-1920. *British Journal of Addiction* 85:1187-1204.

Baumhol J, Room R. 1987. Inebriety, doctors, and the state alcoholism treatment institutions before 1940. In: Galanter M, ed. *Recent Developments in Alcoholism.* Vol. 5. New York: Plenum Press. Pp. 135-174.

Besteman KJ. 1992. Federal leadership in building the national drug treatment system. In: IOM. *Treating Drug Problems.* Vol. 2. Washington, DC: National Academy Press.

Bird HR, Canino G, Rubio-Stipec M, Gould MS. 1988. Estimates of prevalence of childhood maladjustment in a community survey in Puerto Rico. *Archives of General Psychiatry* 45:1120-1126.

BJS (Bureau of Justice Statistics). 1992. *Drugs, Crime, and the Justice System.* NCJ-133652. Washington, DC: Bureau of Justice Statistics.

Bodenheimer T, Grumbach K. 1994. Paying for health care. *Journal of the American Medical Association* 272(8):634-639.

Bridges KW, Goldberg DP. 1985. Somatic presentation of DSM III psychiatric disorders in primary care. *Journal of Psychosomatic Research* 23:563-569.

Bromet EJ, Parkinson DV. 1992. Psychiatric Disorders. In: Last JM, Wallace RB, eds. *Public Health and Preventive Medicine.* Norwalk, CT: Appleton and Lange. Pp. 947-961.

Brook RH, Lohr KN. 1985. Efficacy, effectiveness, variations, and quality: Boundary crossing research. *Medical Care* 23:710-722.

Bunker JP. 1988. Is efficacy the gold standard for quality assessment? *Inquiry* 25:51-58.

Burnam MA. In press. Measuring outcomes of care for substance abuse and mental disorders. In: Steinwachs DM, Flynn L, eds. *New Directions for Mental Health Services: Using Outcomes to Improve Care.* San Francisco: Jossey-Bass.

Caton CLM. 1984. *Management of Chronic Schizophrenia.* New York: Oxford University Press.

Chavaria FR. 1992. Successful drug treatment in a criminal justice setting: A case study. *Federal Probation* 56:48-52.

Committee on Alcoholism. 1956. Hospitalization of patients with alcoholism. *Journal of the American Medical Association* 162:750.

Costello EJ. 1989. Developments in child psychiatric epidemiology. *Journal of the American Academy of Child and Adolescent Psychiatry* 28(6):851-855.

Costello EJ, Costello A, Edelborck C, Burns BJ, Dulcan MK, Brent D, Janiszewski S. 1988. Psychiatric disorders in pediatric primary care. *Archives of General Psychiatry* 45:1107-1116.

Courtwright D, Joseph H, Des Jarlais D. 1989. *Addicts Who Survived: An Oral History of Narcotic Use in America, 1923-1965.* Knoxville, TN: The University of Tennessee Press.

CSAT (Center for Substance Abuse Treatment). 1994. *Managed Healthcare Organizational Readiness Guide and Checklist.* Rockville, MD: Substance Abuse and Mental Health Services Administration, Center for Substance Abuse Treatment.

CSAT. 1995. *Producing Results: A Report to the Nation.* Rockville, MD: Substance Abuse and Mental Health Services Administration, Center for Substance Abuse Treatment.

Dole VP, Nyswander M. 1965. A medical treatment for diacetylmorphine (heroin) addiction. *Journal of the American Medical Association* 193:646-650.

EAPA (Employee Assistance Professionals Association, Inc.). 1996. *Employee Asistance Backgrounder.* Arlington, VA: Employee Assistance Professionals Association, Inc.

Eddy DM. 1990. Variations in physician practice: The role of uncertainty. In: Lee PR, Estes CL, eds. *The Nation's Health.* Boston: Jones and Bartlett. Pp. 347-355.

England MJ, Vaccaro VA. 1991. New systems to manage mental health care. *Health Affairs* 10(4):129-137.

Finn P. 1985. Decriminalization of public drunkenness: Response of the health care system. *Journal of Studies on Alcohol* 46(1):7-23.

Frank RG, McGuire TG. 1996. Introduction to the economics of mental health payment systems. In: Levin BL, Petrila J, eds. *Mental Health Services: A Public Health Perspective.* New York: Oxford University Press.

GAO (U.S. General Accounting Office). 1995. *Block Grants: Characteristics, Experience, and Lessons Learned.* GAO/HEHS-95-74. Washington, DC: General Accounting Office.

Gerstein DR, Johnson RA, Harwood HJ, Fountain D, Suter N, Malloy K. 1994. *Evaluating Recovery Services: The California Drug and Alcohol Treatment Assessment (CALDATA).* Fairfax, VA: Lewin-VHI and National Opinion Research Center at the University of Chicago.

Glaser FB, Greenberg SW, Barrett M. 1978. *A Systems Approach to Alcohol Treatment.* Toronto, Canada: Addiction Research Foundation.

Greenfield S, Nelson EC, Zubkoff M, Manning W, Rogers W, et al. 1992. Variations in resource utilization among medical specialties and systems of care: Results from the medical outcomes study. *Journal of the American Medical Association* 267(12):1624-1630.

Guadagnoli E, McNeil BJ. 1994. Outcomes research: Hope for the future or the latest rage? *Inquiry* 31:14-24.

Hamilton SW. 1944. The history of American mental hospitals. In: Hall JK. *American Psychiatric Association: One Hundred Years of American Psychiatry.* New York: Columbia University Press. Pp. 73-166.

Hankin J, Otkay JS. 1979. *Mental Disordesr and Primary Medical Care: An Analytical Review of the Literature.* No. 5. Washington, DC: National Institute of Mental Health.

Harding CM, Zubin J, Strauss JS. 1992. Chronicity in schizophrenia: Revisited. *British Journal of Psychiatry Supplement* 18:27-37.

Hewitt BG. 1995. The creation of the National Institute on Alcohol Abuse and Alcoholism: Responding to America's alcohol problem. *Alcohol Health and Research World* 19:12-16.

Hubbard RL, Marsden ME, Rachal JV, Harwood HJ, Cavanaugh ER, Ginzburg HM. 1989. *Drug Abuse Treatment: A National Study of Effectiveness.* Chapel Hill, NC: University of North Carolina Press.

Hutt PB. 1967. The recent court decisions on alcoholism: A challenge to the North American Judges Association and its members. In: The President's Commission on Law Enforcement and Administration of Justice. *Task Force Report: Drunkenness.* Washington, DC: U.S. Government Printing Office.

Iglehart J K. 1996. Health policy report: Managed care and mental health. *The New England Journal of Medicine* 334(2):131-135.

Institute for Health Policy, Brandeis University. 1993. *Substance Abuse: The Nation's Number One Health Problem.* Princeton, NJ: Robert Wood Johnson Foundation.

IOM (Institute of Medicine). 1990a. *Broadening the Base of Treatment for Alcohol Problems.* Washington, DC: National Academy Press.

IOM. 1990b. *Treating Drug Problems.* Vol. 1. Washington, DC: National Academy Press.

IOM. 1993. *Employment and Health Benefits: A Connection at Risk.* Washington, DC: National Academy Press.

IOM. 1995. *Federal Regulation of Methadone Treatment.* Washington, DC: National Academy Press.

IOM. 1996. *Primary Care: America's Health in a New Era.* Washington, DC: National Academy Press.

Jaffe JH. 1979. The swinging pendulum: The treatment of drug users in America. In: DuPont RI, Goldstein A, O'Donnell J, eds. *Handbook on Drug Abuse.* Rockville, MD: National Institute on Drug Abuse.

Johnston LD, O'Malley PM, Bachman JG. 1996. *National Survey Results on Drug Use from the Monitoring the Future Study, 1975-1995.* Vol. 1. Ann Arbor, MI: Institute for Social Research, University of Michigan.

Joint Committee of the American Bar Association and the American Medical Association on Narcotics Drugs. 1961. *Drug Addiction: Crime or Disease? Interim and Final Reports.* Bloomington, IN: Indiana University Press.

Jones M. 1953. *The Therapeutic Community—A New Treatment Method in Psychiatry.* New York: Basic Books.

Katon W, Von Korff M, Lin E, Walker E, Simon GE, Bush T, Robinson P, Russo J. 1995. Collaborative management to achieve treatment guidelines: Impact on depression in primary care. *Journal of the American Medical Association* 273:1026-1031.

Kessler RC, McGonagle KA, Shanyang Z, Nelson CB, Hughes M, Eshleman S, Wittchen HU, Kendler KS. 1994. Lifetime and 12-month prevalence of DSM-III-R psychiatric disorders in the United States. *Archives of General Psychiatry* 51:8-19.

King R. 1953. The Narcotics Bureau and the Harrison Act: Jailing the healers and the sick. *Yale Law Journal* 62:735-749.

Kirmayer LJ, Robbins JM, Dworkind J, Yaffe MJ. 1993. Somatization and the recognition of depression and anxiety in primary care. *American Journal of Psychiatry* 150:734-741.

Kurtz NR, Regier M. 1975. The Uniform Alcoholism and Intoxication Treatment Act: The compromising process of social policy formulation. *Journal of Studies on Alcohol* 36:1421-1441.

Lavigne JV, Gibbons RD, Christoffel KK, Arend R, Rosenbaum D, Binns H, Dawson N, Sobel H, Isaacs C. 1996. Prevalence rates and correlates of psychiatric disorders among preschool children. *Journal of the American Academy of Child and Adolescent Psychiatry* 35(2):204-214.

Lewis JS. 1982. Washington report. *Journal of Studies on Alcohol* 43:183-187.

Lewis JS. 1988. Congressional rites of passage for the rights of alcoholics. *Alcohol Health and Research World* 12(4):240-251.

Lohr KN. 1988. Outcome measurement: Concepts and questions. *Inquiry* 25:37-50.

Marmor TR, Gill KC. 1989. The political and economic context of mental health care in the United States. *Journal of Health Politics, Policy, and Law* 14(3):459-475.

McCarty D. 1995. *The Effects of State and Federal Policies and Practices on the Cost and Utilization of Services for Alcohol Abuse and Alcohol Dependence.* Paper prepared for the National Institute on Alcohol Abuse and Alcoholism's National Advisory Council on Alcohol Abuse and Alcoholism, Subcommittee on Health Services Research, Panel on Utilization and Cost. Boston, MA: Institute for Health Policy, Brandeis University.

McCarty D, Argeriou M, Huebner RB, Lubran B. 1991. Alcoholism, drug abuse, and the homeless. *American Psychologist* 46:1139-1148.

McLellan AT, Luborsky L, O'Brien CP, Woody GE. 1980. An improved evaluation instrument for substance abuse patients: The Addiction Severity Index. *Journal of Nervous and Mental Disease* 168:26-33.

McLellan AT, Luborsky L, O'Brien CP, Woody GE, Druley KA. 1982. Is substance abuse treatment effective? *Journal of the American Medical Association* 275(10):761-767.

McLellan AT, Woody GE, Metzger DS, McKay J, Durell J, Alterman AI, O'Brien CP. 1996. Evaluating the effectiveness of addictions treatments: Reasonable expectations, appropriate comparisons. *The Milbank Quarterly* 74(1):51-85.

Minnesota Department of Human Services, Chemical Dependency Division. 1995. *Consolidated Chemical Dependency Treatment Fund: Fiscal Years 1989 through 1994.* St. Paul, MN: Minnesota Department of Human Services, Chemical Dependency Division.

MMWR (Morbidity and Mortality Weekly Report). 1994. Medical-care expenditures attributable to cigarette smoking—United States, 1993. *Morbidity and Mortality Weekly Report* 43(26):469-472.

Morrison EM, Luft HR. 1990. Health maintenance organization environments in the 1980s and beyond. *Health Care Financing Review* 12(1):81-90.

Murtagh JM. 1956. The New York City program for the skid row alcoholic. In: *Institute on the Skid Row Alcoholic of the Committee on the Homeless Alcoholic.* New York: National Committee on Alcoholism. Pp. 6-15.

Musto DF. 1973. *The American Disease: Origins of Narcotic Control.* New Haven, CT: Yale University Press.

Musto DF. 1996. Drug abuse research in historical perspective. In: IOM. *Pathways of Addiction: Opportunities in Drug Abuse Research*. Washington, DC: National Academy Press. Pp. 284-294.

Myerson DJ. 1956. The "skid-row" problem: Further observations on a group of alcoholic patients, with emphasis on interpersonal relations and the therapeutic approach. *The New England Journal of Medicine* 254:1168-1173.

NAMHC (National Advisory Mental Health Council). 1993. Health care reform for Americans with severe mental illnesses: Report of the National Advisory Mental Health Council. *American Journal of Psychiatry* 150(1):1447-1465, October.

NHLBI (National Heart, Lung, and Blood Institute). 1994. *Morbidity and Mortality: Chartbook on Cardiovascular, Lung, and Blood Diseases*. Washington, DC: National Institutes of Health, Public Health Service, U.S. Department of Health and Human Services.

NIAAA (National Institute on Alcohol Abuse and Alcoholism). 1971. *First Special Report to the U.S. Congress on Alcohol and Health*. DHEW Publication No. (HSM) 73-9031. Rockville, MD: National Institute on Alcohol Abuse and Alcoholism.

NIAAA. 1974. *Second Special Report to the U.S. Congress on Alcohol and Health: New Knowledge*. DHEW Publication No. (ADM) 75-212. Rockville, MD: National Institute on Alcohol Abuse and Alcoholism.

NIAAA. 1990. *Alcohol and Health: Seventh Special Report to the U.S. Congress*. DHHS Publication No. (ADM) 90-1656. Washington, DC: U.S. Department of Health and Human Services.

NIJ (National Institute of Justice). 1995. *Drug Use Forecasting 1994: Annual Report on Adult Arrestees*. NCJ 147411. Washington, DC: National Institute of Justice.

NIMH (National Insitute of Mental Health). 1995. Mental disorders in children and adolescents. In: *National Institute of Mental Health: 1995 Budget Estimates*. Rockville, MD: National Institute of Mental Health. Pp. 69-82.

Offord DR, Boyle MH, Racine Y. 1989. Ontario child health study: Correlates of disorder. *Journal of the American Academy of Child and Adolescent Psychiatry* 28:856-860.

Oss ME. 1994. Managed behavioral health programs widespread among insured Americans. *Open Minds Newsletter* 8(3).

Pike TR. 1988. Hearing room dreams and the birth of NIAAA. *Alcohol Health and Research World* 12:268-269.

Plaut TFA. 1967. *Alcohol Problems: A Report to the Nation*. New York: Oxford University Press.

Presnall LF. 1981. *Occupational Counseling and Referral Systems*. Salt Lake City: Utah Alcoholism Foundation.

Regan RW. 1981. The role of federal, state, local, and voluntary sectors in expanding health insurance coverage for alcoholism. *Alcohol Health and Research World* 5(4):22-26.

Regier DA, Narrow WE, Rae DS, Manderscheid RW, Locke BZ, Goodwin FK. 1993. The de facto U.S. mental and addictive disorders service system: Epidemiologic catchment area prospective 1-year prevalence rates of disorders and services. *Archives of General Psychiatry* 50:85-94.

Rice DP. 1995. Personal communication to the Institute of Medicine. University of California at San Francisco. February.

Rice DP, Max W, Novotny T, Shultz J, Hodgson T. 1992. *The Cost of Smoking Revisited: Preliminary Estimates*. Presented at the American Public Health Association Annual Meeting. Washington, DC. November 23. Unpublished.

Rice DP, Miller LS. 1996. *Health Economics and Cost Implications or Anxiety and Other Mental Disorders in the United States*. Presented at Satellite Symposium: X World Congress of Psychiatry. Madrid, Spain. August 25. Unpublished.

Rice DP, Kelman S, Dunmeyer S. 1990. *The Economic Costs of Alcohol and Drug Abuse, and Mental Illness: 1985*. DHHS Publication No. (ADM) 90-1694. Washington, DC: Report submitted to the Office of Financing and Coverage Policy of the Alcohol, Drug Abuse, and Mental Health Administration, U.S. Department of Health and Human Services.

Room R. 1976. Comment on "The Uniform Alcoholism and Intoxication Act." *Journal of Studies on Alcohol* 37:113-144.

Rorabaugh WJ. 1979. *The Alcoholic Republic: An American Tradition.* New York: Oxford University Press.

Rydell C, Everingham S. 1994. *Controlling Cocaine: Supply Versus Demand Programs.* ONDCP/A/DPRC. Santa Monica, CA: RAND Drug Policy Research Center.

SAMHSA (Substance Abuse and Mental Health Services Administration). 1996. *Preliminary Estimates From the 1995 National Household Survey on Drug Abuse.* Rockville, MD: Substance Abuse and Mental Health Services Administration.

Schulberg HC, Burns BJ. 1988. Mental disorders in primary care: Epidemiologic, diagnostic, and treatment research directions. *General Hospital Psychiatry* 10:79-87.

Schulberg HC, Madonia MJ, Block MR, Coulehan JL, Scott CP, Rodriguez E, Black A. 1995. Major depression in primary care practice: Clinical characteristics and treatment implications. *Psychosomatics* 36:129-137.

Schur EM. 1962. *Narcotic Addiction in Britain and America: The Impact of Public Policy.* Bloomington, IN: Indiana University Press.

Scott JE, Greenberg D, Pizarro J. 1992. A survey of state insurance mandates covering alcohol and other drug treatment. *Journal of Mental Health Administration* 19:96-118.

Scrimgeour GJ, Palmer JA. 1976. *Report on the Impact Study of the Uniform Alcoholism and Intoxication Treatment Act.* Washington, DC: Council of State and Territorial Alcoholism Authorities.

Smithers RB. 1988. Making it happen: Advocacy for the Hughes Act. *Alcohol Health and Research World* 12:271-272.

Starr P. 1982. *The Social Transformation of American Medicine.* New York: Basic Books.

Stoil M. 1987. Salvation and sobriety. *Alcohol Health and Research World* 11(3):14-17.

Sturm R, Wells KB. 1995. How can care for depression become more cost-effective? *Journal of the American Medical Association* 273:51-58.

The President's Commission on Law Enforcement and Administration of Justice: Task Force on Drunkenness. 1967. *Task Force Report: Drunkenness.* Washington, DC: U.S. Government Printing Office.

The President's Commission on Mental Health. 1978. *Report to the President From the President's Commission on Mental Health.* Vol. 1. Stock No 040-000-00390-8. Washington, DC: U.S. Government Printing Office.

Van Stelle KR, Mauser E, Moberg DP. 1994. Reductionism to the criminal justice system of substance-abusing offenders diverted into treatment. *Crime and Delinquency* 40:175-196.

Varmus H. 1995. *Disease-Specific Estimates of Direct and Indirect Costs of Illness and NIH Support.* Bethesda, MD: Office of the Director, National Institutes of Health, Public Health Service, U.S. Department of Health and Human Services.

Velez CN, Johnson J, Cohen P. 1989. A longitudinal analyses of selected risk factors for childhood psychopathology. *Journal of the American Academy of Child and Adolescent* 28:861-864.

W Bill. 1957. *Alcoholics Anonymous Comes of Age.* New York: Harper Brothers and Alcoholics Anonymous Press.

Walsh J. 1973. Lexington Narcotics Hospital: A special sort of alma mater. *Science* 182:1004-1008.

4

Structure

Structural measures of quality refer to the resources and capacity of a delivery system to deliver care, including the qualifications of practitioners, the nature of the services and facilities, and certain organizational factors. For practitioners, structural information concerns specialty, licensure, and certification, as well as practice style and setting. The chapter begins with a discussion of these practitioner issues. For facilities and institutions, structural measures include services, size (e.g., number of patients served), location (e.g., number of clinics), licensure and accreditation status, and physical characteristics, such as computer capacity. Traditionally, structural information provides the foundation for quality assurance and accreditation programs.

Analysis of the structure of the behavioral health care service systems requires a review of both public and private service systems for both substance abuse and mental illness. As discussed in Chapter 3, the behavioral health delivery systems involve a complex combination of public and private financing as well as public and private practitioners of care. Public-sector services are financed either with state and federal appropriations or through Medicaid and Medicare coverage, which are discussed first. Next, the public service systems for substance abuse and mental health are examined. Private systems of care have different structures but coexist and often overlap with public-sector services. Workplace service systems (e.g., employee assistance programs [EAPs]) and managed behavioral health care strategies, which have had a stronger influence in the private sector, are also reviewed.

Federally supported service systems developed by the U.S. Department of Defense (DOD) and the U.S. Department of Veterans Affairs (VA) share characteristics of both the private- and public-sector systems of care but represent separate and distinct service systems. Finally, service systems for distinct populations are examined: children, the elderly, Native Americans, and consumers in rural areas.

PRACTITIONER ISSUES

In the field of mental health, training tends to follow a professional, medical model, and state licensing, formal advanced education, and other credentials are typically required for reimbursement. The field consists of several types of professionals, including psychiatrists, psychiatric nurses, psychologists, clinical social workers, and marriage and family counselors. Many mental health treatments (e.g., marital and family counseling, treatment of eating disorders or depression, and group therapy) are offered by more than one type of professional. Medication can only be prescribed by psychiatrists and other physicians, so they sometimes provide medication management while other practitioners provide therapy and counseling. Relatively few health professionals are cross-trained as substance abuse treatment professionals, although this is beginning to change (Josiah Macy Jr. Foundation, 1995).

Substance abuse practitioners include individuals in all of the mental health practitioner categories, as well as substance abuse counselors. Originally, most substance abuse counselors were former substance abusers, because counseling others was seen as an integral part of the recovery model and process. Over the years, many people who are not in recovery have also entered the field. Currently, there is a growing emphasis on credentialing for all substance abuse counselors, and the number of hospital-based treatment units has increased substantially (SAMHSA, 1993). In general, the counseling approach relies on a recovery model and community-based self-help. Counselors are discussed further in a later section of this chapter, Drug Treatment.

Table 4.1 provides an overview of the credentialing involved for all practitioners involved with mental health and substance abuse problems. In managed care networks, an estimated 20 percent of practitioners are psychiatrists, 40 percent are psychologists, and 40 percent are social workers (Iglehart, 1996). The committee is aware of competition and tension among these types of practitioners for philosophical reasons that are largely beyond the scope of this report. However, the committee is not aware of any evidence from outcomes research that any one category of behavioral health practitioner is more or less effective than any other type of practitioner. Moreover, treatment philosophies and strategies vary substantially within professions, as well as across practitioner types, so research would need to take these differences into account.

TABLE 4.1 Profiles of U.S. Practitioners in Behavioral Health Care

Professionals	Responsibilities	Workforce Population
Employee Assistance Professionals (EAPs) (EAPA, 1996)	Counsel employees on personal issues such as health, marital and emotional stress, and drug abuse, which can adversely affect job performance	Approximately 30,000-35,000 EAPs More than 4,000 have become certified employee assistance professionals
Marriage and Family Therapists (AAMFT, 1996)	Counsel people with marital and family issues, as well as those with anxiety, depression, and conduct disorders	Approximately 50,000 marriage and family therapists
Nurses (ANA, 1996a, b)	Provide care, treatment, and other services, including prevention services, to all patients, including those with mental illnesses or substance abuse problems	Approximately 2.2 million registered nurses (RNs) An estimated 1.9 million RNs An estimated 19,145 RNs are state-certified psychiatric and mental health nurses
Physician Assistants (AAPA, 1996; NCCPA, 1996)	Provide support and assistance in the medical care of patients, ranging from surgical assistance to minor diagnostic services	Approximately 25,700 certified physician assistants (PAs)
Primary Care and Other Physicians (AAFP, 1996; ASAM, 1994)	Provide diagnostic, treatment, and prevention services for patients with substance abuse problems and addiction, depression, anxiety disorders, and other behavioral problems	Approximately 2,790 American Society of Addiction Medicine (ASAM)-certified physicians in addiction medicine; most physicians certified by ASAM are psychiatrists, with a few from family and internal medicine

Licensing and Credentialing	Practice Settings	Additional Information
Employee Assistance Professional Association (EAPA) provides certification of EAPs	Workplace	EAPs have no prescription-writing privileges 20,000 EAP training programs
Various states (37) offer licensing, but there is no standardized licensing exam or certification American Association for Marriage and Family Therapy (AAMFT) is lobbying all 50 states to establish standardized licensing and certification regulations for marriage and family therapists	Hospital, private (solo or group) practice, public clinic, and academia	No prescription-writing privileges granted AAMFT has 76 accredited training centers
National Council of State Boards of Nursing licenses RNs and licensed practical nurses (LPNs) administered through state licensing boards American Nurses Credentialing Center certifies nurses in approximately 20 different areas, including addiction and mental health	Hospital, private (solo or group) practice, public clinic, managed care, Veterans' Affairs (VA), correctional facility, academia, and home care	Prescription-writing privileges granted by state; only nurse practitioners (MNS) are usually granted such privileges
Each state licenses PAs through the certification examination offered by the National Commission on Certification of Physician Assistants	Hospital, private (solo or group) practice, public clinic, managed care, military, VA, correctional facility, academia, and home care	Prescription-writing privileges granted by state
ASAM offers a non-American Board of Medical Specialties (ABMS) board certification in addiction medicine to its members; encourages other ABMS boards and the American Medical Association to consider offering certification in addiction medicine American Academy of Family Physicians offers training in substance abuse treatment and prevention	Hospital, private (solo and group) practice, public clinic, managed care, military, VA, correctional facility, and academia	Prescription-writing privileges granted to all physicians (MDs and DOs)

continues on next page

TABLE 4.1 Continued

Professionals	Responsibilities	Workforce Population
Psychiatrists (ABPN, 1996; American Psychiatric Association, 1996)	Provide diagnostic, treatment, and prevention services to patients with mental illnesses and disorders, including substance abuse, through counseling and medical interventions	Approximately 30,000 certified psychiatrists An estimated 1,067 are certified in addiction psychiatry An estimated 1,579 are certified in child and adolescent psychiatry
Psychologists (American Psychological Association, 1995, 1996)	Provide assessment, treatment, and prevention services to patients with mental illnesses and disorders and other individuals seeking counseling for a variety of problems, including substance abuse	Approximately 69,800 licensed and clinically trained psychologists An estimated 950 are certified in substance abuse psychology
Social Workers (AASSWB, 1996)	Counsel people with marital and family issues and behavioral health problems and promote access to social and community-based services	Approximately 300,000 social workers
Substance Abuse Counselors (NAADAC, 1996)	Provide diagnoses, guidance, and treatment for people addicted to drugs, with an emphasis on treatment of specific addictions	Approximately 40,000-50,000 substance abuse counselors

Licensing and Credentialing	Practice Settings	Additional Information
National Board of Medical Examiners licenses all physicians through written examinations taken three times over the course of medical school and residency training American Board of Psychiatry and Neurology (ABPN) of ABMS board certifies psychiatrists Certification of added qualifications in addiction psychiatry and child and adolescent psychiatry is offered through ABPN	Hospital, private (solo or group) practice, public clinic, managed care, military, VA, correctional facility, and academia	Prescription-writing privileges granted to all physicians (MDs and DOs)
Association of State and Provincial Psychology Boards licenses psychologists through state licensing boards American Psychological Association offers certification in several areas, including substance abuse	Hospital, private (solo or group) practice, public clinic, managed care, VA, correctional facility, and academia	No prescription-writing privileges granted, but initiatives are under way to granted limited privileges
American Association of State Social Worker Boards licenses social workers through state licensing boards National Association of Social Workers offers national certification in various areas of social work	Hospital, private (solo or group) practice, public clinic, managed care, military, VA, and correctional facility	No prescription-writing privileges granted
Only six states and the District of Columbia license alcohol and drug abuse counselors National Association of Alcohol and Drug Abuse Counselors offers certification for those with no undergraduate- and graduate-level education; beginning in 1997, all counselors must have at least a baccalaureate degree to be certified	Hospitals, private practice, public clinic, military, VA, and correctional facility, and home visits	No prescription-writing privileges granted

MEDICAID

Background

Medicaid is a public health insurance program jointly funded and administered by federal and state governments. The Medicaid program was created in 1965 as part of the Social Security Act of 1965 to provide medical assistance for eligible poor and low-income populations. Between 1967 and 1995 the number of Medicaid recipients expanded from about 10 million to approximately 36.2 million people, which represents a 262 percent increase (NIHCM, 1996). Dependent children under age 21 accounted for almost half (17.6 million) of the total Medicaid recipients in 1995, an increase of 80 percent since 1985. As of June 1995, 32.1 percent of the 36.2 million Medicaid recipients were enrolled in managed care plans (HCFA, 1996a).

States administer the Medicaid program with guidelines and oversight by the federal Health Care Financing Administration. Financing comes from state funds, with the federal government providing a financial match based on a state's per capita income; the federal share ranges from 50 to almost 80 percent of the total for individual states (GAO, 1991). State Medicaid funding has doubled since 1988 and by 1993 represented 20 percent of many states' budgets (National Association of State Budget Officers, 1995).

Within federal guidelines, states can determine the type, amount, duration, and scope of services and establish eligibility requirements and rates of payment. To be eligible for federal funds, states must provide Medicaid coverage for most of the individuals who receive federally assisted income maintenance payments, including Aid to Families with Dependent Children (AFDC), Supplemental Security Income (SSI), and for some Medicare beneficiaries. States also can choose to provide Medicaid coverage for other "categorically needy" groups, such as aged, blind, or disabled individuals and certain infants and women. Medicaid-eligible children are covered by early and periodic screening, diagnosis, and treatment program (EPSDT), which emphasizes preventive and primary care and which requires comprehensive, periodic health assessments of physical and mental health development.

States can expand Medicaid eligibility to include "medically needy" groups such as children under age 18 or relatives of children other than parents caring for Medicaid-eligible children. Another Medicaid eligibility option addresses those individuals who have medical needs and expenses but may have too much income to qualify as "categorically needy." In this eligibility option, medical or remedial care expenses can offset excess income, allowing individuals or families to "spend down" to Medicaid eligibility.

Medicaid costs depend on many factors, including the size of the eligible and enrolled population, the utilization and availability of services, and the needs of the population. Mandatory Medicaid services that cover mental health and substance abuse care include inpatient and outpatient hospital services, home health care services, nursing facility services, physician services, and EPSDT (Frank and McGuire, 1996; Manderscheid and Henderson, 1995; NIHCM, 1996). An estimated 15 percent of Medicaid funding goes to treatment for mental illness, including skilled nursing facilities, intermediate care facilities, state psychiatric hospitals, and general hospital psychiatric care (Taube et al., 1990). Medicaid supports nearly one-third of community-based mental health programs and is sometimes the only source of funding for community-based support and rehabilitation services (AMBHA and NASMHPD, 1995).

Administration of state Medicaid programs can be based in the health department or social service agency or in a separate agency, depending on whether the state emphasizes eligibility, medical services, or financial accountability. Cost-containment as the Medicaid agency's primary goal can clash with the goals of the public mental health and substance abuse treatment agencies as they seek to maximize access to appropriate care for eligible individuals. Payment practices and the level of collaboration among agencies vary across the states, but Medicaid reform in the 1990s emphasizes managed care. A primary goal of Medicaid managed care is to control the growth in Medicaid expenditures while extending benefits to individuals who are uninsured.

Medicaid Reform Through Managed Care

The Congressional Budget Office estimates that Medicaid expenses will continue to increase at an annual rate of about 10 percent, reaching $260 billion by the year 2000 (CBO, 1995). Faced with increases in the number of recipients and the costs of their care, state and federal Medicaid officials have increasingly turned to managed care to control costs, estimating a 2 to 10 percent savings over fee-for-service care. The savings are projected to come from better coordination of care, shifts from inpatient to outpatient care, and increased emphasis on preventive care.

In 1991, 2.7 million (9.5 percent) of the 28.3 million Medicaid recipients were enrolled in managed care plans. As of June 30, 1995, almost one-third of Medicaid beneficiaries were enrolled in managed care plans (11.6 million of a total of 36.2 million beneficiaries) (HCFA, 1996a). Table 4.2 shows the increase in enrollments in Medicaid, as well as Medicare, from 1991 to 1995.

To implement Medicaid managed care initiatives, states can apply for one of two waivers: 1115 waivers allow program flexibility to research health care delivery alternatives, and 1115(b) "freedom-of-choice" waivers allow managed care delivery systems within specific guidelines. As of August 1996, 49 states have received approval for waivers ranging from small-scale pilot programs to major Medicaid managed care programs, as well as welfare reform projects (HCFA, 1996a). Most of the state initiatives offer acute care, limited benefits for a basic plan and a carve-out for individuals with more intensive needs.

TABLE 4.2   Medicaid and Medicare Total Populations and Number
Enrolled in Managed Care (MC) Plans, 1991–1995

Year	Medicaid Total population (in millions)	MC population (in millions)	Medicare Total population (in millions)	MC population (in millions)
1991	28.3	2.7	34.9	2.2
1992	30.9	3.6	35.6	2.4
1993	33.4	4.8	36.3	2.6
1994	33.6	7.8	36.9	3.1
1995	36.2	11.6	37.6	3.8

SOURCES: HCFA (1991, 1992, 1993, 1994, 1995, 1996a) and HIAA (1996).

To ensure the quality of Medicaid managed care, a Medicaid version of the Health Plan Employer Data Information Set (HEDIS) was developed in cooperation with the National Committee for Quality Assurance. Medicaid HEDIS was released in February 1996, and it adapted the performance measures used by more than 300 plans in the private sector. Medicaid HEDIS was incorporated into the draft version of HEDIS 3.0, which was released for public comment in October 1996, and which integrates measures that are relevant to both publicly and privately insured populations.

MEDICARE

The Medicare program was created by the 1965 Social Security Act as a form of universal health care coverage for all individuals who are age 65 and over and who are eligible for Social Security. In 1972, Medicare was extended to cover disabled individuals, who currently represent about 10 percent of the total Medicare population. Approximately 22 percent of the disabled individuals left the workforce because of mental illness (Lave and Goldman, 1990).

All elderly and disabled Medicare beneficiaries are enrolled in Part A (hospital insurance), which is financed mainly through a payroll tax on earnings that are covered under the Social Security Act (IOM, 1990). Beneficiaries may also voluntarily enroll in Part B (supplementary medical insurance), which covers physician services, including visits in the home, office, and hospital. Part B is financed through a monthly premium that is deducted from the beneficiary's Social Security payment. The division between hospital and physician service coverage is due to historical and political factors in the mid-1960s, and the Medicare program was based on practices and structures in the private sector at that time, particularly Blue Cross and Blue Shield (IOM, 1993).

Medicare has always paid for the evaluation of mental health problems, but it has strict limits on the level of coverage and on the specialty practitioners eligible for reimbursement (Lave and Goldman, 1990). Less than 3 percent of Medicare spending goes to mental health (Frank and McGuire, 1996), and this does not include the social support services and wraparound and enabling services such as employment counseling and child care that other public-sector programs support. However, expenses for mental health services have been rising faster than other Medicare expenses (Frank and McGuire, 1996).

The total costs of the Medicare program approached $185.6 million in 1995 (HCFA, 1995), and federal policymakers have turned to managed care as a means of controlling the increases in costs. As of December 1995, more than 10 percent of Medicare recipients (4 million of a total of 37.6 million recipients) were enrolled in managed care plans (HCFA, 1995) (see Table 4.2). During 1995, the number of managed care plans serving Medicare recipients grew at a rate of more than 25 percent (HCFA, 1995). Nationally, 74 percent of beneficiaries have a choice of one managed care plan, and 53 percent have a choice of two or more managed care plans. The majority of Medicare beneficiaries who are enrolled in managed care plans live in California, Florida, Oregon, New York, and Arizona (HCFA, 1995).

A Medicare version of HEDIS is under development by the Health Care Financing Administration (HCFA) and the Kaiser Family Foundation. The new system will adapt an existing reporting system that will minimize reporting burdens and also standardize the measurement of quality across plans. Beginning in 1997, managed care plans serving Medicare beneficiaries will be required by HCFA to submit data on the HEDIS measures that are relevant to Medicare.

SUBSTANCE ABUSE SERVICE SYSTEMS

Services for the treatment of alcoholism and drug abuse are provided in multiple settings: primary care and acute care facilities, mental health clinics, office-based practices by individual practitioners, and specialty substance abuse treatment programs (see Table 4.3). The National Drug and Alcohol Treatment Utilization Survey (NDATUS) (recently renamed the Uniform Facility Data Set [UFDS]) provides descriptive data on public and private specialty treatment programs. NDATUS began in 1976 as a census of publicly funded drug abuse treatment programs and expanded to include alcoholism treatment services in 1979 (SAMHSA, 1995a). Currently, all public and private programs licensed or approved to provide treatment for alcoholism and drug abuse are surveyed, including units in general hospitals, community mental health centers, and freestanding residential and outpatient addiction treatment services; private practitioners and group practices are generally not included in the census. The National Facility Register was updated and expanded for the 1995 version of UFDS. At present (August 1996), however, the most recent reports are based on data from the 1992

TABLE 4.3   Types of Care in Substance Abuse Treatment

Type of Care	Description
Detoxification services	Detoxification services are designed to guard against medical emergencies that often accompany withdrawal. They frequently serve as the client's introduction to the rest of the publicly funded treatment system.
Inpatient hospital detoxification	Inpatient hospital detoxification services are provided in a 24-hour, supervised medical (hospital) setting. Hospital programs are generally more expensive than traditional programs in a social setting, and research indicates such programs are not generally necessary for less severe cases. Therefore, these services are generally available to publicly funded clients only when they have very serious, life-threatening situations.
Freestanding, residential (nonhospital) detoxification	Inpatient social setting (nonhospital) detoxification services are provided in a 24-hour, supervised (nonhospital) setting. This type of service is used most frequently with publicly funded clients.
Outpatient detoxification	Detoxification services provided in a day (rather than 24-hour, supervised) setting. Infrequently used in the public setting; research indicates that this service may be both clinically effective and cost-effective for many clients. However, this type of service may be too risky for severely addicted patients.
Residential services	Residential services are provided in a 24-hour non-acute care setting. Each residential service setting may provide a variety of clinical services such as individual and group counseling.
Short-term residential services	Short-term services are typically for 30 days or less. Short-term services are usually provided to clients with moderate to severe addiction levels.
Long-term residential services	Long-term services are typically more than 30 days and may include recovery homes or transitional living arrangements such as halfway houses. Long-term services are generally geared to men but are also used for special populations, such as pregnant women and youth, who are considered to be more difficult to treat.
Outpatient/ambulatory services (non-intensive)	Outpatient services generally include individual, family, and group counseling. Pharmacological therapies, such a methadone treatment, may be used as an adjunct to outpatient services.
Intensive outpatient services	Services last 2 or more hours per day for three or more days per week.
Methadone services	Prescribed pharmacological services combined with traditional outpatient counseling services. Methadone clients are generally enrolled in programs for considerable (multiple-year) lengths of stay.

TABLE 4.3 Continued

Type of Care	Description
Outreach services	The goal of outreach programs is to get clients into treatment. Most programs are aimed at special identified populations such as court-adjudicated clients or clients with small children.
Prevention services	Prevention services are aimed at the general population. Some programs are targeted at high-risk groups, such as low-income youth or school dropouts. Programs include a broad range or services such as education, self-esteem enhancement, and the provision of alternative activities.
Wraparound or enabling	Wraparound or enabling services are loosely defined as ancillary services that make it easier for the client to access and stay in treatment or to obtain better outcomes upon discharge from treatment. Examples may include housing assistance, child care, transportation, and employment counseling. In many cases the services are provided within the treatment agency.
EAPs	EAPs attempt to solve alcohol- and other drug-related problems in the workplace. EAPs contain five elements: (1) detection of decrements in job performance, (2) constructive confrontation, (3) referral process, (4) ongoing contact with treatment facility, and (5) intolerance to drug abuse in the workplace.

NDATUS and estimate that 944,880 men, women, and adolescents were in care in 11,316 treatment programs on September 30, 1992 (SAMHSA, 1995a).

The 9,307 facilities that responded to the 1992 survey included 1,650 (17.7 percent) privately funded programs and 332 (3.6 percent) programs within various federal entities (Bureau of Prisons = 73, DOD = 59, VA = 128, and Indian Health Service = 108) (SAMHSA, 1995a). The majority of the respondents were community-based agencies that receive funding from federal, state, or local government (n = 7,325, 78.7 percent). An additional 2,009 agencies were reported as nonrespondents and may include a disproportionate share of private agencies. Nonetheless, it is clear that publicly funded service practitioners predominate in the specialty system for the treatment of alcohol and drug dependence.

More than half of the facilities (56.2 percent) were either freestanding outpatient programs (n = 4,923; 43.5 percent of the respondents) or community-based mental health centers (n = 1,440; 12.7 percent). These two types of outpatient services reported treating 69.2 percent of the patients in care (freestanding = 506,774; community mental health center 146,941). About 15 percent of the respondents were general hospitals (n = 1,181) or specialized hospitals (n = 547), and together these served 118,598 patients (12.5 percent). Residential programs (halfway houses, recovery homes, and residential treatment in therapeutic communities) included 2,474 facilities (21.9 percent) and provided care to 87,494 individuals (9.2 percent). The remainder of the facilities were either correctional programs (n = 312) with 30,658 clients or unknown practitioner types (n = 439) serving 54,413 individuals. Most of the facilities were small, independent agencies; nationally, the mean caseload per facility was 83.5 clients.

The extensiveness of the treatment systems varies substantially from state to state; more than 500 separate services in each of 4 states with large urban centers responded (California = 1,186; New York = 1,001; Michigan = 583; and Florida = 560) and less than 50 programs in each of 13 smaller states responded (Vermont = 17; Idaho = 25; Montana = 29; Alaska = 34; New Hampshire = 40; West Virginia = 40; Wyoming = 40; North Dakota = 41; South Dakota = 43; Delaware = 44; Alabama = 47; Arkansas = 48; and Hawaii = 48). A calculation of the number of clients per capita suggested that nationwide there were 432 clients per 100,000 population; nine states and the District of Columbia had rates that exceeded 600 clients per 100,000 population (Washington, Oregon, California, Alaska, Colorado, New Mexico, Washington, D.C., Maryland, New York, and Rhode Island), and the rate was less than 200 per 100,000 population in nine states (Minnesota, Iowa, Arkansas, Mississippi, Tennessee, Alabama, Georgia, Hawaii, and New Hampshire).

The 1992 NDATUS (SAMHSA, 1995a) analysis suggested that 29 percent of the individuals in care were women. One in 10 were 20 years of age or younger, and less than 1 percent were 65 years of age or older; most (75 percent) were between the ages of 21 and 44 years. Analysis of racial and ethnic characteristics found that 60 percent were white, 22 percent were African American, and 15 percent were Hispanic. Both alcohol and drug dependence was reported by 38 percent of the clients in care, whereas 37 percent were dependent only on alcohol and 25 percent were dependent only on drugs. Private practitioners were more likely to treat white men who were abusing alcohol.

More detail on the men and women treated in publicly funded alcohol and drug abuse programs is provided in the analysis of the Treatment Episode Data Set (TEDS). The Substance Abuse and Mental Health Services Administration (SAMHSA) in collaboration with the state authorities for substance abuse collects and maintains a database (TEDS) on the admissions characteristics of individuals admitted to publicly funded substance abuse treatment services. TEDS provides information on the primary drug of abuse, client characteristics (gender, race or ethnicity, education, and employment status), the presence of health insurance, and the type of treatment service. (Many of the states collect more detailed information, but the national data set is limited to key variables.)

The most recent report from SAMHSA examines admissions during federal fiscal year 1993 (October 1992 through September 1993) and compares current data with data from previous years to speculate about trends in client admissions (SAMHSA, 1995b). The SAMHSA (1995b) report counts 1.4 million admissions to programs in 45 states plus Puerto Rico and the District of Columbia. The admissions included women (28 percent), adolescents (19 years of age and younger, 8 percent), adults (20 to 29 years of age, 30 percent; 30 to 39 years of age, 39 percent; and 40 to 49 years of age, 16 percent), older individuals (50 years of age and older, 6 percent), whites (59 percent), African Americans (28 percent), Hispanics (11 percent), Native Americans (2 percent), and Asian Americans (0.6 percent). Two-thirds (67 percent) were unemployed at admission, 15 percent were homeless, and 63 percent had completed high school. One third (33 percent) of the admissions to publicly funded services were involved with the criminal justice system, and only 1.5 percent were referred by an EAP. Most of the clients (61 percent) were admitted to outpatient services, but 23 percent were in detoxification programs and 16 percent were in short-term (9 percent) or long-term (8 percent) residential services. Alcohol was the primary drug of abuse (58 percent), but cocaine (19 percent) and heroin use were common (13 percent).

Client characteristics vary by drug of choice (SAMHSA, 1995b). Nearly three of four (73 percent) individuals admitted to care for only alcohol abuse were white; 14 percent were African American and 9 percent were Hispanic. Among individuals seeking treatment for heroin abuse, 43 percent were white and more than one in four were African American (27 percent) or Hispanic (28 percent). Clients who reported that crack cocaine was their primary drug of abuse were most likely to be African American (70 percent); one in four (24 percent) were white and about 5 percent were Hispanic. Stimulant (amphetamine) users, on the other hand, were predominantly white (82 percent) or Hispanic (9 percent); only 4 percent were African American. Public treatment programs therefore need to have much sensitivity to racial and cultural patterns of abuse and must be responsive to different cultural needs.

Funding for publicly supported substance abuse treatment services comes from state, local, and federal appropriations. Analysis of data from the 1994 State Alcohol and Drug Abuse Profile (NASADAD, 1996) suggests that for fiscal year 1994 total public funding for substance abuse prevention and treatment services reached nearly $4 billion. State appropriations made up 38 percent ($1.5 billion), the federal Substance Abuse Prevention and Treatment Block Grant added 28 percent ($1.1 billion), other federal funds provided an additional 10 percent ($378 million), local county and municipal governments contributed 6 percent of the total funds ($247 million), and other sources accounted for 18 percent ($723 million) (NASADAD, 1996). Between 1989 and 1994 state funding increased 24 percent, whereas funding from the federal block grant increased 139 percent. In total, state appropriations, however, were still in excess of the funding level from the federal block grant.

MENTAL HEALTH TREATMENT

Mental health services are provided in multiple settings: primary care and acute care facilities, outpatient clinics, office-based practices by individual practitioners and by groups of primary care and specialty practitioners, and nonmedical settings such as the workplace, schools and universities, and community-based settings. Thus, the continuum of care ranges from the most restrictive settings (inpatient hospitalization and residential treatment) to the least restrictive settings (community-based programs and outpatient counseling). Typically, substance abuse treatment is considered a part of mental health treatment because of the similarities in treatment and financing. In this section, the focus is on the treatment of mental health problems.

We have a pluralistic system, and we have great diversity in our service delivery system, which I think is one of its strengths.

Judith Hines
Council on Accreditation of Services
for Families and Children
Public Workshop, May 17, 1996, Irvine, CA

Traditionally, states fund a large proportion of mental health treatment, dominated by inpatient hospitalization. States historically have operated with categorical budgets, with public funds earmarked for specially defined populations, such as runaways or other homeless individuals. Over the years, state mental health agencies have begun to contract with an array of practitioners, including community mental health centers and non-profit community based service agencies (Essock and Goldman, 1995). As discussed in Chapter 3, the public system delivers care for individuals who are uninsured and underinsured and serves a safety net function.

Tables 4.4 and 4.5 display the range of mental health treatment settings, including those in both the public and private sectors.

Because community-based services play an integral part in the delivery system, the next section describes them in more detail.

WRAPAROUND SERVICES

In the public sector, federal and state policies have promoted the development of a coordinated continuum of care. Wraparound or "enabling" services such as transportation to treatment, child care, employment services, legal assistance, and other services have traditionally been an integral part of publicly funded treatment systems for two primary reasons (Institute for Health Policy, 1995). First, the historical evolution of treatment systems for alcoholism and drug dependence has taken place largely outside of medical systems and medical models of care,

TABLE 4.4 Mental Health Treatment Settings

Setting	Description
General Hospital	
Emergency rooms	Evaluation and referral services, most often to psychiatry department. Staffed by nurses, residents, and attending physicians. Paid for by private or public insurance or is uncompensated.
Inpatient psychiatry	Short-term, acute care. Evaluation and referral to long-term or outpatient care. Staffed by psychiatric nurses, psychiatric residents, and psychiatrists. Paid for by private and public insurance. Referrals from emergency room staff, medical staff, private practitioners, and outpatient clinics.
Outpatient psychiatry	Ambulatory care provided by psychiatrists, social workers, psychologists, and psychiatric nurses. Long- and short-term care paid for by private and public insurance.
Specialty Care	
Private psychiatric hospital	Short-term acute care; may specialize in chemical dependency, rehabilitation, children and adolescents. Referrals to outpatient and residential treatment.
State psychiatric hospital	Diagnosis and stabilization for seriously and chronically mentally ill individuals who are experiencing highly symptomatic illnesses. Paid for primarily with state funds.
Community mental health center	Short-term and long-term care for the full range of psychiatric disorders, including rehabilitation, residential treatment, and vocational supports.
Day hospital	High-intensity outpatient treatment for individuals who are symptomatic but who do not need 24-hour inpatient care; may include intensified medication management, treatment, and vocational rehabilitation.
Private practice	Psychiatry, psychology, social work. Solo private practice, preferred provider organization network, or other office-based arrangement.
Nursing homes	Long-term specialty care for individuals with severe disorders and organic mental illness
Community-Based, Nonmedical	
Crisis center	Shelters for those affected by domestic violence, runaways, and individuals who are homeless or need rape counseling. Often staffed by volunteers in donated space, with volunteer professional staff (physicians, nurses, social workers, psychologists, counselors). Funded primarily by donations from charitable organizations and grants. Provide referrals.
Family/social services agencies	Child welfare, foster care, and family reunification programs and case management. Typically staffed by social workers. Include public agencies and private not-for-profit groups.

continues on next page

TABLE 4.4   Continued

Setting	Description
Community-Based, Nonmedical	
Schools and universities	Elementary and high school clinics staffed by nurses. Campus counselors include social workers, psychologists, and psychiatrists. Private insurance or free to students, sometimes to families.
Religious organizations	Counseling by ministers, rabbis, and other clerical personnel
Peer counseling	Social support groups sponsored by hospitals, human services agencies, practitioners, and other volunteers.
Halfway house, transitional living	In combination with outpatient psychotherapy, can help avoid relapse.

relying instead on social services agencies, self-help recovery groups, community-based practitioners, and other nonmedical programs. Second, federal and state policies have supported and encouraged the development of comprehensive program models that facilitated entry to care and support for continued care. These services were identified as "enabling" services in the health plan proposed by President Bill Clinton (White House Domestic Policy Council, 1993).

A portion of the state-managed substance abuse treatment services is funded through the Substance Abuse Prevention and Treatment Block Grant administered by SAMHSA. The block grant and other discretionary funding streams

TABLE 4.5   Comparison of Public and Private Sectors of Care in Mental Health

Characteristics	Public-Sector Mental Health Care	Private-Sector Mental Health Care
Population served	Mostly uninsured, emphasis on the seriously mentally ill	Those with coverage
Funding of care	State general funds, Medicaid and Medicare revenues, local and other funds	Insurance premiums
Locus of treatment responsibility	Local authority (e.g., county government), community mental health center	Insurance plan and/or provider
Predominant services	Case management, medications, housing support, rehabilitation, crisis intervention, and hospitalization	Outpatient therapy, medications, and hospitalization

emphasize comprehensive program models. Moreover, state dollars (added to these systems through general revenue funds) often permit case management and other supportive services. Most states also use Medicaid funds, although the proportion of Medicaid funds supporting alcohol and drug abuse treatment services is relatively small compared with that from other funding sources.

Diagnosis is really an inadequate predictor of the need for services. We need to look both at the functional level at the client, as well as the support system in the environment.

Rita Vandivort
National Association of Social Workers
Public Workshop, April 18, 1996, Washington, DC

If the goal of treatment is long-term recovery from alcohol and other drug abuse, as well as from severe mental illness, wraparound services are often needed to sustain the progress made through medical and psychosocial treatment. Table 4.6 displays many of the wraparound and enabling services used to help individuals with substance abuse and mental health problems. In the movement to managed care, treatment services may be limited to the most essential medical elements; for example, wraparound services that have been developed to support recovery may be eliminated because they are considered "not medically necessary." It is important to recognize that recovery from addiction is not simply a medical issue: complex behavioral factors are intertwined with the medical aspects. Chapter 5, Access, discusses these issues further.

We think we can bring a more comprehensive focus to the ideas of what is necessary—looking beyond narrow definitions of medical necessity to areas of human necessity, which could include having basic income, having help in getting housing, and ongoing support services.

Elizabeth Edgar
National Alliance for the Mentally Ill
Public Workshop, April 18, 1996, Washington, DC

TABLE 4.6 "Wraparound" and "Enabling" Services

Service	Definition	Link to Treatment and Recovery
Cash assistance	Provides income support. Public programs include Supplemental Security Income disability payments, general assistance (welfare), and food stamps.	Without support, most publicly funded clients were unable to complete a treatment regimen. Basic needs, food and shelter, must be met before the client can devote him- or herself to treatment and recovery.
Child care	Provides child care services at no or low cost while parents (generally mothers) attend treatment.	Lack of child care is a barrier to treatment for most women with children.
Domestic violence services	Provides assessment and counseling to clients who have experienced domestic violence or sexual abuse.	The rates of domestic violence and sexual abuse among substance abusers—particularly women—are very high. In many cases, a women's admission to treatment is precipitated by a life-threatening event or crisis.
Education	Provides information as well as direct assistance with enrollment in college/community college or completion of high school/GED programs.	Education contributes to a successful recovery. Education also provides the skills necessary to find work.
Employment counseling	Assists clients in assessing their strengths and weaknesses, learning new job skills, and finding employment.	Without employment, the client is more likely to have trouble living independently or to suffer a relapse.
HIV and TB screening and referral	Provides infectious disease screening, testing, and referral for clients entering and participating in treatment programs.	Reduces risks of infection.
Housing	Assists clients in finding safe and affordable drug-free housing, including recovery homes and halfway houses.	Supported housing enables the client to move out of residential treatment more quickly. A stable living environment is associated with successful treatment and recovery.
Legal assistance	Clients who experience legal problems often receive case management services. Others may be referred to community legal aid programs.	Many substance-abusing, publicly funded clients are referred to treatment in lieu of prosecution or incarceration. Case managers track the client's progress and can assist with Supplemental Security Income disability payments. Seriously mentally ill clients may need legal assistance with civil commitment or other issues.
Parent skills training	Provides parent education and training to help parents function in their family roles during the treatment process.	Mental illnesss and substance abuse disrupts families, which can hinder treatment and recovery.
Transportation	Provides direct transportation information or financial help with public transportation.	Lack of transportation is a barrier to participation in treatment; transportation helps clients continue treatment when they may not have otherwise been able to do so.

NOTE: Other important services that are not wraparound or enabling services include physical health care and vocational rehabilitation. HIV, human immunodeficiency virus; TB, tuberculosis.

THE MANAGED BEHAVIORAL HEALTH CARE INDUSTRY

Background

The organization and financing of mental health and substance abuse treatment have changed dramatically since 1980. The costs of mental health and substance abuse treatment increased faster than both the general rate of inflation and the increases in the costs of the rest of health care in the mid-1980s (about 15 percent a year). By 1991, behavioral health care costs represented 10 to 25 percent of all health care expenditures and became a prime target for cost-containment strategies (Sharfstein and Stoline, 1992; Shore and Beigel, 1996; Sullivan and Miller, 1991).

Psychiatry was excluded from the diagnosis related grouping system in 1983 when it was not clear how to compare mental health services in an equitable way, resulting in a rapid expansion in the number of psychiatric hospitals and the number of inpatient psychiatric beds (Sullivan and Miller, 1991). Between 1980 and 1986 the number of admissions to private psychiatric hospitals increased by 400 percent for adolescents, the average length of stay increased, and per diem costs rose more rapidly than costs in the general medical sector (Jellinek and Newcombe, 1993). Approximately one-third of the increase covered substance abuse treatment (Sullivan and Miller, 1991). Thus, treatment for adolescents and substance abusers was the main component of the cost increases; however, these hospitalizations were not always clinically justified and the results for patients were mixed (England and Goff, 1993).

One consequence of these developments was an increase in for-profit companies contracting to manage behavioral health care benefits. As of January 1995, the combined annual revenue of these companies was estimated to be $2.1 billion; more than half of the amount came from contracts in which the companies were at financial risk (Iglehart, 1996; Oss, 1995). A 1995 survey found that 21.7 million people were enrolled in capitated programs in which behavioral health companies were paid an average of $60 per individual per year (Oss, 1995).

Although managed behavioral health care companies have demonstrated cost savings in the area of behavioral health (Iglehart, 1996), the effects on quality of care are less clear. The trend toward consolidation, mergers, and integrated systems means that there is increasing pressure within the industry to standardize treatment and information systems (CBGP, 1995). There is also more pressure from consumers and other purchasers to demonstrate that appropriate-quality care is being provided efficiently.

Performance Measurement

Two main organizational forces develop standards and measure quality in the behavioral health care industry. One is the American Managed Behavioral

Healthcare Association (AMBHA), the industry membership organization founded in 1995. AMBHA member organizations currently manage mental health and substance abuse care for more than 80 million Americans (AMBHA, 1995). AMBHA works closely with the National Association of State Mental Health Program Directors in developing joint health care policy statements and other collaborative efforts (e.g., AMBHA and NASMHPD, 1995).

In 1995, AMBHA released its first report card, Performance-Based Measures for Managed Behavioral Healthcare Programs (PERMS 1.0). The measures are chosen to be "meaningful, measurable, and manageable" and are classified into three domains: access to care, consumer satisfaction, and quality of care. Measures are based on available data systems, primarily based on existing administrative and reporting data bases. AMBHA has begun field testing of PERMS, and all AMBHA members have agreed to participate (Bartlett, 1996). In Chapter 6, PERMS measures are compared with other current performance measures for behavioral health care.

The Institute for Behavioral Healthcare (IBH) is also influential in the industry, publishing a journal, conducting conferences, and sponsoring other professional development activities in managed behavioral health care. In 1996, IBH released the results of a survey of members of its Leadership Council, a coalition of more than 170 behavioral health care organizations throughout the behavioral health care industry. The survey was completed by 47 percent of these organizations, with representation from four segments of the industry: (1) mental health facilities and integrated delivery systems, (2) community mental health centers and social and rehabilitation service agencies, (3) behavioral group practices, and (4) managed care organizations. The purpose of the survey was to evaluate the current use of a variety of performance indicators and their appropriateness and validity for measuring performance and the feasibility of using these indicators to measure performance (IBH, 1996).

The different segments of the industry, however, varied significantly in types of indicators used to measure access for their clients. For example, the availability of telephone access is frequently used to indicate access to managed care companies but is not used by other organizations that do not possess electronic telephone monitoring systems. The most frequently used indicators of outcomes were symptom reduction, improved functioning, and readmissions to treatment.

Efforts to standardize services and measure performance in managed behavioral health care organizations seem to be a priority for the industry. However, these efforts are in the preliminary stages, and it still is difficult for consumers, employers, and other purchasers of care to compare value and quality across plans.

WORKPLACE SERVICES

The workplace is a primary point of access for health care. An employee's behavior, style, and habits become well known and recognized by coworkers. Changes are frequently recognized in the workplace through declines in the quality of or other changes in work performance. Many times these changes are noticed in the workplace even before they are recognized in the home. Attention to workplace performance can be one of the best means of identifying behavioral problems. Then intervention can occur and the individual can be provided with the help and assistance he or she needs to resolve behavioral health problems. Through prevention, wellness, and early intervention efforts, attention to performance at the workplace facilitates access to health care, contributes to improved health status, and contains costs.

The employee assistance programming field was developed for and has evolved services to assist employers with identifying and resolving behavioral problems and to provide them with a means of intervention (Roman, 1988). Historically, EAP staff worked almost exclusively with individual workers. Organizations now provide assistance with issues related to the productivity, safety, health, and well-being of the entire workforce. This section discusses EAPs, consultation with management, disability management, integrated services, wellness and prevention efforts, training and education, regulatory compliance, demand management, and services for those with special needs, such as those affected by violence and downsizing.

Employee Assistance Programs

An EAP is a worksite-based program designed to assist in the identification and resolution of productivity problems associated with employees impaired by personal concerns including, but not limited to, health, marital, family, financial, alcohol, drug, legal, emotional, stress, or other personal concerns that may adversely affect employee job performance. An EAP is designed to identify problems at an early stage, motivate an employee to seek help, and provide the resources needed to assess and resolve the problem. The program is both a supervisory tool and an employee benefit. An individual can access the service through a referral made by a manager, supervisor, or labor representative, or through self-referral.

EAPs also assist family members. They maintain high levels of confidentiality, focus on early intervention, and are available to employees and family members 24 hours a day. Well-designed EAPs have produced significant outcomes for employers and those that use the services. EAPs are usually evaluated on the basis of the number of employees who use the services as well as the types of problems addressed and the outcomes achieved. Typically, outcomes are defined as improvements in identified problems, access and experience with the resources that were needed, and improved levels of functioning in the individuals who were serviced. Studies have shown that employers, on average, receive a $3 return for every $1 invested in the service (Winslow, 1989). Anecdotal evidence suggests that individuals who use these services realize up to an 80 percent resolution of their presenting problems (Burke, 1996).

The specific core activities of EAPs include the following:

- expert consultation and training to appropriate persons in the identification and resolution of job performance issues related to an employee's personal concerns;
- confidential, appropriate, and timely problem-assessment services;
- referrals for appropriate diagnosis, treatment, and assistance;
- the formation of linkages between workplace- and community-based resources that provide such services; and
- follow-up services for employees who use those services.

Enhanced program services include wellness and health promotion, critical incident (crisis) services, disability management, behavioral health case management, and organizational change management.

Typical program models include the following:

1.   internal: worksite based and staffed by employees of the organization, with or without professional credentialing;
2.   external: may or may not be worksite based and is staffed by outside (outsourced) practitioner or vendor;
3.   mixed: utilizes a combination of both internal and external models.

EAPs have a multitiered relationship with the managed behavioral health care system. They assist with prevention through health promotion and risk reduction activities. They promote the early identification of problems through easily accessed assessment and referral services. They facilitate effective treatment by assisting with the coordination of care, treatment, and workplace support. They assist in controlling costs by addressing gaps or duplication in services, helping deal with barriers to treatment compliance, facilitating return-to-work plans, providing support, advocacy, and follow-up for clients, and serving as liaisons between the treatment community and the workplace.

Management Consultation and Regulatory Compliance

Federal regulations influence the management of employees with behavioral problems, and behavioral health management consultants often assist in the development and implementation of plans for regulatory compliance. The regulations with the most direct impact on the workplace are the Americans with Disabilities Act, the U.S. Department of Transportation, DOD, and Nuclear Regulatory Commission regulations on drug-free workplaces, and the Family Medical Leave Act.

Each set of regulations gives the clearly defined roles and responsibilities related to managing specific behavioral problems. An employer is obligated to establish a plan for implementing each set of regulations and is monitored in its compliance with these regulations. These regulations force employers to pay attention to many problems that affect employees and also increase the likelihood that employees who choose to comply will be given access to well-designed treatment plans.

Workplaces have the potential for violent situations, critical incidents such as a an industrial accident, the sudden death of an employee, or a natural disaster, and increased stress due to change, downsizing, or plant closings. Behavioral consultants with specialized training are becoming more available to managers and supervisors to develop programs that can be used to address these issues. Consultant services include case-by-case consultations, policy design, definition of action plans, proactive planning, and organizational change management (e.g., the orchestration of awareness efforts and other types of training for supervisors, managers, and labor representatives).

Behavioral Health Disability Management

Management of a behavioral disability is an area that has not received much attention. Disability management involves the management of an employer's workers' compensation plan (occupational disability) along with its short-term and long-term disability benefit (nonoccupational disability). Because only a limited number of states allow a behavioral health claim through workers' compensation, the areas that are generally managed are nonoccupational disabilities.

Disability management involves a variety of service components that focus on getting an employee the most appropriate care necessary to enable the employee to return to the workplace in a timely fashion. A behavioral health disability management service is composed of a plan design, specially trained disability case managers, assessment instruments, a specialized practitioner network, and return-to-work protocols.

Behavioral health disability management services are delivered through interactions with the employee, the employer, and the practitioner. Because of the nature of the service provided, the behavioral health disability management service is backed by an appeals process, physician advisers, and an independent medical evaluator network. To minimize the extent of exposure from disability claims, employers implement preventive measures and link the disability program to an EAP.

Integrated Services

Many behavioral health care services overlap and begin to duplicate existing or potentially available services (e.g., the existence of a behavioral managed health care service and an EAP). The existence of these stand-alone services results in the potential for duplication in accessing a practitioner and in the delivery of care. Significant movement, however, has been made toward integrating managed care with EAPs to allow for the blending of the strengths of each service, thus enhancing the overall service delivered in the workplace.

Another motivator for the integration of the two service components is the financial efficiencies that come from managing one rather than two systems. To create financial efficiencies, employers are looking for opportunities to link services and for a "one-stop shopping" opportunity. In an integrated system, the managed care entity focuses on the user of the service and the practitioner. The EAP focuses on the employee and the employer. The linkage of the employee, the employer, and the practitioner enhances the opportunity for the successful treatment of an individual. The EAP can become part of the continuum of care and can provide problem resolution or short-term counseling. Often, the EAP is positioned as the entry point (gateway) to the behavioral health care benefit by providing the assessment and referral to the practitioner network, with ongoing case management provided by the managed care entity.

As purchasers of health care, employers are demanding higher levels of efficiency and cost-effectiveness. These expectations may increase the integration of behavioral health, primary care, and EAP services.

Health Promotion, Wellness, and Prevention

Worksite health promotion is an organized effort supported by an employer to improve employee health, fitness, and well-being. Programs can include health education, behavioral change, occupational health (e.g., workers' compensation and ergonomic training and evaluation), fitness, and recreation services. Most worksites offer health promotion programs because of the possibility of reduced employee health risks, reduced absenteeism, improved employee morale, and controlled costs for health care. At least one-third of employers offer specific health promotion programs, such as smoking cessation, weight control, cholesterol screening, stress management, and exercise programs (EBRI, 1991; Foster Higgins, Inc., 1994).

An employee's use of prevention programs can reduce his or her risk of developing behavioral health problems. Computerized health risk appraisals might be used to identify areas in which an employee might benefit and be interested. Behavioral change programs include programs in such areas as stress management, depression recognition, relationships counseling, assertiveness training, communications skills, and other areas. Programs can be managed through the EAP, with programs held on-site or outsourced to local consultants. Programs also may be associated with health maintenance organizations (HMOs) or managed care plans; for example, health clubs may offer reduced membership rates to enrollees in particular health plans.

Employers implement health promotion programs to enhance employees' quality of life and well-being. In turn, employers can realize savings in corporate health care costs. Some employers reward their employees for healthy behavior by offering discounted health care premiums or rebates or through credits or coupons (IOM, 1993). Employers and health care delivery systems must continue to innovate in areas of prevention and wellness to reduce the prevalence of chronic illness and minimize the financial impacts of these illnesses.

Demand Management

Increasingly, demand management programs are used to educate consumers and prevent serious illness. Demand management provides an array of services including a variety of training and educational programs, ready access to information through toll-free lines that connect an individual to health care professionals, and programs of early detection and self-care. Demand management empowers consumers to be better users of the health care system and to monitor and manage their own health.

Training and Education

Management and labor have valued training and education as a means of providing employees with information that not only assists in self-improvement but that also assists an individual in being more productive in the workplace. Training and education have a proven value and are used frequently. Employers are asking behavioral health care specialists to assist in better informing employees and their family members on areas such as stress, parenting, relationship building, alcohol and drug use, AIDS, caring for the elderly, and communications skills. Behavioral health care specialists conduct training programs so that employees not only gain information but also, many times, use this information as a motivator for accessing the health care delivery system.

Summary of Workplace Issues

The workplace provides one of the best means of accessing health care in the United States. To take full advantage of this potential, it is important that both the employer and the health care industry recognize the power of the workplace. The workplace provides a means of informing and educating the consumer, it provides the financial means for many to access the necessary care, and it serves as a means of early intervention for problems that hold the potential to develop into chronic and costly illnesses.

The field of behavioral health care must recognize the gains that have been made through workplace services and build on that capability. Through the workplace, the potential to gain access to health care will be maximized for the benefit of employees and their family members, employers, and the health care delivery system.

U.S. DEPARTMENT OF DEFENSE AND U.S. DEPARTMENT OF VETERANS AFFAIRS

Background

The federal government has long provided acute and rehabilitative medical services, including mental health care services, for its military personnel. Before World War II, mental health services were limited for active-duty members and were not provided to retirees and their families. With the growth of federally-funded programs during the Depression and World War II, the federal role in providing assistance to state and local governments and its citizens was expanded. The departments of the Navy, Army, and Air Force sustained their medical departments following World War II by building several large tertiary care facilities and obtaining funding for health care programs and personnel. With a large number of injured veterans returning from World War II and the Korean War, the Office of Veterans Affairs (now the Department of Veterans Affairs [VA]) similarly expanded from a modest program providing disability compensation and rehabilitation services to a national system of hospitals and rehabilitation facilities during the 1950s.

With the concurrent growth of other federal programs, both the VA and DOD expanded the scope of their services to include acute and chronic mental health and substance abuse conditions. They aimed to promote professionalism and quality of care through affiliations with medical schools, instituted accredited professional training programs, and made commitments to medical research. With a steady stream of physicians and dentists obligated to military service under the 1933 Selective Services Act, the military was able to medically staff its global system of hospitals and clinics.

Surveys of military personnel leaving the services for civilian work in the 1950s consistently revealed that a major reason for resigning was the limited availability of specialized military or civilian medical services for the families of service members. To bridge this gap, the U.S. Congress enacted in 1964 the Military Medicare Program, later called the Civilian Health and Medical Program of the Uniformed Services (CHAMPUS), to provide health benefits and reimbursements for military family members seeking civilian health care, as well as for retirees and their families. This program was expanded to cover certain health care benefits for disabled veterans under a related program, the Civilian Health and Medical Program of the Veterans Administration (CHAMPVA).

With these new programs in place and a new war in Vietnam that would require even more resources for DOD and VA, the third generation of military health care was under way. With these direct and compensated care systems providing increasing benefits, each program grew substantially in funding and coverage during the next 30 years, and they now cover approximately 20 million eligible citizens.

Mental Health and Substance Abuse Programs

To meet its peacetime and war-related missions, the military provides mental health and substance abuse services to a heterogeneous population that has largely been representative of younger adults in the United States. Although the recruiting and early training processes allow some screening out of individuals who would have difficulty functioning in a military environment because of a mental disorder, many individuals require treatment as the result of biological factors, common life stresses, and the unique and sometimes extraordinary traumas associated with the dangers of military operations.

The families of military personnel are subjected to frequent moves, separations, and threats to the life of the parent or spouse who is a service member. The special needs of military families has resulted in historically high CHAMPUS expenditures for mental health care for family members of active duty and retired personnel. Although some have received "space-available" care by military mental health professionals, the very nature of military family life and the existence of different systems of care (DOD direct care and CHAMPUS), as well as civilian care for spouses with private insurance, complicates the coordination of treatment. An unknown number of these individuals receive care through Medicaid, Medicare, and local charitable and uncompensated sources. Epidemiological studies of this population are incomplete, preventing any meaningful conclusions about the longer-term social impact or health outcomes resulting from this uneven and uncoordinated approach to care.

Special Risk Populations in the Military

Children and Adolescents

Although the Army, Navy, and Air Force have a substantial number of family physicians and pediatricians providing primary care for children, they provide a limited amount of specialized mental health services for children and adolescents. A small number of social workers, especially in the Army and Air Force, provide a core of therapeutic services, especially in remote settings.

Children with special psychiatric and developmental needs are referred to U.S. civilian communities where CHAMPUS-supported residential treatment, special education, and other needed services can be obtained for these "exceptional" family members. When families have children with such needs, they frequently find themselves considering several options: ending their military affiliation to settle in a community that can provide long-term program assistance, accepting the periodic long absences of the service member spouse or parent who can only receive a time-limited special assignment, or accepting an assignment to an area where special services might not be available for the child. The reluctance of many civilian communities to extend public services to military children and the limited military resources available to the family makes this group particularly high risk.

Adults With Chronic Relapsing Conditions

When a service member manifests a chronic relapsing mental health or substance abuse problem, he or she is provided a medical discharge and referred to the VA for follow-up. It is unclear how many drop out of VA care over time because of choice, which may or may not be affected by their perception of need. Many military occupations do not readily convert to civilian work, which creates a barrier to returning to a stable civilian setting. When a spouse is impaired, the service member's absence means a loss of day-to-day support. Although statistics are not available, anecdotal evidence indicates that many of these families dissolve. Ultimately, local communities inherit the responsibility for caring for the single-parent family, which frequently is without health insurance or other economic resources.

Older Adults

Depending on service availability, preferences, and financial abilities, retired military personnel may receive treatment in a military, VA or civilian program, both before and after age 65. Their family members, who are not eligible for care in the VA, may receive some limited care in a military facility, but they generally must count on CHAMPUS, private insurance, or, when eligible, Medicare to support their treatment needs. This multiplicity of sources, which may be variously elected during the course of an illness or even an episode of illness, can make it difficult to coordinate care.

Diversity

The culture of the military population reflects the diversity of cultures of the U.S. population and the cultures of citizens from other countries married to service members. Ethnic and cultural minorities find many opportunities for educational, occupational, and economic advancement in the military, and many consider military work and community life more egalitarian than life in their own communities of origin. Despite the services' successes in equal opportunity, however, cultural factors can result in unique stresses and problems in diagnosis and treatment, particularly when there are language barriers and different cultural approaches for treatment.

A System In Transformation

Recognizing that there are many unique psychological challenges for military personnel and their families, DOD and VA have looked carefully at alternatives to the traditional costly and disconnected systems of care that they provide. The economic forces that have caused such significant restructuring of the private health care financing and delivery systems have also had an effect on public health care budgets, resulting in less money to fund staff and facilities and to provide reimbursements for fee-for-service care under CHAMPUS and CHAMPVA. Like Medicare and Medicaid, DOD and VA have looked at managed care alternatives in recent years. Given the leadership and political sensitivities of the DOD mission, it has been important that federal forays into utilization management and managed care be structured with attention to quality of care and service.

A first major initiative in managing DOD mental health care services quality occurred in 1974, when the U.S. Congress investigated problems associated with residential treatment of children and adolescents. Over the ensuing 7 years, CHAMPUS collaborated with a number of organizations (e.g., the American Psychiatric Association, the American Psychological Association, and the National Institute of Mental Health) to develop residential treatment center certification standards, accreditation, and admission and treatment criteria. These were followed by targeted programs in San Diego, California, and the tidewater area of Virginia, that structured care for persons with depressive disorders and schizophrenia.

In 1981, CHAMPUS launched a national peer review program with the American Psychiatric Association and the American Psychological Association to better account for quality and costs in inpatient and outpatient settings through structured record reviews. This program migrated to commercial insurers and eventually promoted the development of a number of private managed behavioral health care companies during the mid-to-late 1980s. During this same period, DOD established contracts for a targeted mental health demonstration project in the Tidewater area and for a comprehensive managed care program in California and Hawaii, the CHAMPUS Reform Initiative.

These and a number of other pilot programs and demonstrations, such as a joint DOD and state of North Carolina child mental health project at Ft. Bragg, provided a mounting case for structured managed care arrangements to meet DOD goals of reducing avoidable costs and accounting for quality of care. During this same period, VA was considering various complementary managed care approaches, but it was constrained by political concerns about reducing veterans' access to centralized care in VA medical centers.

With the experience of several years of experimenting with options and considering cost and quality issues in contracting with private managed care firms, DOD has now embarked on a major initiative, termed "TriCare." DOD is using a combination of pooling of Army, Navy, and Air Force personnel and facilities with local targeted contracting to provide regional systems of care. Consumers (beneficiaries) are given the option of choosing direct military care when available, a point-of-service option, and where available, HMO and preferred provider organization options, with variable cost-sharing for beneficiaries of different status (i.e., active duty versus retired). Copayments are comparable for primary care and behavioral health care.

DOD will be accounting for quality in these systems through a combination of licensing, accreditation, certification, reporting and auditing, and grievance and appeal requirements. Since this initiative is so new, it is unclear whether it will solve DOD's problems, create new ones, or begin to address the problems in disconnected care that has plagued the military health care system for so long. In the mass of uncertainty is how mental health and substance abuse services for both active duty personnel and active and retired military families will be affected.

CARE AND SERVICES FOR CHILDREN AND ADOLESCENTS

Different Needs

Children and adults have different health care needs, and this becomes especially important in mental health and substance abuse services. Children are continually growing, developing, and changing, sometimes with unpredictable results. The pace of physical, emotional, mental, and social development during childhood and adolescence requires ongoing assessment within the context of what is culturally appropriate for the family.

Children with emotional disorders are in all kinds of families—wealthy, middle class, poor, some with insurance, some with no insurance, some eligible for public sector financing and programs.

Sybil Goldman
Georgetown University
Public Workshop, April 18,1996, Washington, DC

Children are dependent on adults for protection and promotion of their well-being, including having the ability to recognize and seek assistance for health problems. Parents and other caregivers provide access to care through insurance coverage and other means, so children from low-income families can be at risk of being uninsured or underinsured and, thus, of having less access to care. Similarly, children whose parents or caregivers are impaired by substance abuse or other problems require additional supports and may be at higher risk of developing similar problems themselves. More than three-fourths of all foster children have parents who are addicted to drugs or alcohol or both (Children's Defense Fund, 1994).

One of the best indicators of children's health status is performance in school, which is also one of the more consistent ways in which children are assessed and provided with care. In a recent population-based survey known as the Great Smoky Mountains Study of Youth, approximately 20 percent of the children met the criteria for a diagnosis of a mental health problem. Of those who had received care, most (70 to 80 percent) received services from practitioners who worked in schools, primarily guidance counselors and school psychologists. Approximately 12 percent had received services in the general medical sector, usually in combination with other kinds of services (Burns et al., 1995).

Child and Adolescent Service Systems

Nature and Extent of the Problem

An estimated 12 million children—20 percent of all children—experience some mental health or substance abuse problems while they are growing up, including attention deficit hyperactivity disorder, severe conduct disorder, depression, and alcohol and other drug abuse and dependence problems (CMHS, 1996; DHHS, 1991; IOM, 1989; OTA, 1986). An estimated 3.5 million children have serious emotional disturbances (CMHS, 1996). In 1990, state agencies fielded more than 1.7 million reports of child abuse affecting approximately 2.7 million children (National Center for Child Abuse and Neglect, 1992). By the age of 11, 1 in 5 children has smoked cigarettes and 1 in 11 children has had their first drink of alcohol (AMA, 1994; Johnston et al., 1995).

Pediatricians and other primary care practitioners are often the first health care professionals to be consulted when behavioral problems and emotional disturbances are noticed by parents or teachers. Guidelines have been developed to assist in the evaluation and treatment of mental health and substance abuse problems in adolescents, including psychosocial adjustment, eating disorders, use of alcohol and other drugs, depression, learning disorders, and emotional, physical, and sexual abuse (AMA, 1994). In Medicaid's early and periodic screening, diagnosis, and treatment program for Medicaid-eligible children under age 21, states are required to provide or arrange for "comprehensive, periodic assessments of their physical and mental health and follow-up services to diagnose and treat any problems discovered as part of the screening process" (NIHCM, 1996, p. 3). The extent of implementation of the guidelines, however, is not known.

Fragmentation in Financing

Once a problem has been identified, publicly financed care for children and adolescents comes from a variety of categorical programs, including Medicaid, the

Maternal and Child Health Block Grant (part of Title V of the Social Security Act), mental health programs, social services, foster care, substance abuse services, school-based clinics, special education, recreation programs, and the juvenile justice system. Given the multiplicity of funding streams and fragmentation of responsibilities among these agencies, the coordination of care across all systems is almost impossible (Burns et al., 1995; England and Cole, 1995; Newacheck et al., 1995). Studies have shown that only about one-third of children with severe problems get the needed services (Brandenburg et al., 1990; DOE, 1993; Knitzer, 1982; Stoul et al., 1994).

Managed behavioral health care plans serving children and their families face the added challenge of providing family-centered services that need to interface with the multitude of systems that serve children.

Michael Faenza
National Mental Health Association
Public Workshop, April 18, 1996, Washington, DC

National policy for children's mental health services promotes "systems of care," based on principles and values of the Child and Adolescent Service System Program (CASSP). Initiated in 1984 through the National Institute of Mental Health, CASSP was the first federally funded initiative responding to the needs of children and adolescents with serious emotional disturbances. Although in 1993 it was renamed the Planning Systems Development Program, the CASSP principles have wide support among state agencies, professional organizations, and advocacy groups concerned with children and adolescents. These principles include (SMHRCY, 1995):

- case management;
- coordination of care;
- individualized treatment on the basis of need;
- culturally competent services;
- active involvement of families and surrogate families (e.g., foster care) in the development of treatment plans;
- commitment to providing the least restrictive, most normative environment that is clinically appropriate.

Adolescent Treatment Issues

A unique challenge exists in providing developmentally appropriate services to adolescents with alcohol and drug abuse problems. Because of the historic fragmentation of public services to children, a comprehensive approach to serving the needs of adolescents has not evolved. Adolescent clients are served in a variety of settings, with treatment paid for by a variety of funds. Often, clients are served simultaneously in several systems or are referred from one system to another until they reach adulthood. In the absence of clinically coordinated treatment, the severity of the addiction often progresses.

During the 1970s, models of early intervention for alcohol- and drug-abusing youth evolved simultaneously in different locales. Private insurance often paid for traditional 28-day inpatient treatment for adolescents. Programs supported by a variety of funds attempted to develop unique approaches to intervening at the early-onset stages of substance abuse. With cutbacks in funds, many of these early efforts were ended, despite their promising results. There is a need to further evaluate what services should appropriately be developed to address adolescents with problematic substance abuse. Perhaps models from other adolescent interventions could be applied, for example, peer counselors, who are an important part of many teen pregnancy prevention models.

There was a young person who was not successful on any kind of inpatient treatment or intensive outpatient treatment or any of the programs. And we finally got him into a group home situation. The health plan paid for it and then they did a cost-benefit analysis. And they found that not only was it clinically effective, but it was incredibly cost effective.

Susan Goldman
John Hancock
Public Workshop, April 18, 1996, Washington, DC

The 1994 Institute of Medicine study *Reducing Risks for Mental Disorders* recommended further research on the effectiveness of interventions for children and adolescents and also recommended that the research efforts be coordinated. There is little research on the structural characteristics and components of interventions that serve children and adolescents, that is, child-serving and teen-friendly interventions, and that seem to produce the most favorable results (IOM, 1994). Much remains to be learned.

CARE AND SERVICES FOR SENIORS

Contrary to stereotypes, most senior citizens view their health status in a positive way. A 1987 survey found that close to 70 percent of older adults living in the community viewed their health as excellent, very good, or good compared with the health of others their own age; the percentage reporting poor health was about 30 percent (NCHS, 1989). However, the incidence and prevalence of chronic illness do increase with age. More than four of five older persons have at least one chronic medical condition, although they do not necessarily experience significant limitations in their daily activities because of that condition (U.S. Senate, 1988).

An estimated 15 percent of older persons have symptoms of primary depression (U.S. Senate, 1988). This estimate does not include secondary depression, which can result from medication side effects or physical causes. Thus, depression may be far more prevalent than suggested by these estimates. Suicide is a more frequent cause of death among elderly individuals, particularly among elderly men, than among individuals in any other age group (IOM, 1990).

For seniors with multiple problems, such as medical and mental health problems, there is a great need for coordination of care. Demonstration programs such as the social HMO programs and the Program for the All-Inclusive Care of the Elderly pool Medicare and Medicaid funding and funding from private sources to coordinate medical and other services (IOM, 1995). These programs build on a team approach with primary care physicians, nurse practitioners, social workers, nutritionists, and others who participate in the joint planning and delivery of care.

With the increasing movement of Medicare populations into managed care plans, the Health Care Financing Administration has undertaken a project with the United Seniors Health Cooperative to help seniors become more informed consumers. In the words of Sarah Gotbaum (1996), a sociologist who directs the project:

> Whether or not to join a Medicare HMO, which one to join, whether to remain in one, transfer to another, or return to fee-for-service—these are among the overwhelming concerns of millions of older Americans faced with entering the foreign world of managed care. The elderly, burdened with the aging process, increased illnesses, decreased incomes, decreasing family supports, changing lifestyles and security, are even more unprepared to identify what they must know in judging a plan, what questions to ask, whom to go to for unbiased, relevant information, whom to trust, what offering is best suited to their personal needs. Most health care choices made today are made on the basis of benefits and price. Consumers know little or nothing about the internal workings of managed care plans with respect to access, appeals, complaints, service denials, benefit restrictions, disenrollments, consumer satisfaction, quality of care. Consumers shopping for a plan should be able to compare HMOs on these dimensions (Gotbaum, 1996).

In 1996, more than 37 million Americans over the age of 65 were enrolled in the Medicare program, and about 10 percent of these individuals were in managed care plans (HCFA, 1996b). Many of the concerns of Medicare-covered individuals entering managed care plans are unique to the concerns of the elderly. As Dr. Gotbaum pointed out in her testimony to the committee, however, many of the concerns are shared by other purchasers: how to balance costs and benefits with the quality of services provided.

INDIAN HEALTH SERVICE

The Indian Health Service (IHS) was established in 1787 under Article I of the U.S. Constitution. An agency of the U.S. Public Health Service, IHS is responsible for providing health care to approximately 1.4 million American Indians and Alaska Natives residing in remote, isolated areas in 34 states. Services are provided through either IHS- or tribally-operated hospitals and clinics or through urban Indian projects. Only members of federally recognized Indian tribes and their descendants are eligible to receive the services provided by IHS (IHS, 1996a).

With a current annual appropriation of approximately $2.2 billion, IHS, like other public and private health care practitioners, must address the soaring costs of delivering health care. This mission is compounded by the lack of a health care infrastructure in the remote areas being served and by the fact that the overall health status of American Indians and Alaska Natives lags far behind that of other Americans (IHS, 1996a). For example, among American Indians and Alaska Natives the infant mortality rate in 1990-1992 was 9.4 per 100,000, compared with a rate of 7.3 per 100,000 among all other races in the United States (IHS, 1996b). For 1990-1992, the mortality rate from accidents among American Indians and Alaska Natives was nearly 2.7 times the age-adjusted rate among all races in the United States (83.2 compared with 31.0 per 100,000), and age-adjusted mortality from alcoholism was nearly six times that for the rest of the U.S. population (37.2 compared with 6.8 per 100,000) (IHS, 1996b).

To serve the American Indian and Alaska Native populations better, IHS has formed partnerships with tribal governments and other Indian organizations. As of March 1996, 64 health centers, 50 health stations, 37 hospitals, 34 urban health projects, and 5 school health centers formed the basis of the IHS system. The total clinical staff consists of approximately 2,580 nurses, 840 doctors, 380 dentists, and 100 physician assistants (IHS, 1996a).

Following the national trend, IHS is increasingly becoming an outpatient care delivery system, with ambulatory care visits increasing and hospital admissions declining. In 1993, outpatient visits totaled more than 5.5 million, compared with total IHS and tribal hospital admissions of 69,000 (IHS, 1996b). As patients become sicker and have more complex problems, such as complications from diabetes, IHS hospitals are seeking to develop referral relationships with non-IHS tertiary care facilities. For example, in some locations, IHS hospitals have developed cooperative agreements with Veterans Administration hospitals (Cedar Face, 1996).

As of January 1995, all IHS- and tribally-operated hospitals and eligible IHS-operated health centers were accredited by the Joint Commission on Accreditation of Healthcare Organizations (IHS, 1995). In combination with the accreditation process, total quality management guidelines are requiring IHS facilities to restructure the ways in which they are organized and deliver services. Staffing patterns and the ratios of health professionals to patients at some clinics are being reevaluated to improve efficiency and cost-effectiveness.

With escalating health care costs, a growing population requiring services, and declining resources, IHS and its partners have committed themselves to the concept of managed care to ensure the delivery of cost-effective and high-quality health care. Although no comprehensive system has been established among the IHS- and tribally-operated hospitals and clinics, several communities have enacted aspects of managed care that have reduced costs, expanded services, and improved the quality of care. Some communities have established pharmaceutical cost-containment programs, day hospitals for mentally ill individuals, clinical prevention programs, practice management initiatives, telemedicine, and quality improvement programs (IHS, 1995).

One example of the role that managed care is having on IHS involves California's 1992 Managed Care Expansion Plan, which would bring managed health care to an additional 13 counties, including counties that serve thousands of American Indians. In 1993, the California Indian Managed Care Task Force was established to work with the state of California in expanding managed care into American Indian populations. Working with tribal leaders and 638 contract and urban Indian clinic administrators, the task force agreed to the following:

• recognition of the concept of Indian tribal sovereignty, allowing Indian clinics to negotiate directly with the state on the extension of managed care;
• acknowledgment, under P. L. 102-573, of the Indian clinics' right to provide health care first and foremost to American Indians and Alaska Natives;
• recognition of the need of Indian clinics to provide culturally sensitive health care; and;
• acknowledgment of the Indian clinics' federally qualified health center status—and, therefore, agreement to reasonable-cost reimbursement to the clinics—and acceptance of the automatic enrollment of Indian patients into Indian health clinics (IHS, 1995).

This task force has also begun negotiations with the state of California concerning managed care reform plans in the areas of dental and mental health. Working closely with the Health Care Financing Administration, the task force is addressing the issues of Native American health care rights and the way in which the state or managed care plan will be reimbursed in these and other areas (IHS, 1995). Managed care and the role of quality assurance and accreditation guidelines have certainly become an integral part of IHS in providing both quality and cost-effective care to American Indians and Alaska Natives.

CULTURAL COMPETENCE

The United States is becoming increasingly multicultural: racial and ethnic minorities are the fastest-growing groups in the population of the United States. In 1990, Hispanics, Asians, and Pacific Islanders made up 19.7 percent of the total population, and by the year 2000 it is estimated that the proportion will have increased to 25 percent of the population (BOC, 1990). Thus, cultural differences between patients and practitioners are becoming more common, and these differences can have crucial implications for the quality and outcomes of care. For example, studies have indicated that there are ethnically based differences in treatment for pain (Todd et al., 1993) and disparities in health status between racial and ethnic minorities and the rest of the U.S. population (DHHS, 1991).

The literature, the science, and the body of knowledge about the effect of culture in providing mental health services or in being able to diagnose mental health problems is very important.

Raphael Metzger
National Coalition of Hispanic Health and Human Services
    Organizations
Public Workshop, April 18, 1996, Washington, DC

Cultural competence is a term that refers to the sensitivity, cultural knowledge, skills, and actions of practitioners that meet the needs of patients from diverse backgrounds (AMA, 1994). Cultural competence can be demonstrated in many ways, for example, by including cultural factors in history-taking and diagnosis, addressing language barriers by having multilingual staff or interpreters, and changing communication patterns to recognize cultural beliefs, practices, and roles, such as deference to elders (Oösterwal, 1994).

> We put on the referral form the numbers the staff could call
> so we could provide translation while the patient was there. I
> realize these things are mundane, but this is the level you
> have to think at if you are talking about being able to provide
> for diverse patients.
>
> *Grace Wang*
> *Association of Asian Pacific Community Health*
>   *Organizations*
> *Presentation to the Committee, June 29, 1996*
>   *Washington, DC*

Several models and guides have been developed to promote cultural competence in service delivery to particular racial and ethnic groups. For example, the Association of Asian Pacific Community Health Organizations developed a manual on culturally competent managed care for Asians and Pacific Islanders, with support from the Bureau of Primary Health Care (AAPCHO, 1994). The manual describes the Language Access Project, a model that has been developed in community health centers serving predominantly Asian and Pacific Islander populations. The emphasis is on helping individuals with limited English proficiency to access health care services.

The National Coalition of Hispanic Health and Human Services Organizations has developed a manual for practitioners in the delivery of preventive services to Hispanic groups (COSSMHO, 1990), with funding from the U.S. Office of Disease Prevention and Health Promotion in the Office of the Assistant Secretary for Health. The manual provides background on general health characteristics of the Hispanic population, describes beliefs and practices that influence health status, and offers strategies for effective interactions between practitioners and patients.

Managed care raises issues regarding the determination of when steps need to be taken to provide culturally competent care. Known operationally as the "threshold" issue, these determinations can be made on the basis of the number of individuals who have language barriers or the percentages in the population (AAPCHO, 1994). In communities in which particular racial and ethnic groups are concentrated, the threshold issue may need to be approached differently than in multicultural communities, but there are no standards in this area.

In cities like New York or Los Angeles, there are up to 150 language groups. Requiring each health care entity to be responsible for all of those languages is a real problem. Seattle has created a community interpreter service program for a variety of different languages, and interpreters can be dispatched to hospitals on scheduled or on-call basis. They hire Spanish-speaking providers or interpreters as staff, and then rely on the interpreter pool for the less frequently used languages.

Julia Puebla Fortier
Resources for Cross-Cultural Health Care
Presentation to the Committee, June 29, 1996
Washington, DC

A culturally-competent system of care values diversity, has the capacity for cultural self-assessment, is conscious of the dynamics inherent when cultures interact, has institutionalized cultural knowledge, and has developed adaptations to diversity.

Grace Wang
Association of Asian Pacific Community Health
Organizations
Presentation to the Committee, June 29, 1996
Washington, DC

California's MediCal managed care system moved from determining thresholds on a percentage basis to using absolute numbers (AAPCHO, 1994). One guide for California's strategic plan for the MediCal conversion to managed care was a study supported by the Health Resources and Services Administration, which identified the ways in which bilingual and bicultural practitioners change their practice patterns when they serve non-English-speaking Latino and Chinese patients (Tirado, 1995). The study distinguished between *cultural competence*, "a level of knowledge and skills to provide effective clinical care to patients from a particular ethnic or racial group" and *cultural sensitivity*, "a psychological propensity to adjust one's practice styles to the needs of different ethnic or racial groups" (Tirado, 1995, p. 1).

In some communities, community-based racial and ethnic groups form coalitions to develop resource networks. For example, the Latino Coalition for a Healthy California, the Asian Pacific Islander Health Forum, and the California Black Health Network are part of California's Multi-Cultural Health Information Project, which is developing a database of health care experts and resources. The desire for contact with a practitioner of similar racial and ethnic background is difficult to satisfy, since racial and ethnic minorities are underrepresented among health care professionals (COSSMHO, 1990).

We are hearing more and more now that managed care organizations are really seeing linguistically and culturally diverse populations as a niche they can approach within the marketplace.

Julia Puebla Fortier
Resources for Cross-Cultural Health Care
Presentation to the Committee, June 29, 1996
Washington, DC

A general discussion such as this one cannot begin to capture the richness and variation among and within this country's racial and ethnic groups. However, it is clear that the diversity provides a significant challenge to managed care organizations in being responsive to cultural preferences among the populations that they serve.

RURAL HEALTH AND MANAGED CARE

According to the U.S. Bureau of the Census, a rural area is defined as a county without a central city or two cities of 50,000 or more in population or as a county or town with areas of open country or fewer than 2,500 people. Nearly 23 percent of the U.S. population live in rural areas (BOC, 1988, 1989). Health care delivery and financing in these areas are often confronted with low numbers of physicians, financially fragile hospitals, low incomes, and low population densities. Although the extent and number of managed care delivery systems in place in rural areas is unknown, that number is growing. Managed care plans in rural areas are hoping to help improve health care availability and affordability.

Managed care plans in rural areas appear to be more successful when they are built around physicians instead of hospitals, since practitioners usually control both the hospital and specialist referrals in such an area. Physicians often feel overworked and underpaid in rural areas, but they will enroll in managed care networks to maintain their patient base. Point-of-service plans and HMOs may provide rural physicians with the greatest market share benefits, because managed care plans offer additional benefits to employees to use their designated primary care physicians (NRECA, 1991).

Managed health care plans in rural areas provide communities with opportunities to reduce health care costs, enhance the financial viability of practitioners, and overcome distances and isolation that can reduce the quality of health care in these areas. Within managed care plans, health professionals are selected on the basis of their credentials and ongoing performance, ensuring that the outcome and the impact of care on the patients indicate that the care is of the highest quality (Christianson, 1989; NRECA, 1991).

However, other factors, such as the enhanced role of primary care physicians, the focus on the cost-effectiveness of care, and the changes that have been made at both the state and federal levels, have also led the way in fostering changes in rural medical practice. Issues surrounding the uninsured, the relative scarcity of practitioners, low population densities, and low incomes still need to be addressed in relation to rural health care. Such factors do not generally restrict the usefulness of managed care, but managed care can provide opportunities and alternatives to overcome those problems (Korczyk, 1989; NRECA, 1991.)

SUMMARY OF STRUCTURAL ISSUES

This review of system structures illustrates the complex organization and financing systems required to provide mental health and substance abuse services, documents the presence of multiple autonomous but overlapping systems of care (public, private, DOD, and IHS), and recognizes the fragmentation inherent in developing services for distinct populations (e.g., children, adults with chronic problems, various cultural groups, and consumers in both urban and rural areas).

Standards of care, accreditation guidelines, and quality improvement mechanisms that address system integration are one way to overcome fragmentation in the delivery of care. Integrated delivery systems are transforming the delivery of care in the public and private sectors in different ways and are also creating new needs for quality measurement systems that keep pace with evolving structures and other new developments in the delivery of care.

REFERENCES

AAFP (American Academy of Family Physicians). 1996. *Family Medicine Online*. [http://www.aafp.org]. October.

AAMFT (American Association of Marriage and Family Therapy). 1996. *A Consumer's Guide to Marriage and Family Therapy*. Washington, DC: American Association of Marriage and Family Therapy.

AAPA (American Academy of Physician Assistants). 1996. *AAPA Homepage: General Information*. [http://www.aapa.org]. September.

AAPCHO (Association of Asian Pacific Community Health Organizations). 1994. *Culturally Competent Health Service Delivery Under Managed Care for Asians and Pacific Islanders.* Oakland, CA: Association of Asian Pacific Community Health Organizations.

AASSWB (American Association of State Social Work Boards). 1996. *Social Work Laws and Board Regulations: A State Comparison Study.* Culpeper, VA: American Association of State Social Work Boards.

ABPN (American Board of Psychiatry and Neurology). 1996. *Information for Applicants for Added Qualifications, 1996.* Deerfield, IL: American Board of Psychiatry and Neurology, Inc.

AMA (American Medical Association). 1994. *AMA Guidelines for Adolescent Preventive Services (GAPS): Recommendations and Rationale.* Baltimore, MD: Williams and Wilkins.

AMBHA (American Managed Behavioral Healthcare Association).1995. *Performance Measures for Managed Behavioral Healthcare Programs.* Washington, DC: American Managed Behavioral Healthcare Association.

AMBHA (American Managed Behavioral Healthcare Association) and NASMHPD (National Association of State Mental Health Program Directors). 1995. Public mental health systems, Medicaid re-structuring, and managed behavioral healthcare. *Behavioral Healthcare Tomorrow* September/October:63-69.

American Psychiatric Association. 1996. *Psychiatric News Homepage: Newspaper of the American Psychiatric Association.* [http://www.appi.org/pnews]. October.

American Psychological Association. 1995. *Profile of All APA Members: 1995.* Washington, DC: American Psychological Association.

American Psychological Association. 1996. Personal communication to the Institute of Medicine. Washington, DC. June 4.

ANA (American Nurses Association). 1996a. *ANA Homepage: About the American Nurses Association.* [http://www.ana.org]. September.

ANA. 1996b. *ANA Homepage: American Nurses Credentialing Center.* [http://www.ana.org/ancc/ancc.htm]. September.

ASAM (American Society of Addiction Medicine). 1994. *Subspecialization in Addiction Medicine.* Presentation at the American Medical Association's Council on Medical Education. Rosemont, IL. August 27.

Bartlett J. 1996. *PERMS: The American Managed Behavioral Health Care Association.* Presentation at Public Workshop held by the IOM Committee on Quality Assurance and Accreditation Guidelines for Managed Behavioral Health Care. Washington, DC. April 18.

BOC. (U.S. Bureau of the Census). 1988. *County and City Data Book 1988.* Washington, DC: U.S. Government Printing Office.

BOC. 1989. *County Business Patterns, 1987.* Washington, DC: U.S. Government Printing Office.

BOC. 1990. *Statistical Abstract of the United States: 1990.* Washington, DC: U.S. Department of Commerce.

Brandenburg NA, Friedman RM, Silver S. 1990. The epidemiology of childhood psychiatric disorders: Recent prevalence findings and methodologic issues. *Journal of the American Academy of Child and Adolescent Psychiatry* 29:76-83.

Burke J. 1996. Personal communication to the Institute of Medicine. October 8.

Burns BJ et al. 1995. Children's mental health service use across service sectors. *Health Affairs* 14(3):147-159.

CBGP (Council of Behavioral Group Practice). 1995. Position statement: Principles and priorities. Standardization of operations, measurement, and communications in behavioral healthcare. *Behavioral Healthcare Tomorrow* September/October:56-57.

CBO (Congressional Budget Office). 1995. *CBO December Preliminary Baseline: Medicaid.* Washington, DC: Congressional Budget Office. December 14.

Cedar Face R. 1996. *Coordination of Services for Native Americans.* Presentation to the IOM Committee on Quality Assurance and Accreditation Guidelines for Managed Behavioral Health Care. Washington, DC. June 30.

Children's Defense Fund. 1994. *The State of America's Children*. Washington, DC: Children's Defense Fund.

Christianson JB. 1989. Alternative delivery systems in rural areas. *Health Services Research* 23:849-890.

CMHS (Center for Mental Health Services). 1996. *Child, Adolescent, and Family Programs*. Washington, DC: National Mental Health Services Knowledge Exchange Network.

COSSMHO (National Coalition of Hispanic Health and Human Services Organizations). 1990. *Delivering Preventive Health Care to Hispanics: A Manual for Providers*. Washington, DC: National Coalition of Hispanic Health and Human Services Organizations.

DHHS (U.S. Department of Health and Human Services). 1991. *Healthy People 2000*. DHHS Publication No. (PHS) 91-50212. Washington, DC: U.S. Government Printing Office.

DOE (Department of Education). 1993. *Together We Can: A Guide for Crafting a Profamily System of Education and Human Services*. Washington, DC: U.S. Government Printing Office. April.

EAPA (Employee Assistance Professionals Association, Inc.). 1996. *Employee Assistance Backgrounder*. Arlington, VA: Employee Assistance Professionals Association, Inc.

EBRI (Employee Benefits Research Institute). 1991. Health promotion: Its role in health care. *Issue Brief* No. 120.

England MJ, Cole R. 1995. Children and mental health: How can the system be improved? *Health Affairs* 14(3):131-138.

England MJ, Goff VV. 1993. Health reform and organized systems of care. *New Directions in Mental Health Services* 59:5-12.

Essock SM, Goldman HH. 1995. States' embrace of managed mental health care. *Health Affairs* 14(3):34-44.

Foster Higgins, Inc. 1994. *Managed Behavioral Healthcare: Quality and Access Survey Report*. Washington, DC: American Managed Behavioral Healthcare Association.

Frank RG, McGuire TG. 1996. Introduction to the economics of mental health payment systems. In: Levin BL, Petrila J, eds. *Mental Health Services: A Public Health Perspective*. New York: Oxford University Press.

GAO (U.S. General Accounting Office). 1991. *Medicaid Expansions: Coverage Improves But State Fiscal Problems Jeopardize Continued Progress*. GAO/HRD-91-78. Washington, DC: U.S. General Accounting Office.

Gotbaum S. 1996. Testimony to IOM Committee on Quality Assurance and Accreditation Guidelines for Managed Behavioral Health Care. Washington, DC. June 26.

HCFA (Health Care Financing Administration). 1991. *Medicare Managed Care Report: December, 1991*. Baltimore, MD: Health Care Financing Administration.

HCFA. 1992. *Medicare Managed Care Report: December, 1992*. Baltimore, MD: Health Care Financing Administration.

HCFA. 1993. *Medicare Managed Care Report: December, 1993*. Baltimore, MD: Health Care Financing Administration.

HCFA. 1994. *Medicare Managed Care Report: December, 1994*. Baltimore, MD: Health Care Financing Administration.

HCFA. 1995. *Medicare Managed Care Report: December, 1995*. Baltimore, MD: Health Care Financing Administration.

HCFA. 1996a. *Medicaid Managed Care Enrollment Report: Summary Statistics*. Baltimore, MD: Health Care Financing Administration.

HCFA. 1996b. *Medicare Managed Care Report: June, 1996*. Baltimore, MD: Health Care Financing Administration.

HIAA (Health Insurance Association of America). 1996. *Source Book of Health Insurance Data: 1995*. Washington, DC: Health Insurance Association of America.

IBH (Institute for Behavioral Healthcare). 1996. *Performance Indicator Survey*. Tiburon, CA: Institute for Behavioral Healthcare.

Iglehart JK. 1996. Health policy report: Managed care and mental health. *The New England Journal of Medicine* 334(2):131-135.

IHS (Indian Health Service). 1995. *Successful Strategies for Increasing Direct Health Care Quality, Accessibility, and Economy for American Indians and Alaska Natives.* IHS Publication No. 95-85016. Rockville, MD: Indian Health Service.

IHS. 1996a. *Indian Health Services Homepage: Fact Sheet.* [http://www.ihs.gov/9vision/This Facts.html]. September.

IHS. 1996b. *Trends in Indian Health, 1995.* Rockville, MD: Indian Health Service.

Institute for Health Policy. 1995. *Enabling Support Services Within Mental Health and Substance Abuse Services.* Paper submitted to the Substance Abuse and Mental Health Services Administration.

IOM (Institute of Medicine). 1989. *Controlling Costs and Changing Patient Care? The Role of Managed Care.* Washington, DC: National Academy Press.

IOM. 1990. *Medicare: A Strategy for Quality Assurance.* Vol. 1. Washington, DC: National Academy Press.

IOM. 1993. *Employment and Health Benefits: A Connection at Risk.* Washington, DC: National Academy Press.

IOM. 1994. *Reducing Risks for Mental Disorders.* Washington, DC: National Academy Press.

IOM. 1995. *Real People, Real Problems: An Evaluation of the Long-term Care Ombudsman Program of the Older Americans Act.* Washington, DC: National Academy Press.

Jellinek MS, Newcombe B. 1993. Two wrongs don't make a right: Managed care, mental health, and the marketplace. *Journal of the American Medical Association* 270(14):1737-1739.

Johnston LD, O'Malley PM, Bachman JG. 1995. *National Survey Results on Drug Use from the Monitoring the Future Study, 1975-1994.* Vol. 1. Ann Arbor, MI: Institute for Social Research, University of Michigan.

Josiah Macy Jr. Foundation. 1995. *Training About Alcohol and Substance Abuse for All Primary Care Physicians.* New York: Josiah Macy Jr. Foundation.

Knitzer J. 1982. *Unclaimed Children: The Failure of Public Responsibility to Children and Adolescents in Need of Mental Health Services.* Washington, DC: Children's Defense Fund.

Korczyk SM. 1989. *Health Care Needs, Resources, and Access in Rural Health.* Washington, DC: National Rural Electric Cooperative Association.

Lave JR, Goldman HH. 1990. Medicare financing for mental health care. *Health Affairs* 9(1):19-30.

Manderscheid RW, Henderson MJ. 1995. *Speaking With a Common Language: The Past, Present, and Future of Data Standards for Managed Behavioral Healthcare.* Rockville, MD: Center for Mental Health Services.

NAADAC (National Alcoholism and Drug Abuse Counselors). 1996. *NAADAC Homepage: What is NAADAC?* [http://www.naadac.org]. September.

NASADAD (National Association of State Alcohol and Drug Abuse Directors). 1996. *State Resources and Services Related to Alcohol and Other Drug Problems for Fiscal Year 1994: An Analysis of State Alcohol and Drug Abuse Profile Data.* Washington, DC: National Association of State Alcohol and Drug Abuse Directors.

National Association of State Budget Officers. 1995. *1994 State Expenditure Report.* Washington, DC: National Association of State Budget Officers.

National Center for Child Abuse and Neglect. 1992. *Working Paper 1, 1990 Summary Data Component.* DHHS Publication No. (ACF) 92-30361. Washington, DC: U.S. Department of Health and Human Services.

NCCPA (National Commission on the Certification of Physician Assistants). 1996. *NCCPA: 1995 Update and General Information.* Atlanta, GA: National Commission on Certification of Physician Assistants.

NCHS (National Center for Health Statistics). 1989. *Health, United States, 1988.* DHHS Publication No. (PHS) 89-1232. Washington, DC: U.S. Government Printing Office.

Newacheck P, Hughes D, Brindis C, Halfon N. 1995. Decategorizing health services: Interim findings from The Robert Wood Johnson Foundation's Child Health Initiative. *Health Affairs* 14(3):232-242.

NIHCM. 1996. *Assuring Quality of Care for Children in Medicaid Managed Care—EPSDT in a Time of Changing Policy.* Washington, DC: National Institute for Health Care Management.

NRECA (National Rural Electric Cooperative Association). 1991. *Managed Care Plans in Rural America.* Washington, DC: National Rural Electric Cooperative Association.

Oösterwal G. 1994. *Community in Diversity.* Barrier Springs, MI: Andrews University Center for Intercultural Relations.

Oss M. 1995. More Americans enrolled in managed behavioral health care. *Open Minds* March:12.

OTA (Office of Technology Assessment). 1986. *Children's Mental Health: Problems and Services.* OTA-BP-H-33. Washington, DC: U.S. Government Printing Office, December.

Roman P. 1988. Growth and transformation in workplace alcoholism programming. In: Galanter M, ed. *Recent Developments in Alcoholism.* Vol. 6. New York: Plenum Press. Pp. 131-158.

SAMHSA (Substance Abuse and Mental Health Services Administration). 1993. *State Methadone Treatment Guidelines.* Treatment Improvement Protocol (TIP) Series 1. Rockville, MD: Substance Abuse and Mental Health Services Administration.

SAMHSA. 1995a. *Overview of the National Drug and Alcoholism Treatment Unit Survey (NDATUS): 1992 and 1980-1992.* Advance Report No. 9. Rockville, MD: Substance Abuse and Mental Health Services Administration, Office of Applied Studies. January.

SAMHSA. 1995b. *Client Admissions to Specialty Substance Abuse Treatment in the United States: Treatment Episode Data Set (TEDS), Fiscal Year 1993.* Advance Report Review Draft. Rockville, MD: Substance Abuse and Mental Health Services Administration, Office of Applied Studies. September.

Sharfstein SS, Stoline AM. 1992. Reform issues for insuring mental health care. *Health Affairs* 11(3):84-97.

Shore MF, Beigel A. 1996. The challenges posed by managed behavioral health care. *The New England Journal of Medicine* 334(2):116-118.

SMHRCY (State Mental Health Representatives for Children and Youth). 1995. *Successful Integration of System of Care Development with Managed Behavioral Healthcare Technologies in Public Children's Mental Health.* Alexandria, VA: National Association of State Mental Health Program Directors.

Stoul BA, Pires SA, Katz-Leavy JW, Goldman SK. 1994. Implications of the Health Security Act for mental health services for children and adolescents. *Hospital and Community Psychiatry* 45(9):877-882.

Sullivan CG, Miller JE. 1991. *The Evolution of Mental Health Benefits.* Washington, DC: Health Insurance Association of America.

Taube CA, Goldman HH, Salkever D. 1990. Medicaid coverage for mental illness: Balancing access and costs. *Health Affairs* 9(1):5-18.

Tirado MD. 1995. *Tools For Monitoring Cultural Competence in Health Care.* Presentation to the Office of Planning and Evaluation, Health Resources and Services Administration. San Francisco, CA. January 31.

Todd KH, Samaroo N, Hoffman JR. 1993. Ethnicity as a risk factor for inadequate emergency department analgesia. *Journal of the American Medical Association* 269(12):1537-1539.

U.S. Senate. 1988. *Aging America: Trends and Projections, 1987-1988 Edition.* Washington, DC: U.S. Department of Health and Human Services.

White House Domestic Policy Council. 1993. *Health Security: The President's Report to the American People.* New York: Simon and Schuster.

Winslow R. 1989. Spending to cut mental health costs. *The Wall Street Journal,* 13 December, A1.

5

Access

Donabedian's (1966, 1980, 1982, 1984, 1988a, b, c) approach to quality assessment examines structure, process, and outcome. Access is typically considered part of the structural component of quality measurement. The committee, however, has special concerns about access to managed care, particularly for vulnerable and high-risk populations, and believes that a separate discussion about access is warranted.

Managed care reduces the expense of health care, in part, by restricting the use of some services. Gatekeeping, utilization management, and treatment guidelines are designed to ensure that the levels and amounts of care are appropriate for the severity of the clinical condition and to inhibit the delivery of unnecessary amounts or types of services (IOM, 1989, 1992). Sometimes, however, the procedures used to manage costs are perceived as barriers to access rather than as mechanisms that facilitate efficient care. Plans may restrict the choice of providers to only those practitioners who are willing to accept discounted fees and may implement copayments to discourage the overuse of services. Capitated practitioners and health plans, moreover, may have financial incentives to avoid the use of expensive services and to limit the amount of care provided. Access to care therefore becomes a critical issue in the analysis, evaluation, and management of managed care plans.

Managed behavioral health care produces savings in several ways, including paying lower prices to providers; reducing the use of inpatient care, especially for substance abuse treatment; and reducing the length of outpatient treatment. A study of mental health and substance abuse in the Massachusetts Medicaid program found that utilization of care changed in accordance with an incentive structure that was designed to reduce costly inpatient admissions while allowing more use of less expensive outpatient treatment (Callahan et al., 1994). Typically, however, such incentives are not in place, and there are no protections to ensure that individuals are able to receive the most appropriate care that is available to them. The committee believes that access to care must be monitored carefully to ensure that individuals in need of mental health and substance abuse services receive prompt and appropriate care. Because private insurance and health plans often limit benefits for mental health and substance abuse services and because public systems of care serve individuals with high levels of disability and vulnerability, access to services must be monitored in both systems.

The reasons for monitoring access to care within managed care plans are outlined in this chapter. Current approaches to the measurement of access are also reviewed. Finally, the need for a broader approach to the measurement and evaluation of access is examined.

IMPORTANCE OF ASSESSING ACCESS

Historically, either a lack of coverage for mental health and substance abuse services or limited benefits restricted access to and the utilization of treatment for mental health and substance abuse problems (Frank and McGuire, 1996; McGuire, 1981, 1989; Rogowski, 1992, 1993; Scott et al., 1992). Although some states passed legislation that required that commercial group health care plans include coverage for mental illness and alcoholism, the benefits were limited and many states simply required that coverage be offered (Scott et al., 1992). Services for drug abuse and dependence were rarely specifically included in health plans (Rogowski, 1993), although plans tended to extend coverage for alcoholism treatment to other drugs of abuse.

Even in the public sector, Medicaid coverage for mental health and substance abuse treatment tends to be limited (Horgan et al., 1994; Larson and Horgan, 1994; Solloway, 1992). Copayments have also been used to discourage service utilization. Moreover, a large portion of the population and a disproportionate number of individuals with mental health and substance abuse problems are uninsured and dependent on publicly funded services. Public systems of care limit access through the use of strict eligibility criteria: individuals must be categorically eligible for Medicaid and must usually meet "most-in-need" criteria for serious mental illness to receive care in state mental health systems. Access to mental health and substance abuse benefits was therefore problematic even before the introduction of managed care.

Even more threats to limit access may exist within a managed care environment. Self-insured employers can design benefits packages without regard to state mandates for mental health and substance abuse coverage. Capitated health plans and practitioners may have incentives to deny access to expensive levels of care and even to deny care (Woolhandler and Himmelstein, 1995). Utilization management procedures can be used to restrict access to certain levels and types of care and to pressure practitioners to limit lengths of stay (Schlesinger et al., 1996). These practices and incentives not only reduce expenses but also exert both subtle and overt pressures on individuals with mental health and substance abuse problems to leave or disenroll from the plan. Critics of managed behavioral health care plans often focus on the potential for reduced access and undertreatment (Boyle and Callahan, 1995; NCQA, 1996).

The stigma associated with mental illness and substance abuse also contributes to the potential for undertreatment and insufficient access to care (Mechanic et al., 1995). Individuals with mental health and substance abuse problems may be reluctant to publicly acknowledge their illnesses and seek care. In addition, when they seek care for other medical problems, the relevance of mental health and substance abuse problems may not be evaluated. As discussed in Chapter 2, primary care practitioners in general are not trained to identify the need for mental health and substance abuse treatment and may not be comfortable making interventions and referrals if they suspect a problem. Thus, the characteristics of these illnesses increase the susceptibility of individuals with mental health and substance abuse problems to being underdiagnosed and undertreated.

Men, women, and children who suffer from mental illness and substance abuse tend to be vulnerable in several ways. Individuals who have a serious mental illness or a dependence on alcohol and other drugs are likely to have inadequate economic and social supports, may have difficulty in advocating for their own health care needs, and are at high risk of disease, injury, and death. A lack of access to behavioral health services can aggravate their needs for acute and chronic medical care and may increase the cost of health care. More generally, mental illness and substance abuse problems and the costs associated with treating those problems also place large burdens on families, communities, and the criminal justice system (Mechanic et al., 1995). Inadequate care for mental illness and substance abuse increases the strains that families and employers experience and shifts the burden of intervention from the medical system to the criminal justice system and may affect public safety. Access to treatment for mental health and substance abuse treatment therefore has direct implications for employers, communities, and the public authorities for the Medicaid, mental health, substance abuse, and criminal justice systems.

The issue of parity of coverage for mental health and medical care achieved widespread national attention during the summer and fall of 1996, when Congress debated amendments to the Kassebaum-Kennedy bill on job-to-job coverage. The Senate version of the bill included a provision advocating parity of mental health coverage with medical coverage but the provision was dropped from the final version of the bill passed by Congress and signed by President Bill Clinton. House and Senate negotiators later agreed to a compromise version that requires parity for existing lifetime or annual limits but does not mandate mental health services. The provision does not include substance abuse or chemical dependency, and it exempts small businesses with 2 to 50 employees. The compromise version was passed as part of the annual appropriations bill for the Departments of Housing and Urban Development and Veterans Affairs in October 1996 and additional parity proposals are likely in the future.

In 1993, the Institute of Medicine went on record supporting universal access to insurance and health care (IOM, 1993, p. 7) by saying, "All or virtually all persons—whether employed or not, whether ill or well, whether old or young—must participate in a health benefits plan." The present committee agrees with this goal and recognizes that the absence of a national strategy for universal coverage means that the responsibility lies with the states.

The committee therefore adopted a broad perspective on access to mental health and substance abuse treatment and prevention services. The committee defines *access* as the extent to which those in need of mental health and substance abuse care receive services that are appropriate to the severity of their illness and the complexity of their needs. Too often indicators of access reflect merely the availability of services or the delivery of any service rather than the delivery of services that respond effectively to the needs. In fact, an analysis of the measures used to assess access suggests that they often merely reflect prompt attention rather than the amount and level of care delivered.

MEASURES OF ACCESS

Managed behavioral health care organizations, purchasers, and accreditation organizations are using a variety of measures of access. Box 5.1 compares some of the existing measures.

A survey of performance indicators used in mental health facilities, community mental health centers, behavioral group practices, and managed care organizations examined 11 measures of access and assessed current use, appropriateness of use, perceived validity, and measurement feasibility (IBH, 1995). The assessment found that the organizations were most likely to monitor access using utilization and penetration rates: (1) days and number of visits per 1,000 population, (2) average length of stay, and (3) number of sessions per episode of care. More than 90 percent of the respondents rated measures of patient satisfaction with access, waiting time for emergency visits, and geographical convenience as useful measures. Patient satisfaction, however, was perceived as the least valid measure, and only 55 percent of the respondents monitored geographical convenience; waiting time was rated as useful by 70 percent of the respondents. Finally, managed care organizations rated telephone access highly. The overall impression is that relatively little attention has been given to the development of systems and measures to monitor access.

Analysis of the access standards proposed for the National Committee on Quality Assurance's Health Plan Employer Data and Information Set version 3.0 (HEDIS 3.0), and of those currently used by Digital Equipment Corporation and

BOX 5.1
Sample Access Standards and Measures for
Behavioral Health Care

HEDIS 3.0 (NCQA, 1996)

Waiting time

• Waiting time (in hours) for an appointment for mental health care and chemical dependency care for routine, nonurgent, urgent, and emergency or crisis care; plans report their standard and the percentage within the standard.
• Waiting time (in seconds) for the telephone to be answered within clinical services (separate reports for mental health and substance abuse), claims, and customer service departments; plans report their standard and the percentage within the standard.

Availability of mental health and chemical dependency providers

Plans report:
1. the number and percentage of mental health and chemical dependency providers who serve commercial patients, Medicaid patients, and Medicare patients;
2. the number and percentage of providers who accept new members in each category with no restrictions;
3. the number and percentage of providers who accept new members in each category with some restrictions; and
4. the number and percentage of providers who do not accept new members in each category.

AMBHA (1995)

Penetration rate

• Overall: The percentage of enrollees who have a mental health or chemical dependency claim within a 1 year period.
• By age and diagnostic category: The percentage of enrollees with a claim by age and diagnostic category.
• By treatment setting, age, and diagnostic category: The percentage of enrollees with a claim by treatment setting (place of service), age, and diagnostic category.
• By clinician type: The percentage of enrollees with a claim by type of clinician (psychiatrist, psychologist, master's-level clinician, or chemical dependency or alcohol counselor other than one of the above).

Utilization

Outpatient
1. average number of outpatient visits per patient with a claim by age and diagnostic category; and
2. average number of outpatient visits per 1,000 covered lives by age and diagnostic category.

Inpatient
1. inpatient discharges by age and diagnostic category;
2. average length of stay by age and diagnostic category; and
3. inpatient days per 1,000 covered lives by age and diagnostic category.

Intensive alternatives to inpatient care

Patient encounters per 1,000 covered lives for intensive alternatives to inpatient care by age and diagnostic category.

Cost data for severely and persistently mentally ill (for patients with psychotic or bipolar diagnoses only)

1. inpatient expenses divided by total expenses;
2. outpatient expenses divided by total expenses;
3. intensive alternatives expenses divided by total expenses; and
4. residential expenses divided by total expenses.

Call abandonment rate

The average call abandonment rate.

National Association of County Behavioral Health Directors
(The Evaluation Center@HSRI, 1996)

Cultural competence

• Percentage of staff who have attended training on cultural competency in the last two years.
• Percentage of service recipients who reported not seeking services because of perceptions of incompatibility related to ethnicity, language, culture, and age.
• Degree to which direct service staff characteristics represent enrollee characteristics (number of services recipients belonging to each ethnic category per 100,000 population of that same ethnic group).

Geographic access

Percentage of individuals receiving services who live within a 15-mile radius or a 30-minute travel time.

Waiting time for appointments

Percentage of individuals referred for mental health services who are seen within a specified period of time, given the urgency of the request (emergent = 8 hours, urgent = 48 hours, routine = 7 days).

Perceived access

Percentage of individuals indicating that services were easily obtainable in a self-report interview or survey.

Convenience

• Percentage of individuals indicating that service sites were convenient in a self-report interview or survey.
• Percentage of individuals indicating that the time of day or evening for their appointments was convenient in a self-report interview or survey.

Responsiveness

Program provides 24-hour access to professional help.

the American Managed Behavioral Healthcare Association (AMBHA) confirm that initial impression. Prompt attention is measured and assessed more often than the fit between the service provided and the level of need. HEDIS 3.0, for example, only requires monitoring of appointment waiting time, telephone access time, and the number of mental health and chemical dependency providers available to plan members (NCQA, 1996). Digital Equipment Corporation's (1995) standards reflect HEDIS 3.0 but specify the performance expected. AMBHA's (1995) Performance-Based Measures for Managed Behavioral Healthcare (PERMS 1.0), perhaps because the AMBHA membership specializes in the management of mental health and substance abuse services, disaggregate penetration and utilization rates by age and diagnostic category but do not assess the overall need for services and whether the services are appropriate for the needs. Thus, the current measures of access used in commercial arenas appear to be insufficient for monitoring access in a more comprehensive fashion.

The National Association of County Behavioral Health Directors recommended a broader set of access measures in their review of performance outcome indicators (The Evaluation Center@HSRI, 1996). Their measures reflect the broader mission of public systems of care and include cultural competencies training for staff, consumer reports of language and cultural barriers to using services, cultural similarities between staff and consumers, geographic access to care, and consumer reports that services were accessible and convenient, in addition to measures of waiting time. These measures of access begin to monitor some of the more subtle barriers to care and should be more widely disseminated and adopted. There is still no information, however, on the level of need for care in the enrollee population and the degree to which the need is being met.

NEED AND ACCESS

The committee believes that purchasers and plan managers should be encouraged to expand their monitoring of access. The indicators promoted for use in county behavioral health programs illustrate strategies for monitoring more subtle influences on access. Population measures of need, however, must still be developed and integrated into the access monitoring systems. A managed care program, for example, might be satisfied with a penetration rate of 10 percent for mental health and substance abuse services. If information on need, however, suggested that 20 percent of plan members were in need of services, a 10 percent penetration rate would be less satisfactory.

Population-based measures of health status and needs assessment, in fact, are major components in the development of effective integrated systems of care (Shortell et al., 1994). Close linkages are required with public health and social service systems so that health status can be assessed and monitored. Managed systems of care must improve their ability to assess the needs of their enrollees and collect primary data on the populations that they serve, especially those at greatest risk for health and mental health and substance abuse problems: individuals in poverty, racial and ethnic groups, and others with special needs (Shortell et al., 1994).

The measurement of access is an extremely important area of concern for purchasers and for consumers. No valid and reliable technology exists to measure access, which is assessed in a variety of ways: access to clinicians, to initial and follow-up appointments, to appointments with clinicians of choice, at time of day of choice, and so on. Satisfaction with access is one important source of information, but additional measures need to be conceptualized, developed, tested, and implemented.

NEEDS OF SPECIAL POPULATIONS

Gender Differences

Considering the fit between service need and access also means taking into account variations in need among different groups, particularly differences associated with gender and race or ethnicity. The issue of fitting special services to special needs is particularly relevant to ethnic and gender subgroups. Utilization of services in general and of particular types of services varies by gender and ethnic groups according to treatment and national survey data, but it is not known if this is due to discrimination (e.g., selective screening at admission, including insurance criteria that exclude those without proper health profiles), to a lack of interest and denial of the problem, or to the fact that appropriate services that would attract such groups are not made available to them.

Different population groups have different problem profiles, are differentially represented, and have different treatment needs and issues related to access. For example, women's substance abuse treatment needs often differ from men's (De Leon et al., 1982; Reed, 1987), particularly because of their higher rates of childhood sexual and physical abuse and victimization (Wallen, 1992) and also because women may have fewer economic resources and social supports available (Anglin et al., 1987; Harrison and Belille, 1987; Weisner, 1993; Weisner and Schmidt, 1992). Drug addicts who are pregnant have been identified as a group that could become involved in the prevention of chronic medical conditions in children (Weisner, 1996).

Ethnic and Racial Differences in Substance Abuse

It is also important to consider ethnic and racial differences when examining availability and access to services. Ethnic minorities are overrepresented in the public system and are underrepresented in the private system, and this poses special considerations as the public system increasingly contracts with managed care organizations. Rates of need for services differ by age, socioeconomic status, and gender within ethnic groups (Anglin et al., 1988; Caetano and Herd, 1988). For example, African American men have higher rates of drug problems than do African American women, and the men and women also differ with regard to type of drug used (McNagny and Parker, 1992; NIAAA, 1990; NIDA, 1991).

Studies of Hispanic populations have found similar important differences by gender and type of drug (Caetano and Mora, 1988; De La Rosa et al., 1990; Hser et al., 1987). For example, use of illegal drugs and the utilization of drug treatment facilities varies widely with the type of drug used across and within the subgroups of the Hispanic population (De La Rosa et al., 1990). To underline the vast heterogeneity within ethnic groups, the rates of drug use are also affected by factors such as acculturation for Hispanics (Caetano, 1983, 1987, 1993a; De La Rosa et al., 1990) and by migration patterns and urban versus rural location for African Americans (Herd, 1989, 1990, 1994).

As with health care in general, differences in the availability of mental health and substance abuse treatment, as well as type of program, are affected by the geographic distribution of services, particularly urban versus rural status (IOM, 1990). There is also evidence that availability differs by state, since the balance between private and public sectors in the services that they provide, need levels, general availability, and program type vary greatly by state (IOM, 1990; Weisner et al., 1995a).

In addition to different courses of service in the public- and private-sector systems, large disparities have been found in the type of service provision across the states, especially in the allocation of services; per capita funding (public and federal combined) ranges from $23.54 to $2.36 across the states (IOM, 1990). The extent of private services across the states is not well correlated with the amount of public services. Neither is there any relationship between need in a state (measured by cirrhosis mortality or per capita consumption) and the amount of service provided (IOM, 1990).

There is some variation across states in terms of program philosophy and the type of public substance abuse treatment program that is funded (e.g., the use of 28-day programs by the public sector in Minnesota and the support of social model programs in the public sector of California). It has also been suggested that the merging of alcohol and drug treatment programs may affect access to treatment in that the balance of treatment capacity for primary alcohol abuse treatment compared with that for a drug problem may shift (Weisner, 1992). Similar concerns have been expressed with regard to the merging of alcohol and drug treatment within mental health systems.

Combined drug and alcohol use is increasingly characteristic of substance abusers (Clayton, 1986; Hubbard, 1990). In addition, many chronic substance abusers use more than one drug and also have diagnosable mental health problems. In this regard, the Epidemiologic Catchment Area data found the proportion of individuals who met the criteria for a lifetime prevalence of alcohol dependence to be 24 percent of those meeting the criteria for schizophrenia, 52 percent of those with antisocial personalities, 12 percent for those with any anxiety disorder, 12 percent for those with phobia disorders, 22 percent for those with panic disorders, and 17 percent for those with obsessive-compulsive disorders (Regier et al., 1993). For these individuals, the entry point to the specialized alcohol and drug treatment system is often through the mental health system or emergency rooms and sometimes the criminal justice or welfare systems.

Although young drug and alcohol users are at risk for chronic problems, their problematic use patterns are appropriately addressed through prevention or early intervention treatment services. Although rates of substance abuse are greatly affected by type of substance, gender, and ethnicity (Anglin et al., 1987; Hser et al., 1987; Kandel and Yamaguchi, 1985), roughly 30 to 40 percent of those who begin using alcohol or drugs early continue the use past adolescence and become chronic users (Robins and Przybeck, 1985). Those who do continue are at great risk of developing future problems. They are most likely to enter the specialized treatment system through the criminal justice or educational systems or emergency rooms rather than through the primary health care system. A system monitoring chronicity might track high-risk status for adolescents (ages 12 to 17) with alcohol and drug use problems coming into contact with the systems listed above.

Young and middle-age adults who are at risk for chronic problems often began using drugs or alcohol during adolescence and are currently dependent. Others begin using drugs or alcohol later as adults, but meet the criteria for severe dependence. Both groups are most likely to enter the treatment system through the workplace and employee assistance programs, the criminal justice system for alcohol or drug-related arrests, the mental health system (for comorbid problems), or emergency rooms for alcohol- and drug-related injuries. They can be identified by screening for long use or the severity of their dependence and the frequency of their polydrug use. Medical complications may or may not be present.

Middle-age or elderly individuals who have substance abuse disorders generally have long drinking and/or drug use histories and meet the criteria for severe dependence. The symptoms of individuals in this group also are often characterized by the presence of chronic medical conditions and often by repeated admissions for alcohol or drug abuse treatment. This group may also enter treatment programs through the criminal justice system through a variety of alcohol- or drug-related arrests, including arrests for public intoxication. They may also enter the system through workplace programs, although many may no longer be employed, or through emergency rooms and the primary health care system. Relapse management for chronic abusers is an important part of treatment as well as the rehabilitation and aftercare stages of treatment (Curry et al., 1988; Leukefeld and Tims, 1986, 1990; Marlatt and Gordon, 1985).

A range of services needs to be available for these groups of individuals and treatments may need to be repeated. Longer or more intensive treatment stays may also be required for chronic substance abusers. Ideally, individuals would be assessed, and appropriate levels and modalities of services could be provided. These services are likely to involve the specialized treatment system as well as the primary health care system. Different assessment tools are available, including the Addiction Severity Index (McLellan et al., 1992) and the Patient Placement Criteria developed by the American Society on Addiction Medicine (CSAT, 1994).

MEASURING ACCESS TO SERVICES WITHIN MANAGED CARE ORGANIZATIONS

National data sets and data sources available at the community level can be used to assess the prevalence of substance abuse problems and the services needed within health plans. Information on the chronic medical conditions resulting from alcohol and drug use or abuse is mainly available from hospital discharge surveys and death certificates (NIAAA, 1990). The major strength of these measures is their availability at the county level. The causes of death that the National Institute on Alcohol Abuse and Alcoholism (NIAAA) argues are actual measures of chronicity are cirrhosis (including chronic liver disease and cirrhosis and portal hypertension), alcohol dependence syndrome, and alcohol-related psychoses.

Data are also available on the deaths due to alcohol-related incidents, such as drunk driving. In using such alcohol-related mortality measures, NIAAA notes that factors in addition to mortality rates should be considered (NIAAA, 1991). Such indicators include the size of the population; the existing treatment capacity, including the geographic dispersal of that capacity; the amount of financial support per treatment modality; the level of urbanization; the sociodemographic characteristics of the population, such as ethnicity and age; and the existence of waiting lists for treatment programs. NIAAA claims that the data can be used to project population estimates of need by linking data on current resources with these types of data listed above in multivariate models (NIAAA, 1991). The major usefulness of adapting large data systems to measure chronicity is their potential usefulness in providing ratios of the number of cases to the overall prevalence, adapted for differences in population characteristics.

It is important to note the differences between the results drawn from data collected from the general population and those collected from populations in treatment systems (Corty and Ball, 1986; Rounsaville and Kleber, 1985; Weisner et al., 1995b). Although both data sources are crucial to estimating need and to developing systems for monitoring the care of chronic substance abusers, they cannot answer the same questions. Systems that track the prevalence of substance abuse in the general population provide both prevalence estimates and the need for services in the population as a whole. Data from treatment agencies provide information on trends in the group receiving the services and the needs of the individuals in that group.

The preferred data for measuring prevalence and monitoring the effectiveness of managed care organizations in responding to substance abuse problems involves epidemiologic surveys. However, these are expensive, and it is not feasible for many managed care organizations to conduct such surveys. However, with managed care organization membership data on age, sex, and basic socioeconomic status, it is possible to make reasonable estimates of need for services within the membership from several surveys conducted every few years. The rates of alcohol and drug abuse problems by age, sex, and socioeconomic status are quite consistent, particularly when they are adjusted by region of the country.

SUMMARY

Managed behavioral health care organizations define access and accessibility using utilization (e.g., penetration rates and the use of specific services) and telecommunication (e.g., on-hold time and call abandonment rates) measures (AMBHA, 1995; Digital Equipment Corporation, 1995; NCQA, 1996). Purchasers, however, may prefer to view access more broadly and include reductions in barriers to care and improvements in benefits (e.g., reductions in copayments, increases in hours of service, reductions in travel time, and expanded eligibility for specific services or populations) (IOM, 1990).

The nature of managed care and the nature of mental health and substance abuse problems combine to make access a critical issue. Well-developed public and private health care and behavioral health care plans will promote access to mental health and substance abuse services. Enrollees who access the available care promptly and early in their illness episodes may require less intensive care, and with appropriate continuing support, they may be less likely to experience relapses.

Access enables quality, which is a treatment plan focused on recovery. Quality informs innovation, reducing to the irreducible minimum the time between the discovery of a treatment or service that works and the implementation of that service in the field.

Donald Galamaga
State of Rhode Island
Public Workshop, April 18, 1996, Washington, DC

Measures of access, however, must go beyond telephone answering time and must begin to reflect the real and perceived barriers to care, including cultural differences, geographic distance, inconvenient locations and times, and care that is less intensive than needed. Moreover, the purchasers of health care plans and plan administrators must begin to assess the adequacy of current access to their plans. Information on the ambient level of need in a health plan is required to truly assess the adequacy of the plan in meeting the demand and need for care.

REFERENCES

AMBHA (American Managed Behavioral Healthcare Association).1995. *Performance Measures for Managed Behavioral Healthcare Programs.* Washington, DC: American Managed Behavioral Healthcare Association.

Anglin MD, Hser YI, Booth MW. 1987. Sex differences in addict careers. 4. Treatment. *The American Journal of Drug and Alcohol Abuse* 13(3):253-280.

Anglin MD, Booth MW, Ryan TM, Hser YI. 1988. Ethnic differences in narcotics addiction. II. Chicago and Anglo addiction career patterns. *The International Journal of Addictions* 23(10):1011-1027.

Boyle PJ, Callahan D. 1995. Managed care and mental health: The ethical issues. *Health Affairs* 14(3):7-22.

Caetano R. 1983. Drinking patterns and alcohol problems among Hispanics in the U.S.: A review. *Drug and Alcohol Dependence* 12(1):37-59.

Caetano R. 1987. Acculturation, drinking and social settings among U.S. Hispanics. *Drug and Alcohol Dependence* 19(3):215-226.

Caetano R. 1993a. Priorities for alcohol treatment research among U.S. Hispanics. *Journal of Psychoactive Drugs* 25(1):53-60.

Caetano R. 1993b. The association between severity of DSM-III-R alcohol dependence and medical and social consequences. *Addiction* 88:631-642.

Caetano R, Herd D. 1988. Drinking in different social contexts among white, black, and Hispanic men. *The Yale Journal of Biology and Medicine* 61(3):243-258.

Caetano R, Mora ME. 1988. Acculturation and drinking among people of Mexican descent in Mexico and the United States. *Journal of Studies on Alcohol* 49(5):462-471.

Callahan JJ, Shepard DS, Beinecke RH, Larson M, Cavanaugh D. 1994. *Evaluation of the Massachusetts Medicaid Mental Health/Substance Abuse Program.* Submitted to the Massachusetts Division of Medical Assistance, Mental Health Substance Abuse Program. Waltham, MA: Institute for Health Policy, Brandeis University.

Clayton RR. 1986. Multiple drug use: Epidemiology, correlates, and consequences. *Recent Developments in Alcoholism* 4:7-38.

Corty E, Ball JC. 1986. What can we know about addiction from the addicts we treat? *The International Journal of Addictions* 21(9-10):1139-1144.

Curry SJ, Marlatt GA, Gordon J, Baer JS. 1988. A comparison of alternative theoretical approaches to smoking cessation and relapse. *Health Psychology* 7(6):545-556.

CSAT (Center for Substance Abuse Treatment). 1994. *Treatment Improvement Protocol: The Role and Current Status of Patient Placement Criteria in the Treatment of Substance Abuse Disorders.* Rockville, MD: Center for Substance Abuse Treatment.

De La Rosa MR, Khalsa JH, Rouse BA. 1990. Hispanics and illicit drug use: A review of recent findings. *The International Journal of Addictions* 25(6):665-691.

De Leon G, Wexler HK, Jainchill N. 1982. The therapeutic community: Success and improvement rates 5 years after treatment. *The International Journal of the Addictions* 17(4):703-747.

Digital Equipment Corporation. 1995. *HMO Performance Standards: 1995.* Maynard, MA: Digital Equipment Corporation.

Donabedian A. 1966. Evaluating the quality of medical care. *The Milbank Quarterly* 44:166-203.

Donabedian A. 1980. *Explorations in Quality Assessment and Monitoring: The Definition of Quality and Approaches to its Assessment.* Vol. 1. Ann Arbor, MI: Health Administration Press.

Donabedian A. 1982. *Explorations in Quality Assessment and Monitoring: The Criteria and Standards of Quality.* Vol. 2. Ann Arbor, MI: Health Administration Press.

Donabedian A. 1984. *Explorations in Quality Assessment and Monitoring: The Methods and Findings of Quality Assessment and Monitoring, An Illustrated Analysis.* Vol. 3. Ann Arbor, MI: Health Administration Press.

Donabedian A. 1988a. Quality assessment and assurance: Unit of purpose, diversity of means. *Inquiry* 25:173-192.

Donabedian A. 1988b. The quality of care: How can it be assessed? *Journal of the American Medical Association* 260:1743-1748.

Donabedian A. 1988c. Monitoring: The eyes and ears of healthcare. *Health Progress* 69:38-43.

Frank RG, McGuire TG. 1996. Introduction to the economics of mental health payment systems. In: Levin BL, Petrila J, eds. *Mental Health Services: A Public Health Perspective.* New York: Oxford University Press.

Harrison PA, Belille CA. 1987. Women in treatment: Beyond the stereotype. *Journal of Studies on Alcohol* 48(6):574-578.

Herd D. 1989. The epidemiology of drinking patterns and alcohol-related problems among U.S. blacks. *NIAAA Research Monograph No. 18.* Rockville, MD: National Institute on Alcohol Abuse and Alcoholism.

Herd D. 1990. Subgroup differences in drinking patterns among black and white men: Results from a national survey. *Journal of Studies on Alcohol* 51(3):221-232.

Herd D. 1994. Predicting drinking problems among black and white men: Results from a national survey. *Journal of Studies on Alcohol* 55(1):61-71.

Horgan C, Larson MJ, Simon L. 1994. Medicaid funding for drug abuse treatment: A national perspective. In: Denmead G, Rouse BA, eds. *Services Research Monograph No. 1: Financing Drug Treatment Through State Programs.* NIH Publication No. 94-3543. Rockville, MD: National Institute on Drug Abuse.

Hser YI, Anglin MD, McGlothlin W. 1987. Sex differences in addict careers. 1. Initiation of use. *The American Journal of Drug and Alcohol Abuse* 13(1-2):33-57.

Hubbard RL. 1990. Treating combined alcohol and drug abuse in community-based programs. *Recent Developments in Alcoholism* 8:273-283.

IBH (Institute for Behavioral Healthcare). 1995. *Performance Indicators in Behavioral Healthcare: Measures of Access, Appropriateness, Quality, Outcomes, and Prevention.* Tiburon, CA: Institute for Behavioral Healthcare.

IOM (Institute of Medicine).1989. *Controlling Costs and Changing Patient Care? The Role for Utilization Management.* Washington, DC: National Academy Press.

IOM. 1990. *Treating Drug Problems.* Vol 1. Washington, DC: National Academy Press.

IOM. 1992. *Guidelines for Clinical Practice: From Development to Use.* Washington, DC: National Academy Press.

IOM. 1993. *Employment and Health Benefits: A Connection at Risk.* Washington, DC: National Academy Press.

Kandel DB, Yamaguchi K. 1985. Developmental patterns of the use of legal, illegal, and medically prescribed psychotropic drugs from adolescence to young adulthood. *NIDA Research Monograph No. 56.* Rockville, MD: National Institute on Drug Abuse. Pp. 193-235.

Larson MJ, Horgan C. 1994. Variations in state Medicaid program expenditures for substance abuse units and facilities. In: Denmead G, Rouse BA, eds. *Services Research Monograph No. 1: Financing Drug Treatment Through State Programs.* NIH Publication No. 94-3543. Rockville, MD: National Institute on Drug Abuse.

Leudefeld CG, Tims FM. 1986. Relapse and recovery: Some directions for research and practice. *NIDA Research Monograph No. 72.* Rockville, MD: National Institute on Drug Abuse. Pp. 185-190.

Leukefeld CG, Tims FM. 1990. Compulsory treatment for drug abuse. *The International Journal of Addictions* 25(6):621-640.

Marlatt GA, Gordon JR, eds. 1985. *Relapse Prevention: Maintenance Strategies in the Treatment of Addictive Behaviors.* New York, NY: The Guilford Press.

McGuire TG. 1981. *Financing Psychotherapy: Costs, Effects, and Public Policy*. Cambridge, MA: Ballinger Publishing.

McGuire TG. 1989. Financing and demand for mental health services. In: Taube C, Mechanic D, Hohmann A, eds. *The Future of Mental Health Services Research*. DHHS Publication No. (ADM) 89-1600. Rockville, MD: National Institute on Mental Health.

McLellan AT, Cacciola J, Kushner H, Peters R, Smith I, Pettinati H. 1992. The fifth edition of the Addiction Severity Index: Cautions, additions, and normative data. *Journal of Substance Abuse Treatment* 9(5):461-480.

McNagny SE, Parker RM. 1992. High prevalence of recent cocaine use and the unreliability of patient self-report in an inner-city walk-in clinic. *Journal of the American Medical Association* 267(8):1106-1108.

Mechanic D, Schlesinger M, McAlpine DD. 1995. Management of mental health and substance abuse services: State of the art and early results. *The Milbank Quarterly* 73:19-55.

NCQA (National Committee for Quality Assurance). 1996. *HEDIS 3.0: Health Plan Employer Data and Information Set*. Washington, DC: National Committee for Quality Assurance.

NIAAA (National Institute of Alcohol Abuse and Alcoholism). 1990. *Alcohol and Health: Seventh Special Report to the U.S. Congress*. DHHS Publication No. (ADM) 90-1656. Washington, DC: U.S. Department of Health and Human Services.

NIAAA. 1991. *U.S. Alcohol Epidemiologic Data Reference Manual: County Alcohol Problem Indicators, 1979-1985, 3rd Edition*. Vol. III. DHHS Publication No. (ADM) 91-1740. Washington, DC: U.S. Department of Health and Human Services.

NIDA (National Institute on Drug Abuse). 1991. *Drug Abuse and Drug Abuse Research: The Third Report to Congress from the Secretary, Department of Health and Human Services*. DHHS Publication No. (ADM) 91-1704. Washington, DC: U.S. Department of Health and Human Services.

Reed BG. 1987. Developing women-sensitive drug dependence treatment services: Why so difficult? *Journal of Psychoactive Drugs* 19(2):151-164.

Regier DA, Narrow WE, Rae DS, Manderscheid RW, Locke BZ, Goodwin FK. 1993. The de facto U.S. mental and addictive disorders service system: Epidemiologic catchment area prospective 1-year prevalence rates of disorders and services. *Archives of General Psychiatry* 50:85-94.

Robins LN, Przybeck TR. 1985. Age of onset of drug use as a factor in drug and other disorders. *NIDA Research Monograph No. 56*. Rockville, MD: National Institute on Drug Abuse. Pp. 178-192.

Rogowski JA. 1992. Private versus public sector insurance coverage for drug abuse. *Health Affairs* 11(3):137-148.

Rogowski JA. 1993. *Private Versus Public Sector Insurance Coverage for Drug Abuse*. Santa Monica, CA: RAND Drug Policy Research Center.

Room R, Greenfield T. 1993. Alcoholics anonymous, other 12-step movements and psychotherapy in the U.S. population, 1990. *Addiction* 88(4):555-562.

Rounsaville BJ, Kleber HD. 1985. Untreated opiate addicts: How do they differ from those seeking treatment? *Archives of General Psychiatry* 42:1072-1077.

Schlesinger M, Dorwart RA, Epstein SS. 1996. Managed care constraints on psychiatrists' hospital practices: Bargaining power and professional autonomy. *American Journal of Psychiatry* 153:256-260.

Scott JE, Greenberg D, Pizarro J. 1992. A survey of state insurance mandates covering alcohol and other drug treatment. *Journal of Mental Health Administration* 19:96-118.

Shortell SM, Gillies RR, Anderson DA. 1994. New world of managed care: Creating organized delivery systems. *Health Affairs* 13(4):46-64.

Solloway MR. 1992. *A Fifty-State Survey of Medicaid Coverage of Substance Abuse Services*. Washington, DC: Intergovernmental Health Policy Project, The George Washington University.

The Evaluation Center@HSRI. 1996. *Candidate Indicators for County Performance Outcomes Project.* Rockville, MD: Center for Mental Health Services.

Wallen J. 1992. A comparison of male and female clients in substance abuse treatment. *Journal of Substance Abuse Treatment* 9(3):243-248.

Weisner C. 1992. A comparison of alcohol and drug treatment clients: Are they from the same population? *The American Journal of Drug and Alcohol Abuse* 18(4):429-444.

Weisner C. 1993. The epidemiology of combined alcohol and drug use within treatment agencies: A comparison by gender. *Journal of Studies on Alcohol* 54:268-274.

Weisner C. 1996. Social indicators of chronic alcohol and drug abuse. In: *Chronic Care Social Indicator Project Monograph.* Princeton, NJ: Robert Wood Johnson Foundation.

Weisner C, Schmidt L. 1992. Gender disparities in treatment for alcohol problems. *Journal of the American Medical Association* 268(14):1872-1876.

Weisner C, Greenfield T, Room R. 1995a. Trends in the treatment of alcohol problems in the U.S. general population, 1979 through 1990. *American Journal of Public Health* 85(1):55-60.

Weisner C, Schmidt L, Tam T. 1995b. Assessing bias in community-based prevalence estimates: Towards an unduplicated count of problem drinkers and drug users. *Addiction* 90(3):391-405.

Woolhandler S, Himmelstein DU. 1995. Extreme risk: The new corporate proposition for physicians. *The New England Journal of Medicine* 333:1706-1708.

6

Process

In general terms, measurement of the quality of health care is driven by different forces in the private and public sectors. In the private sector, quality measurement is a reflection of the requirements of the accreditation process and, increasingly, is also a response to the demands of employers and other purchasers through contracting, report cards, and other means. In the public sector, performance measurement is the primary tool of accountability for spending public funds on health care (DHHS, 1995; IOM, 1989a).

This chapter begins with a general discussion of quality and accountability in the private sector, an overview of methods of quality improvement, and a comparison of current quality improvement methods in managed behavioral health care. Next is a discussion of performance measurement, model standards, and related developments in the public sector. The chapter then provides an overview of the accreditation process, including the development of standards and descriptions of five organizations currently in the accreditation industry. The chapter concludes with a discussion of the role of government in quality assurance.

QUALITY AND ACCOUNTABILITY

Background

Health care purchasers are caught in a dilemma created over the past 50 years and for which there is no easy resolution. Following World War II, the U.S. economy was strong and its industry dominated the world marketplace. Jobs were plentiful, and employers competed for skilled workers. The American ethic of a benevolent employer was firmly reinforced by years of unions' struggles with management and by a healthy economy under which employers could afford to offer generous health benefits.

For years, the health insurance contract offered ever-increasing benefits, freedom of choice, and first-dollar coverage (few copayments or deductibles). Employers trusted their employees and providers. Although consumers and providers struggled for many years to develop more adequate mental health and substance abuse benefits, most people were happy with the health care system. Furthermore, the U.S. Congress initiated the Community Mental Health Centers Act, Medicare, Medicaid, Hill-Burton, and other programs (see Chapter 3), which contributed greatly to the growth of the health care industry. With these investments, the public and private sectors created health care access and resources that were unparalleled in world history.

Fueled by scientific prowess and expanding financial commitments, the health care system appeared to have no limits in its potential capacities to provide health care. However, unlimited growth could not continue. With the rising costs of health care services threatening the financial stability of their budgets, private and public payers increasingly turned to methods that make health care accountable and affordable and that prevent cutbacks in previously reimbursed health benefits. The widespread initiation of utilization management, health maintenance organizations (HMOs), and other managed care methods during the past quarter century has emphasized cost accountability (IOM, 1989a).

These programs have cumulatively evolved into an industry and have become a strong force in the health care system. Consumers and providers who believe that autonomous health resource decisions on the basis of tradition and the health care contract are consequently in conflict with such policies. The tensions over cost controls have increasingly focused concerns about cost-containment efforts on quality issues such as the following:

- qualifications of and consumers' geographic access to a comprehensive range of providers;
- prevention of avoidable illness and provision of timely and focused treatment interventions;
- availability of services, on the basis of urgency of need;
- courtesy, convenience, and comfort of services;
- compassion and kindness of care;
- competence of providers to institute most appropriate evaluations and treatments, which would result in services that would result in the least risk to the patient and with the best health status outcome; and
- administrative efficiencies of health care services that promote quality through effective communications, consumer and provider education, decision support, and quality management, treatment coordination, and other systems.

The interest in quality is reinforced by consumer demand and empowerment, professional ethics, legal and regulatory interpretation of citizens' rights, and attempts by businesses to satisfy and keep customers in a competitive health care marketplace. For public purchasers who are accountable for public funds, it is important to demonstrate that health care has good value and is worth the investment. The next section will give an overview of different methods for assessing quality.

Methods for Quality Assessment

Accreditation

One of the more traditional methods of quality assessment, accreditation of hospitals and managed care organizations, has evolved over the past 60 years to include highly specialized and involved accreditation of facilities, programs, and systems by numerous national accrediting entities, both voluntary and governmental. In addition, many managed behavioral health care organizations have developed "certification" methods based on various quality parameters and sources to establish the qualifications of various institutional and professional providers that are contracted into their networks. Managed care accreditation has become increasingly popular for public- and private-sector health programs because it is viewed as the best current system for creating accountability and quality, even though there is limited evidence to support the relationship between adherence to quality standards and improvements in patients' health status. Accreditation will be discussed more fully in a later section of this chapter.

Professional Review of Care

Review of care by peers or other qualified health professionals has been practiced extensively, especially in professional case conferences and for granting credentials and privileges. Peer review has become more institutionalized, detailed, and systematically applied in recent years with the evolution of the utilization management and quality assurance movements. Concerns by payers, courts, and facilities about the medical appropriateness of care have led to broader applications of professional review to prospectively, concurrently, and retrospectively validate clinical decisions made by clinicians for individual patient care and care for populations of patients.

Licensing

States have licensed physicians and nurses for many of the past 75 years through examinations and the recognition of professional training in accredited programs. Licensing has expanded substantially to other health care practitioners and has become more prescriptive regarding the scope of practice limits in many jurisdictions. In addition, it has been tied in recent years to continuing education requirements, proof of competence, and both sanctions and supervision in instances in which impairment is established. Licensing of facilities has likewise become a major state function, involving monitoring of numerous and varying requirements established by state legislatures and regulatory agencies.

Credentialing and Privileging

Health care programs provide risk and quality management through a number of approaches. They and accreditation organizations have established standards of practitioner competence based on such factors as training in accredited health professional programs, possession of a current state license, professional certification, demonstration of specific technical skills under expert supervision, evidence of liability coverage and acceptable prior malpractice experience, and attestation to the existence of no current health conditions that would expose patients to risks. Programs now commonly have dedicated resources to establish primary source verification of practitioners' qualifications, to conduct initial and ongoing peer review of practitioners' skills, and to restrict a clinician's practice and to report defined infractions to various state agencies and national data banks.

The complexities and multiple requirements imposed on providers to account to many agencies and managed care organizations and managed behavioral health care organizations has caused credentialing-privileging to become a costly and time-consuming enterprise for both organizations and individual practitioners. The evolution of integrated credentialing systems could substantially reduce these burdens and maintain protection for the public.

Physicians who have contracts with multiple organizations tell us that they can have as many as 20 or 30 reviews in a year, each of which looks at similar but just a little bit different criteria.

Linda Bresolin
American Medical Association
Public Workshop, April 18, 1996, Washington, DC

Auditing

A number of quality-focused activities have evolved from purchasers' needs to account for costs and regulators' needs to account for risks. The Health Care

Financing Administration (HCFA) regularly conducts audits of the Medicare and Medicaid programs using both staff financial auditors and professional reviewers, including evaluations from state peer review organizations. Explicit survey standards and procedures are followed in these evaluations of agencies' and providers' statutory responsibility to provide services that are of acceptable cost, quality, and risk. Other agencies are substantially involved in developing standards affecting quality of care (e.g., the Substance Abuse and Mental Health Services Administration [SAMHSA] and the Agency for Health Care Policy and Research [AHCPR]) and in inspecting health care providers for compliance with quality-related requirements (e.g., the Occupational Safety and Health Administration).

In the private sector, a number of health benefits consulting firms have hired clinicians, including mental health professionals, to develop clinical services standards, auditing instruments and methods, and quality improvement programs for their customers, which include purchasers and provider organizations. Of any single institution, these consulting firms have collectively had one of the most profound and least publicized impacts on managed care. Their influence over the managed care purchasing decisions of health plans, through the promotion of their performance requirements, selection of managed care organization and managed behavioral health care organization vendors, and auditing of managed care operations, has been a major contributor to the development of monitoring standards and systems embraced by other organizations (e.g., American Managed Behavioral Healthcare Association [AMBHA] and the National Committee for Quality Assurance [NCQA]).

Courts

The legal system, guided by tort principles and case law, provides an uneven but sometimes effective means of regulation in situations in which a lack of attention to quality of care can result in risk or harm to patients. Legal mechanisms serve as an arbitrator and financial compensator in situations in which grievances or harm are established to be the result of neglect or malpractice by the health care provider. The substantial growth of risk management programs in health care plans, initially propelled by the need for liability control, has also been accentuated by their incorporation into quality improvement activities.

Clinical Practice Standards and Guidelines

The opportunities for high-quality clinical care are enhanced when providers follow steps in evaluation and treatment that have evolved over years through scientific research and clinical experience. Clinical texts by authoritative specialists and published articles in reputable peer-reviewed journals represent a traditional source of clinical standards. In recent years, expert consensus panels have proliferated to guide clinicians toward optimal decisions through their promulgation of specialized standards for a variety of conditions and medical technologies.

A variety of published and unpublished standards, criteria, guidelines, indicators, and protocols have flooded the landscape of health care, resulting in sometimes differing views about medical appropriateness by various expert panels. Nevertheless, empirically and experientially based clinical standards constitute an essential method by which clinical decisions can be independently evaluated through professional review and indicator-based measurements.

Consumer Satisfaction

Concern about the satisfaction of patients and patients' families with health services by providers or regulators was uncommon until recent years. The growing power of consumers in a competitive market economy has migrated from other areas of business to health care, underscoring the essential importance of routinely assessing what consumers think and feel about their health benefits and services. Health services research has shown that patient satisfaction is one of the most relevant markers for quality, even if it is not always a sensitive indicator. Significant resources are being allocated to refine specific methods of assessing quality through consumer evaluation and to systematically seek customers' opinions in designing clinical services and improving the quality of clinical services.

National and local newspapers and magazines provide consumers with information by comparing different health plans, including the results of consumer satisfaction surveys and other data available from report cards. The media also cover stories about provider "gag rules," denials of services, problems with care, HMO profits, and other information that have unmeasured effects on disenrollment or other indications of dissatisfaction.

QUALITY MANAGEMENT IN BEHAVIORAL HEALTH CARE

Quality management activities in behavioral health care services have evolved over the past 30 years. They originated with the academic and professional bases of medical quality assurance (Mattson, 1992; Rodriguez, 1988), and have blended with traditional local practice (e.g., clinical privileging), state regulatory (e.g., licensing), and tort interventions to provide implicit and explicit oversight of health care quality.

One of the major initiatives in the accountability of behavioral health care quality was instituted by the U.S. Department of Defense in 1975 to provide explicit oversight over psychiatric residential treatment for child and adolescent services under the Civilian Health and Medical Program of the Uniformed Services (CHAMPUS). As noted in Chapter 4, this national initiative was the first by a national payer to establish specialized program standards and admission-treatment criteria for mental health services. Its evolution into a national peer review program (Rodriguez, 1985) for inpatient psychiatric and outpatient psychiatric and psychological services became the foundation for private health plans' rapid embrace in the early 1980s of commercial utilization and quality management programs.

In the latter part of the 1980s, indemnity health plan administrators realized that utilization management approaches such as retrospective and concurrent review had limited impacts on both costs and quality. Utilization management and employee assistance program vendors were encouraged to develop contracted networks of mental health providers to allow for mixed reimbursements and capitation of services and to better promote network-based quality management. In less than 10 years this phenomenon grew to the point that now more than 120 million people with insured or entitled behavioral health care benefits receive care in one of these managed care arrangements (HIAA, 1996).

Employers as Purchasers of Behavioral Health Care

Managed behavioral health care organizations have encouraged the documentation of efforts to account for quality of care and services. Xerox, IBM, GTE, and Digital Equipment Corporation have led the way in establishing quality specifications for their managed behavioral health care organization vendors. Through the imposition of contract guarantees, corporate purchasers reward quality and penalize poor service.

Employers are increasingly concerned about the quality of care that's being provided to their employees, and they want to gather more data on it. It's not self-reported through the health plans, so they need to look to groups that have the market power as well as the relationships with the health plans to gather that data collaboratively and in an audited format.

Catherine Brown
Pacific Business Group on Health
Public Workshop, May 17, 1996, Irvine, CA

Contract-based performance standards have become the base for industry and voluntary accreditation organization standards, notably those developed by AMBHA (1995) and NCQA (1996a, b). Some payers have developed their own explicit requirements for HMOs that provide care under their health benefits plan for such areas as member services and satisfaction, administrative services, organizational structure and philosophy, provider credentialing and performance monitoring, clinical services management, clinical delivery support systems, and confidentiality. Digital Equipment Corporation, for example, has specific requirements for the behavioral health services that it purchases:

- benefit design,
- access,
- triage,
- treatment approach,
- case management,
- alternative treatment settings,
- outcomes measurement,
- quality management, and
- prevention and early intervention.

Table 6.1 compares some of the more widely used behavioral health care standards.

Trends in Quality Standards in the Private Sector

Because so many purchasers' efforts to become involved in prescribing methods and outcomes goals for quality accountability are in the early stages and because the state of population-based measurement systems is not refined, quality management in behavioral health and other clinical services is in the early stages but is evolving rapidly. As with most evolutions, an experimental phase precedes consensus about what constitutes the best approach.

In addition to the standards listed in Table 6.1, numerous employer coalitions, both local and national, are now embarked on efforts to establish performance requirements for managed care. Examples include the Managed Health Care Association, the Employer Consortium, the National HMO Purchasing Coalition, the Minnesota Buyers Healthcare Action Group, and the Pacific Business Group on Health. Many of these coalitions have significant participation by health services consumers and their representatives, such as unions, advocates, organizations, and insurance commission agencies.

The Foundation for Accountability (FACCT), representing a broad coalition of public and private purchasers and others, has begun to develop and test tools that will allow documentation of population-specific functioning, quality of life, satisfaction with services, and risk reduction for a number of medical conditions commonly seen in health plans, such as diabetes, asthma, breast cancer, coronary artery disease, and low back pain (FACCT, 1995). Mood and anxiety disorders represent other conditions whose prevalence and direct and indirect

TABLE 6.1 Cross-Comparison of Managed Behavioral Health Care Performance Indicators

Indicator	AMBHA: PERMS	Digital Equipment Corporation	NCQA: HEDIS (Medicaid and 3.0 Draft)	SAMHSA: MHSIP
Population	Populations served by carve-out behavioral health care organizations; mostly employed individuals, and their dependents	Employed population and their dependents in an HMO	Employed population and their dependents; publicly supported populations including children	Employed populations and their dependents; publicly enrolled populations including children and the disabled
Access to care: Time frames	Patient satisfaction with access experience: First appointment • Intake process • Call abandonment rate • On-hold time • Call answer time	Establish the following time frames for access: • Nonurgent, 10 days • Urgent office visit within 48 hours • Emergency, within 48 hours • Telephone response: 90 percent in 20 seconds and not more than 5 percent abandoned call rate	1. Waiting time to appointment 2. Specific minimum time frames for access to emergency care within 4 hours, urgent care within 24 hours, and nonurgent care within 5 days 3. Waiting time for telephone to be answered	1. Average length of time from request to first face-to-face meeting with mental health professional 2. Convenient location of services 3. Convenient appointment times 4. Easy-to-reach providers
Access to Care: Range of services	Penetration approach 1. Percentage receiving services by age and diagnostic category 2. Percentage receiving services by treatment setting, age, and diagnostic category 3. Percentage receiving services by clinician type 4. Overall rate of receiving services	1. Ratio of health professionals not less than 45:1,000 2. Number of providers in each specialty service: eating disorders, children, adolescents, elderly, dually diagnosed, culturally appropriate, psychotropic medication management 3. Geographic disbursement of alternative services (halfway houses, respite care, etc.)	1. Percentage of mental health providers who have Medicaid beneficiaries in their panel and those whose panels are open to new Medicaid beneficiaries 2. Report units of transportation services Availability of mental health/chemical dependency providers:	Full range of services, with benchmarks for: 1. Average resources spent on mental health 2. Proportion of services that are consumer-run 3. Proportion of services provided in natural settings (home, school, and work) 4. Proportion for whom services are readily available

Access to care: Demographically (ethnic, language, and culture) appropriate services	Not stated	1. Who accept new members with no restrictions (open panels) 2. Who accept new members with some restrictions 3. Who accept no new members (closed panel)	1. Defines plan beneficiaries' demographic characteristics by contact subtypes (i.e., SSI, AFDC, regular, etc.) 2. Defines and reports the number of culturally-competent providers	1. Percentage who report that staff are sensitive to ethnicity, language, culture, and age 2. Percentage who had only one contact in a year 3. Percentage of SSI and SSDI recipients who received services
Access to care: Barriers to service	Covered by other categories	1. EAP direct referral to providers 2. Direct referral in a closed HMO system by triage, primary care, EAP, and self	Report units of transportation services	Percentage for whom cost is an obstacle to service utilization
Measurement of appropriateness of treatment	1. Availability of medication management: number of cases of schizophrenia in last year with (1) ≤3 medication review visits and (2) ≥4 medication review visits 2. Frequency of family visits for children age 12 and under 3. Appropriate utilization of resources for adjustment	1. Triage performed by appropriately credentialed staff 2. Criteria for treatment are based on clinical research and acceptable industry standards 3. Established criteria for determining the need for case management	1. Mental health discharge rate per 1000 enrollees and average length of stay 2. Percentage receiving any inpatient day/night or ambulatory mental health services by age and gender 3. Number of enrollees hospitalized for major affective disorder and percent readmitted within 90 and 365 days	1. Percentage who actively participate in treatment decisions 2. Percentage who feel coerced into treatment options or services 3. Proportion of inpatient admissions that are involuntary 4. Proportion of services that promote recovery

continues on next page

TABLE 6.1 Continued

Indicator	AMBHA: PERMS	Digital Equipment Corporation	NCQA: HEDIS (Medicaid and 3.0 Draft)	SAMHSA: MHSIP
	disorder cases in categories of ≤10 and ≥10 individual sessions		4. Ambulatory follow-up within 30 days post-hospitalization for major affective disorder	5. Proportion of people who receive ambulatory services within 7 days of discharge from inpatient treatment 6. Proportion of people who receive ambulatory services within 3 days of discharge from emergency care 7. Percentage who change their primary mental health professional
Treatment outcome measures	Effectiveness measures 1. Chemical dependency treatment retention measured by number and distribution of detoxification patients who had no additional detoxifications for 90 days and those with one or more detoxifications within 90 days 2. Continuity of care: distribution of post-discharge mental health/chemical dependency cases with no follow-up, follow-up contact, contact plus read-mission, or readmission only	1. Measure functional capacity 2. Measure treatment outcome 3. Analyze aggregated data for quality 4. Conformance with HEDIS	Effectiveness and utilization measures: 1. Availability of mental health/chemical dependency providers 2. Descriptions of pediatric mental health network (Medicaid only) 3. Utilization of inpatient and ambulatory care Measures in testing: 1. Substance abuse counseling for teens 2. Continuity of care for substance abuse 3. Medication management for schizophrenia	1. Percentage who are connected to primary care 2. Differential evidence of mortality due to medical causes 3. Average level of involuntary movements from psychotropic medications 4. Decreased level of psychological distress 5. Increased sense of personal dignity 6. Reduced level of impairment 7. Increase in productive activity and competitive employment

Efficiency measures:

3. Follow-up status from any inpatient discharge from psychiatric setting or substance abuse detoxification

4. Use of psychotherapeutic agents
5. Continuation of treatment for depression
6. Treatment failure substance abuse
7. Patient-reported behavioral health measure
8. Family visits for children in treatment

8. Average change in days of work lost
9. Increase in level of school performance
10. Extent to which alcohol, drugs, or mental problems interfere with productive activity
11. Percentage of children with severe emotional disturbances placed outside the home
12. Percentage of adults with severe mental illness living in residences they own or lease
13. Percentage whose housing situations improve after treatment
14. Percentage with increased level of functioning
15. Percentage in jail in the past year
16. Percentage involved in self-help activities
17. Percentage of inpatient readmissions within 30 days of discharge
18. Percentage who report positive changes after treatment
19. Percentage who have increased activities with family, friends, neighbors, and social groups

continues on next page

TABLE 6.1 Continued

Indicator	AMBHA: PERMS	Digital Equipment Corporation	NCQA: HEDIS (Medicaid and 3.0 Draft)	SAMHSA: MHSIP
Consumer rights/ involvement/ satisfaction	Satisfaction survey examining behavioral health experience in access, intake, clinical care, outcome, and global satisfaction	1. Has guidelines for patients' rights, appeals, grievances, and time frames for all steps 2. Clear printing of grievance procedure 3. Annual reporting of the number, type, and percent of grievances and summary status/outcome report of resolutions	1. Annual member health care survey examining acceptability of care 2. Measures of informed health care choices: (a) new member orientation, including grievance procedures (b) materials available in different languages	1. Percentage who serve on planning and development groups or hold paid staff positions in the health plan 2. Percentage who get adequate information to make informed choices
Quality of care	1. Ambulatory follow-up post-discharge for major depressive disorder 2. Chemical dependency treatment failure	1. Behavioral health departments have active involvement in HMO quality activities 2. Written description of quality structure annually 3. Report annually on progress toward reaching goals 4. Appropriate process for credentialing and recredentialing of providers 5. Number of board-certified physicians	1. CD discharges and length of stay 2. Readmissions 3. Use of prescription drugs	1. Percentage of treatment that follows accepted best practices guidelines (Also see appropriateness above)

| Prevention/ education/ early intervention | 1. Cost breakdowns for severely and persistently mentally ill (psychotic or bipolar diagnoses) | 1. Evidence that printed materials on behavioral health issues were given to members within 6 months
2. Evidence of seminars/ workshops on health and prevention in last 6 months
3. Examples of specialized behavioral health prevention programs
4. Examples of case managers facilitating promotion, prevention, and education | Core measure on well-care pediatric visits with mental health and developmental handicap screening | 1. Expenditures per enrollee on preventive information
2. Percentage who participate in preventive programs |

NOTE: AFDC, Aid to Families with Dependent Children; CD, chemical dependency; EAP, Employee Assistance Program; HEDIS, Health Plan Employer Data and Information Set; HMO, health maintenance organization; MHSIP, Mental Health Statistics Improvement Program; PERMS, Performance-Based Measures for Managed Behavioral Healthcare Program; SSDI, Social Security Disability Insurance; and SSI, supplemental security income.

SOURCES: AMBHA (1995), Digital Equipment Corporation (1995), NCQA (1996a, b), and SAMHSA (1996).

costs and for which there are problems in the quality of evaluation and treatment are of great concern.

FACCT evolved during 1995 because of the interests of several major private and public purchasers, as well as consumer groups, for public-measurement systems that account for outcomes related to quality such as patient satisfaction, health-related quality of life, and functional status. Their wish to expedite the development of outcomes and methodologies and systems was spurred by Paul Ellwood's long-standing promotion of the national goal of a patient-centered and integrated outcomes management system. To date, FACCT has released measurement methods for a number of conditions (e.g., diabetes, asthma, and breast cancer) and is planning the development of similar tools and pilot programs for behavioral health conditions such as depression. The application and evolution of FACCT methods will be influenced by the amount of funding that is available and how meaningful the collected information will be to consumers and purchasers.

Many purchasers are now prodding their contracted managed care organizations and a few are requiring their contracted managed care organizations to collect and publicly report their Health Plan Employer Data and Information Set (HEDIS) results. This and other public report cards constitute a major trend in health care and are being actively supported by consumers who want meaningful data on which they can make personal health care and health plan selection decisions. Managed care organizations are concerned about the risk adjustment problems with some measures, the cost of collecting data, the high-stakes business risks that can follow questionable performance, and the plethora of reporting requirements that are being imposed under multiple reporting systems. The evolution of other potentially large systems, such as the Joint Commission on Accreditation of Healthcare Organizations (JCAHO), NCQA, Utilization Review Accreditation Commission (URAC), and Council on Accreditation of Services for Families and Children (COA), adds to their concerns about their abilities to simultaneously meet the market's demands for improved accountability and lower premiums.

From these early efforts to establish quality standards and tools that can be used to measure quality, several views are emerging:

• Standards and measures for quality-related components of structure (e.g., state licensure and national accreditation), process (e.g., provider adherence to clinical policies), and outcomes (e.g., level of functioning and patient satisfaction with clinical care) are relevant to conclusions about quality.
• Routine and consistent measurement of specific health conditions and illnesses should be conducted for individuals in a health plan and for the population.
• Risk adjustments, based on individual and population variables, are critical in reaching conclusions about the process and outcomes of health care.
• Health status (physical functioning, role capacities, and objective and

subjective well-being) should be consistently evaluated in determining the effectiveness of health care interventions.

• Generic population and disease-specific health measures are relevant to the management of a population's health.

• Plans need to evaluate systematically individual and population health risk behaviors in developing targeted interventions that could reduce avoidable health costs and increase the likelihood of positive health status over time.

• Accreditation, licensing, quality auditing, performance monitoring, and other accountability mechanisms have limited impacts when they are instituted in a piecemeal or uncoordinated fashion. For example, external oversight processes may adequately monitor the overall quality of care, but oversight tends only to identify problems rather than to help solve them, especially when the solutions may involve changes in the internal procedures of an organization.

• Quality of care requires cooperative commitments to quality-related goals by payers, practitioners, consumers, regulators, and managed care organizations, as well as a common and practical system for measuring and analyzing quality-related information.

Purchasers share with responsible managed care organizations and consumers a unifying goal of creating a more responsive health care delivery system, that is, one that is both more efficient and more effective. Over time it is probable that a best practices system will emerge that monitors, measures, and reports on the relevant information needed to determine effectiveness in sensitive, reliable, specific, and valid terms. The process of developing best practices will be facilitated if purchasers and managed care organizations include a variety of stakeholders in the discussions, including practitioners, administrators, researchers, accreditation organizations, public agencies, and the general public.

The quest for best practices and affordable systems is one of the current megatrends in health care, spawning a new industry that may provide the tools that stakeholders in the U.S. health care system need to make quality-based decisions. During the next few years of systems experimentation and consensus development, quality-related accountability will continue to develop in a variety of ways and will require leadership (Ellwood, 1988). It is now unclear by what means payers, providers, consumers, managed care organizations, and other stakeholders will come together to develop consensus about the systems that promote gains in personal health and the public good. Leadership will be needed to guide each step in this development and consensus-building process.

PERFORMANCE MEASUREMENT IN THE PUBLIC SECTOR

Performance measures are used to monitor progress made by agencies in reaching public health goals. Information from performance measures sometimes is used by agency administrators to justify the use of public funds. In addition, the information infrastructure needs to be developed to support state and local performance measurement systems and to standardize information across agencies, making it easier to aggregate and to analyze trends at the state level and then at the national level.

Standardization of information is a current priority of the U.S. Department of Health and Human Services. In addition to this report, the DHHS is sponsoring two other studies relevant to performance measurement. One study is being conducted by the National Research Council at the request of the Office of the Assistant Secretary for Health, to examine the technical issues involved in adopting performance measures in mental health and substance abuse, as well as other areas (human immunodeficiency virus infection, sexually transmitted diseases, tuberculosis, chronic disease, immunization, prevention of disabilities among children, rape prevention, and emergency medical services). That study will make recommendations for the specific performance measures that should be used over the next 3 to 5 years. DHHS also asked the Institute of Medicine (IOM) to convene the Committee on Using Performance Monitoring to Improve Community Health. That committee will develop prototypical sets of indicators for use by communities in monitoring the performance of public health agencies and personal health care services. One of the indicator sets addresses depression. The committees performing both studies are scheduled to issue reports in 1997.

The present committee is aware that many other efforts to develop performance measures are being undertaken by the states and cannot be addressed in this report. The section that follows will describe key efforts and lead agencies in the development of performance measures at the federal level.

Healthy People 2000

In 1979, the U.S. Public Health Service (PHS) initiated a process of setting objectives and measurable targets for health promotion and disease prevention. Now known as *Healthy People 2000*, this U.S. Public Health Service process adapted the private-sector "management by objectives" approach and set objectives for improvements in health status, risk reduction, public and professional awareness of prevention, health services, and protective measures. There are now 300 objectives in 22 priority areas addressing health promotion, health protection, preventive services, and data systems (DHHS, 1995).

The development of *Healthy People 2000* was directed by the Office of Disease Prevention and Health Promotion, under the leadership of J. Michael McGinnis, in response to a Congressional mandate. The national objectives were developed by 22 expert working groups, a consortium of more than 300 national membership organizations, 56 state and territorial health departments, the IOM, and public review and comment involving more than 10,000 individuals (DHHS, 1990, 1992).

Dissemination of these objectives has been widespread in the public health community through coordination with the American Public Health Association, the Association of State and Territorial Health Officials, the National Association of County and City Health Officials, and other groups. Regular reports describing the national progress toward meeting the objectives are issued, and there is general agreement that the objectives encourage the systematic measurement of needs, the setting of targets, the monitoring of the progress that has been made, and the evaluation of outcomes in public health (IOM, 1989a).

Substance Abuse and Mental Health Services Administration

Managed Care Initiative

SAMHSA is the lead federal agency for behavioral health care. SAMHSA's three centers (Center for Substance Abuse Treatment, Center for Mental Health Services, and Center for Substance Abuse Prevention) work in partnership with the states to improve prevention, treatment, and rehabilitation services for individuals with mental illness and substance abuse disorders.

In April 1995, SAMHSA began a managed care initiative to assist administrators and providers in adapting to the national shift to managed care delivery systems. Through its three centers, SAMHSA is supporting the development of activities that will help to consolidate information on managed care with regard to individuals with serious mental illness and chronic substance abuse disorders. SAMHSA also provides technical assistance to states and local providers concerning managed behavioral health care systems, including the development of performance-monitoring systems that include consumers and families, and the negotiation and management of contracts with managed behavioral health care organizations.

Mental Health Statistics Improvement Program

Public mental health programs have recently experienced several transformations concurrently with the development of managed behavioral health care systems. One of the most important is the emergence of the mental health consumer movement, with an increasing emphasis on consumer satisfaction with the quality of care and on the assessment of quality of life and other outcomes of mental health treatment.

In 1993, the Mental Health Statistics Improvement Program of the Center for Mental Health Services initiated the first phase of its report card project. The effort was a reflection of the emphasis on consumer choice during the Clinton Administration's health care reform proposals, and it converged with the growing mental health consumer movement to develop a collaborative effort with many stakeholders, including mental health consumers, state agency directors, and researchers.

The first phase of the report card project identified the domains and general concerns of stakeholders. The second phase involved the development of indicators for these domains, and in the spring of 1996, a report describing measurable indicators for the domains of access, appropriateness, outcomes, satisfaction, and prevention was released. In the summer of 1996, the Center for Mental Health Services announced that it will provide funding for field testing in up to 25 states, in which a combination of administrative data, clinical information such as medical records, and consumer self-reports will be used to prepare the report cards (CMHS, 1995; Cody, 1996).

The report card is a consumer-oriented prototype. It was designed to help mental health consumers, advocates, health care purchasers, providers, and state mental health agencies compare and evaluate mental health services in the areas of access, appropriateness, outcomes, and prevention. It is unique in the field because of the involvement of consumers in every stage of its development, the focus on serious mental illness, and the emphasis on outcomes in mental health treatment.

Health Care Financing Administration

HCFA, which administers the Medicare and Medicaid programs, is the largest single purchaser of managed care in the United States and currently provides direct or financial support to 15.5 million people (Valdez, 1996). As of June 30, 1996, about 11.5 million Medicaid beneficiaries were enrolled in managed care programs, representing about a 140 percent increase in managed care enrollment since 1993. Currently, 10 percent of the Medicare population is enrolled in about 278 managed health care plans across the country, representing about a 67 percent increase since 1993 (Valdez, 1996).

In the area of quality assurance (referring to plan structure and processes), in 1991 HCFA began its Quality Assurance Reform Initiative, which was designed to monitor and improve the quality of managed care for Medicaid recipients. The initiative has developed a guide that includes specific criteria for the design of internal quality assurance programs by managed care plans. Over the long term, HCFA plans to move toward a single set of quality assurance standards for both Medicaid and Medicare beneficiaries within managed care environments (Valdez, 1996).

In the area of performance measures, HCFA worked with NCQA in the development of the Medicaid version of HEDIS and has included Medicaid HEDIS in its Quality Improvement Primer, which has been developed for state Medicaid agencies. In addition, HCFA has worked with NCQA to develop HEDIS 3.0 and by 1997 will require health plans serving the Medicare population to use some of the HEDIS measures. HCFA also is working with FACCT to develop outcome measures for plan performance.

Agency for Health Care Policy and Research

The Agency for Health Care Policy and Research (AHCPR), a U.S. Department of Health and Human Services agency, was established in 1989 with a Congressional mandate to generate and disseminate information that would be useful to consumers, practitioners, and other audiences. The majority of AHCPR's activities are aimed at improving the quality of health care. Accordingly, the agency works with several organizations, including the Foundation for Accountability, the Joint Commission on Accreditation of Healthcare Organizations, the National Committee for Quality Assurance, and the American Medical Association, to help to provide a science base for quality measurement, and to assist in translating research findings to quality measures.

Through its Center for Quality Measurement and Improvement, AHCPR conducts and supports research on the measurement and improvement of the quality of health care, including consumer surveys and satisfaction with health care services and systems. The agency has produced and disseminated clinical practice guidelines in a variety of formats to meet the needs of health care practitioners, the scientific community, educators, and consumers. A clinical practice guideline on the detection, diagnosis, and treatment of depression was released in 1993.

AHCPR sponsors a Computerized Needs-Oriented Quality Measurement Evaluation System (CONQUEST), a prototype system for collecting and evaluating clinical performance measures. The system includes two linked data bases, one on conditions and one on measures, to help clinicians, providers, managed care organizations, and purchasers find clinical performance measures that match their needs. Information is included on approximately 1,200 measures developed by public- and private-sector organizations. Among these are measures for the following conditions: affective disorder, alcohol abuse, bipolar disorder, depression, drug abuse, dysthymic disorder, panic disorder, suicidal ideation, and suicide (mortality).

AHCPR has supported research on the implementation of guidelines in a variety of settings, including HMOs and group practice, and examining a variety of strategies, including incentives and individualized feedback. Other areas of AHCPR-supported research include factors that affect costs, premiums, and choice of health plans; clinical and effectiveness research in HMOs; and managed care in rural areas.

ACCREDITATION

Ideally, accreditation is a process that surveys health care delivery organizations to determine whether the services provided have met a set of recognized standards for that domain. During the last ten years, accreditation has become an important vehicle to review and monitor the inner structure of organizations that deliver health care. As discussed in other parts of this report, a growing trend among many state licensure/certification boards is to require accreditation from JCAHO, NCQA, the Rehabilitation Accreditation Commission (CARF), COA, or URAC to become licensed or certified in that state. The domains of the various accreditation agencies are different but sometimes overlap.

Accreditation Organizations

The committee reviewed accreditation materials from five organizations that accredit behavioral health plans, programs, and services: CARF, COA, JCAHO, NCQA, and URAC. Representatives of these organizations were invited to make presentations at the committee's two public workshops. This section briefly describes each of the organizations, which are further compared in Table 6.2.

The Rehabilitation Accreditation Commission (formerly the Commission on Accreditation of Rehabilitation Facilities) (CARF)

CARF accredits programs that serve individuals with disabilities and others who need rehabilitation. The organization was developed in 1966 through efforts of the American Rehabilitation Association and the Association of Sheltered Workshops. In CARF's first 2 years, it received administrative support from JCAHO, and the two organizations are developing a "recognition initiative" that eventually will recognize the other's accreditation standards and thus eliminate the need for dual accreditation.

CARF currently accredits more than 11,000 programs in the United States and Canada, including alcohol and drug programs, mental health programs, and community-based rehabilitation programs that are primarily designed for the chronically and persistently mentally ill. CARF has a consumer-centered philosophy that actively encourages consumer involvement in assessing community needs, planning services, participating in governance activities, and collaborating in the development of individual treatment plans. CARF also requires that programs have a plan to reduce barriers to care, including cultural, architectural, attitudinal, and other barriers (Slaven, 1996).

Council on Accreditation of Services for Families and Children (COA)

COA was founded in 1977 and currently accredits about 1,000 behavioral health programs and 3,000 social service programs in the United States and Canada. COA has developed standards for more than 50 services, including outpatient mental health and substance abuse services, day treatment, foster care and day care for children, services for persons with developmental disabilities, services for victims of domestic violence, adoption services, vocational and employment services, and others.

COA has developed a set of core standards that apply to all organizations that it accredits, such as financial management, quality assurance, and record keeping, as well as service-specific standards, such as foster care, residential care, and so on. The behavioral health accreditation overlaps somewhat with those of CARF and JCAHO, but most of the other services are not addressed by any other accreditation organization. Also, in contrast to the other accreditation organizations, the programs accredited by COA are largely community-based programs more closely related to a social services than to a medical model of treatment.

Joint Commission on Accreditation of Healthcare Organizations (JCAHO)

JCAHO is the oldest and largest of the accreditation organizations. In 1951, the Joint Commission on Accreditation of Hospitals (JCAH) was formed in cooperation with the American College of Surgeons, the American College of Physicians, the American Medical Association, and the Canadian Medical Association. The new organization formalized hospital standards that had been under development since the 1920s and 1930s by the American College of Surgeons. In the 1970s, JCAH began to develop additional accreditation programs for psychiatric facilities, substance abuse programs, community mental health programs, and ambulatory care facilities. In 1987 the name was changed to JCAHO to reflect the new activities and to anticipate a new activity, accreditation of managed care organizations (SAIC, 1995)

Accreditation of HMOs is now a relatively small proportion of JCAHO's accreditation activities. JCAHO, however, has accreditation guidelines for networks, including independent practice associations, integrated health care delivery systems, HMOs, managed care organizations, physician-hospital organizations, preferred provider organizations, provider-sponsored networks, and specialty service systems (JCAHO, 1996). Another set of accreditation guidelines address mental health, chemical dependency, and mental retardation/developmental disabilities services.

National Committee for Quality Assurance (NCQA)

NCQA was formed in 1979 by two managed care associations, the Group Health Association of America and the American Managed Care and Review Association (now merged and renamed the American Association of Health Plans). The original purpose of NCQA was to perform quality care reviews for a former federal agency, the Office of Health Maintenance Organizations. From the beginning, NCQA established collaborative relationships with industry, including large employers such as Xerox and GTE, insurers, such as Prudential, and managed care plans, such as Harvard Community Health Plan (now Harvard Pilgrim Health Plan) and Kaiser Permanente.

In 1989, with a grant from the Robert Wood Johnson Foundation, NCQA began to develop a performance monitoring system now known as HEDIS. The

TABLE 6.2   Cross-Comparison of Selected Accreditation

Features	CARF	COA
Accreditation domains	Behavioral health care programs and community providers	Providers of more than 60 types of behavioral health care and social services programs
Mission/purpose statement	To promote the delivery of high-quality services in rehabilitation	To define expectations regarding the high quality of management and service delivery
Behavioral health-specific standards	Behavioral health provider-specific standards	Behavioral health-specific standards and standards for community-based, therapeutic providers
Approach to Quality: Structure, governance, and process	1. Identifiable governance structure 2. Written goals and objectives 3. Inclusion of ethnic representation in governance 4. Improvement of efficiency/effectiveness and satisfaction 5. Cultural sensitivity 6. Systematic information collection 7. Reviews of fiscal management 8. Reviews for sufficient resource allocation 9. Emphasis on CQI and outcomes evaluation	1. Inclusion of governing body/advisory board and management in formal process 2. Written goals and mission 3. Systematic information monitoring 4. Emphasis on review of service compatibility with the cultural needs of the population served 5. Reviews of termination, grievance, and risk areas 6. Has thresholds for review of functions 7. Review leads to changes in policy intervention

Organizations in Managed Behavioral Health Care

JCAHO	NCQA	URAC
Health care networks; HMOs, IPAs, PPOs, PHOs, MCOs, integrated delivery systems, networks (e.g., behavioral health, rehabilitation)	HMOs, POS, PPOs with defined populations, credentialing organizations, MBHOs (in 1997)	HMOs, PPOs, PHOs, IPAs, POS, single specialty networks, other managed care systems; Provider networks providing services for Medicare, Medicaid, and Workers Compensation
To improve the quality of care provided to the public; to develop a patient-centered approach to accreditation	To provide information that enables purchasers and consumers to distinguish plans on the basis of quality	To encourage efficient and effective managed care processes and to provide a method of evaluation and accreditation of provider networks and managed care programs
1. Patient rights, including access to care and participation in treatment decisions 2. Assessment and reassessment, including clinical and physical evaluations 3. Care of patients specific to needs 4. Education of patients and families 5. Continuity of care among practitioners and over time	New behavioral health standards for carve-out companies and HMOs with behavioral health services carved in. Measures on substance abuse, depression, use of medications, and family visits, are being evaluated for inclusion in future reporting sets. Current measure: follow-up after hospitalization and discharge	Networks shall establish and implement criteria that address quality of care, quality of service, professional qualifications, availability and accessibility needs for these types of providers, and the business needs and goals of the network
1. Leadership determines approach and sets priorities 2. System-wide approach 3. Emphasis on plan design of systems and processes, measurement, assessment of data, and improvement in a cycle of continuous improvement and innovation 4. Systematic processes to collect data and to measure health outcomes, functional status, satisfaction, access, appropriateness effectiveness, and financial stability	1. Identifiable governance accountability and structure 2. Written program plan outlining structure, accountability, and projects 3. Emphasis on quality studies 4. CQI integrative process encourages involving multiple departments 5. Must demonstrate service and clinical improvement and clinical effect on a large portion of the population	1. Identifiable committee structure and responsibility 2. Written plan with goals and objectives 3. Staff development 4. Reviews, studies, and surveys of enrollees/pro-viders, access, complaints, and provider performance 5. Reviews for disease management, acute/chronic care, treatment outcome, and preventive care 6. Corrective action plan 7. Reporting of complaints 8. Mechanism for identifying or monitoring poor quality provider

continues on next page

TABLE 6.2 Continued

Features	CARF	COA
Approach to utilization	No identifiable UM section, but similar areas covered elsewhere are 1. Accessibility review of barriers 2. Record/information management, and confidentiality 3. Emphasis on record documentation 4. Emphasis on specific qualifications by service type 5. Emphasis on use of case managers to coordinate, assist, and assess needs	Utilization management addressed under specific standards: 1. Written procedure for review 2. UR conducted confidentially 3. Reviewers not in conflict of interest 4. Focus on appropriateness and effectiveness 5. UR at least every 90 days 6. Measurable criteria 7. UR of applicable services is conducted
Credentialing	1. Human resource approach 2. Sufficient staffing 3. Credentialing based on establishing qualifications and review of documents 4. Credentials must be relevant to the needs of those served 5. Credential verification requested 6. Evaluate job performance 7. Staff input into personnel policies	1. Human resource approach 2. Job description for each job 3. Equal opportunity employer 4. Personnel reflect the population serviced 5. Specific requirements for administrative personnel 6. Professional staff have advanced degrees and appropriate licensure/certification

JCAHO	NCQA	URAC
5. Improvement priorities reflect needs, expectations, and priorities of patients and staff 6. Must affect large portion of the population served or the population must be at high risk 7. Emphasis on teamwork and collaboration 8. Co-leadership between administration and clinical leaders		
1. Emphasis on continuum of care process 2. Care is assessed on the basis of patient need for a level or type of care 3. Process to allow patients to make knowledgeable decisions 4. Coordination and continuity of care, with smooth transition to new care	1. Identifiable governance structure 2. Accessibility defined by telephone access, geographic distance, and treatment and triage personnel credentials 3. UM criteria are based on clear and updated scientific evidence 4. Process to assess interpreter reliability 5. Qualifications of the reviewers 6. Timely reviews 7. Clear/complete documentation justifying decision 8. Assessment of new technology/prescribing skill practices	1. Confidentiality of patient-specific information obtained during utilization management process 2. Scope of responsibility for accreditation 3. Qualification for UM staff including physician director 4. Outlines levels of reviews and reviewers 5. Requires second-level review by peer structure 6. Use of explicit criteria 7. Review of reviewers 8. Review of UM accessibility and on-site review 9. Information collection process requirement 10. Appeals/ grievance management
1. Applicable to licensed practitioners, whether employed, contractual, or independent 2. Heavy emphasis on privileging and on assessing and demonstrating staff competency by: a. peer review b. demonstration of specific capabilities in documentation requirements	1. Define mandatory credentials for professionals 2. Documents for review 3. Primary verification 4. Time limitation for process 5. Recredentialing processes 6. Evidence of provider performance with recredentialing 7. Site visits	1. Define staff qualifications and job expectations 2. List of nine areas for review 3. Primary verification 4. Outlines a specific privileging process 5. Recredentialing process 6. Record/site review for unaccredited sites

continues on next page

TABLE 6.2 Continued

Features	CARF	COA
Rights	Defines areas of rights to protect and promote consumer rights: 1. Consumer participation in treatment planning 2. Consumer involvement in governing structure 3. Inform consumers of their rights 4. Timely management of complaints and grievances 5. Right to protection from physical and emotional abuse and provision of a safe environment, ethical services, etc.	Defines areas of consumer rights: 1. Involvement in treatment plan 2. Voluntary consumer board 3. Free from architectural barriers/harm 4. Rights to have language/ linguistic needs addressed 5. Service specific, chooses least restrictive; preserve integrity of families
Records	Records management in an organization; 20-item checklist and standards on accessibility, time frames for data entry, and confidentiality	Records on a provider level that address content, nature, and source information; timeliness; confidentiality; and record access
Unique areas	Specific standard for the following services: 1. Alcohol/drug services 2. Mental health services	Standards emphasize consumer orientation and require measurement of outcomes: 1. Social advocacy

JCAHO	NCQA	URAC
c. performance against a specific expectation 3. Specific requirements for providers in the fields of CD, child/adolescent forensic, and MR/DD 4. Primary verification required for the credentialing process 5. Avoid duplication of existing credentialing		
Defines areas of member rights and implies mechanism to detect: 1. Member participation in treatment planning 2. Compliance with state/ federal regulations and stated mission 3. Families/caregivers inclusion 4. Member conflict resolution 5. Obtain informed consent 6. Right to pastoral services 7. Complaint/grievance information reported to governance structure 8. Prohibition of gag clauses 9. Organization has code of business ethics 10. Mechanisms to protect integrity of clinical decision-making	Defines areas and measurement of member rights and responsibilities: 1. To participate in treatment planning 2. Receive information on services available, practitioners, guidelines, UM protocols, etc. 3. Families/support input 4. Member complaint/timely resolved/monitor and trend 5. Member responsibility to provide information 6. Member to follow agreed plans 7. Member participation in understanding behavioral problems	Define areas, responsibilities of organization, and processes: 1. Consumer participation in treatment planning 2. Receive medically necessary/appropriate care 3. Clear/understandable information 4. Provider/staff courteous/ respectful 5. Obtain input via surveys/ telephone lines 6. Complaint/grievance process summarized 7. Confidential management of consumer information
Information management for networks. Areas addressed are planning, confidentiality, and security; definition and capture of data/information; aggregate data and information; knowledge-based information; and comparative data information	Medical records on an organizational level with emphasis on record audits against organizational standards including prevention areas; a 21-item checklist audit during survey process	Implementation of a policy on confidentiality that assures compliance with applicable laws, release of information to authorized agents and appropriate authorities, procedures for storage and retention
1. Education standards to promote patient/family education to improve health status	Prevention services. MBHOs are expected to: 1. Screen for prevalence of behavioral health disorders	*continues on next page*

TABLE 6.2 Continued

Features	CARF	COA
	3. Community rehabilitation 4. Employment services Components of service reviewed: case management, detoxification, outpatient services, residential housing, inpatient services, crisis intervention, partial hospitalization, psychosocial rehabilitation	2. Information and referral to emergency shelter 3. Domestic violence 4. Runaways/homeless 5. Resettlement 6. Immigration/citizenship assistance 7. Child day care 8. Volunteer relationship 9. Social development 10. Family education 11. Financial management 12. Case management 13. Homemaker/in-home 14. Protective service 15. Employee vocational services 16. Support services for older adults 17. Day treatments 18. Therapeutic wilderness programs

NOTE: CD, chemical dependency; CQI, continuous quality improvement; HMO, health maintenance organization; IPA, independent practice association; MBHO, managed behavioral health organization; MCO, managed care organization; MR/DD, mentally retarded and developmentally disabled; PHO, physician hospital organization; POS, point of service plan; PPO, preferred provider organization; QI, quality improvement; UM, utilization management; and UR, utilization review,

SOURCES: CARF (1996), COA (1996a, b), JCAHO (1995, 1996), NCQA (1996a, b), and URAC (1996).

first version, known as HEDIS 1.0, was released in 1991, HEDIS 2.0 was released in 1993, and HEDIS 3.0 was released in the summer of 1996. NCQA has worked in collaboration with HCFA to develop a Medicaid version of HEDIS, which was released in July 1995, and in the spring of 1996 NCQA released a set of behavioral health performance measures for testing, based in part on the performance measurement system (PERMS) developed by the American Managed Behavioral Healthcare Association and on other sources.

Now in its third evolution, HEDIS 3.0 is a voluntary reporting set of managed care quality measures that have evolved over the past 5 years under the aegis of NCQA but with inputs from broad range of experts from a variety of public and private organizations. Although only one specific behavioral health measure has

JCAHO	NCQA	URAC
2. Educational skill is assessed by patient display of knowledge 3. Information management-review of timeliness, accuracy, levels of security, design to reduce work and enhance care delivery 4. Leadership process, including planning, directing, implementing and improving skills 5. Emergency preparedness plan 6. Education about disenrollment 7. Annual independent audit 8. Strategic and operational plans 9. Plan to integrate activities and member services 10. Plan and design for information management 11. Standard format for information	2. Develop/adopt programs with participation of members, behavioral health providers, other medical providers, and community agencies 3. Programs reflect age, sex, ethnic, economic, and risk factors 4. Informs members about preventive services 5. Monitor the use of preventive programs 6. Reports results of preventive services to behavioral health providers and primary care providers 7. Takes action to improve the use of preventive services programs by population	

been part of earlier reporting sets (ambulatory follow-up after hospitalization for major affective disorder), a number of other measures have recently been proposed as a test set that will promote the refinement of these measures over time and the possible evolution of some measures toward the next HEDIS reporting set. Although HEDIS data collection is not required for NCQA accreditation, managed care organizations regularly institute HEDIS measures.

Utilization Review Accreditation Commission

URAC was formed in 1990 after a series of meetings with the American Managed Care and Review Association and utilization review industry representatives indicated that there was a need for standards for utilization review and an independent accreditation organization. URAC currently accredits the utilization and quality management systems of 150 managed care programs that provide services for more than 120 million individuals. URAC also works closely with state regulators to address managed care regulatory issues, and nine states deem URAC accreditation in lieu of licensure. URAC has implemented a Network Accreditation Program and will be implementing a Workers' Compensation Utilization Management Accreditation program.

Changing Environment of Accreditation

There has been a proliferation and growth of accreditation organizations to match the structural changes in the industry. As described above, new accreditation organizations form to review any structure devised in managed care. Some organizations are unique, whereas others overlap in their accreditation domains but have a slightly different focus. For example, JCAHO and NCQA both accredit HMOs. JCAHO's accreditation process focuses on a staff model delivery system, whereas NCQA's process is focused on the HMO structure. Also, NCQA standards tend to focus at the highest level of an organization, whereas JCAHO, CARF, and COA are geared more toward particular programs or facilities that may be a division of a larger organization or may be free-standing or independent.

Currently, major purchasers of care may require accreditation for a health care delivery system to be eligible for contracts. In addition, many state insurance boards and employer groups have mandated that HMOs have NCQA or URAC accreditation to operate in their state or to be offered to employees, respectively. However, because of the complexities of health care structures, mandatory accreditation can impose a tremendous burden. Accreditation requirements often overlap in national managed care companies or health care delivery systems that perform multiple functions (e.g., a staff model HMO that is also a provider network). Many times, organizations must obtain more than one type of accreditation to satisfy employers, states, and other stakeholders. A behavioral health care carve-out company, for example, may operate in a state that requires URAC accreditation, whereas a multi-state employer group operating within that state may require NCQA accreditation.

The costs of achieving accreditation are also burdensome. The actual cost of the accreditation survey is only part of the burden. The personnel costs and time involved in preparing for accreditation also can also be extensive, and may be prohibitive for smaller organizations. For community-based organizations, the cost of COA accreditation is done on a sliding scale, with a graduated scale based on total agency revenue (COA, 1996a, b).

Cost certainly makes accreditation prohibitive for many small organizations; it also makes the issue of multiple accreditations unrealistic, despite the demands of states and employer groups. Thus, questions are raised about the utility and validity of accreditation. The accreditation industry is faced with pressure to focus its standards on the relevant issues, collaborate with similar organizations, and consolidate the multitude of accreditation standards to reduce overlap and redundancy.

The Accreditation Process

The accreditation process entails generating standards and then comparing the actual delivery of care with the standards. There are at least seven distinct steps:

1. Measures of performance, also known as parameters, are identified and recommended as standards.
2. A process of review leads to acceptance of the standards.
3. The standard is generally tested internally ("alpha" tested) and then tested on a external site ("beta" tested).
4. After testing, the standards are incorporated into a review process.
5. Organizations desiring to be accredited apply to be surveyed.
6. A site review is performed by peer surveyors who examine the inner workings of the organizations against the standards.
7. Finally, a process of scoring is developed to determine the organization's degree of compliance with each standard and whether the aggregated results reached the threshold for granting accreditation.

These steps are described in the following section.

A *standard,* according to Donabedian (1982), is a professionally developed expression of the range of acceptable variation from the norm. A standard has also been defined as the desirable and achievable (rather than the observed) performance or value with regard to a given parameter (Slee, 1974).

A *parameter* is an objective, definable, and measurable characteristic of the process or the outcome of care (e.g., access to behavioral health care within 5 days of a request in a nonurgent situation). Each parameter has a scale of possible values. For example, a geographic access parameter might require outpatient mental health services to be available within 30 minutes of a consumer's home or workplace. Variables would include, for example, traffic patterns in a busy urban setting where traveling 5 miles could take 1 hour during rush hour. Another variation might be in a rural setting, where there is a scarcity of consumers and services and travel time may be longer because of distance.

The development of the current accreditation standards is based on professional consensus. The extent and diversity of opinions into the consensus process vary from agency to agency, as well as from standard to standard. Some agencies use a wide range of experts and elicit public participation, whereas others may use a closed panel of experts and a board review-editing procedure to develop a standard. The scope and relevancy of the standards by this process are dependent on the input and consensus from all the affected parties. The process of standardizing different views from participants in the development of a standard is not clearly outlined in the public information provided by CARF, COA, JCAHO, NCQA, or URAC.

Unless the accreditation process incorporates principles of quality in establishing standards and the survey process, there is a danger of inconsistency, variance, and unreliability. There are many opportunities in the accreditation process for variance in measures, interpretations, and dispositions, leading to disparate outcomes. The process of accreditation is heavily dependent on the strength of the standard as described, the surveyor's interpretation of the standard, and the applicability of the standard to a real situation.

Accreditation standards written with admirable intentions may not lead to consistent interpretation and/or applicability to the real world. For example, COA has included a standard to define the scope of an agency's mission. It states that the primary purpose of an agency is to provide services to meet the needs of the community for protection, maintenance, strengthening, or enhancement of individual and family life and social and psychological functioning (COA, 1996a). This standard demonstrates responsible intentions but is subject to much variation in interpretation by reviewers and variability in what is considered to be the supporting evidence. During the training of surveyors, it would be important to outline the different variables in this standard. Reviewers should be familiar with the variations to the standard so they are able to assess during a review whether the nuances of the agency comply within the boundaries of the standard.

Therefore, the accreditation label is only as good as the process of accreditation, from the development of the standards through the process of scoring. It is important in the accreditation process that:

1.   Standards are developed through a rigorous process of extensive peer consensus, a review of scientific evidence when applicable, and reevaluations of normative data to determine the true range of acceptable variations.

2.   Standards are objective, measurable parameters specific enough to minimize variations in interpretations by reviewers and the public.

3.   Standards are reviewed for their relevance and importance to the goal of accreditation and the integrative needs of the public.

4.   The validity and reliability of a standard must be known and reflective in the scoring, such that those standards with much variability are given less value than those for which there is stronger consensus.

5.   The implementation process is updated frequently, and there is a clear and recurrent process for establishing inter-rater reliability among reviewers.

6.   The final accreditation dispositions are compared with (trended against) acceptable parameters, that is, informed public perception, as a strong indicator of the competency of the accreditation process.

INFORMATION INFRASTRUCTURE FOR QUALITY MEASUREMENT

Administrative data sets are frequently a basis for quality-of-care assessments and are used in systems such as HEDIS 3.0 (NCQA, 1996a) and Performance-Based Measures for Managed Behavioral Healthcare Program (AMBHA, 1995). The data sets include claims data, records on visits and procedures, and, with the introduction of computerization, medical records. These information systems generally include relatively large pools of individuals and therefore permit analyses of specific practitioners and facilities (profiling), examinations of selected conditions and diagnoses, and changes in patient status over time. Because the data are collected for ongoing management functions (e.g., billing), they provide a relatively inexpensive source of information.

Unfortunately, the value of the data sets for assessments of quality are limited because they are designed for management functions like billing and claims payment and may not include sufficient detail to facilitate analyses of quality of care (Garnick et al., 1994). Garnick et al. (1994) have noted that quality-of-care assessments require information on the utilization of care (e.g., visits, services, procedures, site of service, diagnoses, and outcomes), patient characteristics (e.g., age, gender, race, and employment status), and health plan descriptors (e.g., benefit structure, copayments). Many systems, however, do not include all utilization information and may not contain detail on the services provided. Plans with high deductibles and/or copayments may not record service utilization if it does not exceed the deductible, and high copayments may discourage individuals from seeking care. Plans may also fail to record the use of services when utilization exceeds the maximum benefit either because the individual seeks services outside the plan or the plan does not track self-paid services. Claims data are often insufficient to identify specific service dates (especially when multiple services are provided within a short period of time), procedure codes may not reflect the actual services provided, and diagnostic codes may be inaccurate or incomplete. Finally, commercial data sets often include limited information on patient characteristics and may not provide accurate information on the numbers of individuals enrolled at a point in time. Public-sector data sets often have more patient information because public policy requires the tracking of the services provided by age, race, and gender.

These limitations are particularly problematic in the assessment of the quality of behavioral health care. Out-of-plan utilization is a major source of potential bias. The benefits for the substance abuse and mental health care and services provided within a plan are limited. Individuals with such problems often require more than the benefits offer, and turn to publicly-funded programs for additional care. Thus, a review of the services provided to an individual may suggest that he or she received one episode of care from the health plan for a short duration and no readmissions. If it were known, however, that the individual had received additional public services, the assessment of that plan's quality might change substantially. Moreover, procedure codes for ambulatory services may not differentiate mental health and substance abuse care (NCQA, 1996a, b). For example, new admissions for mental health problems can be misinterpreted as readmissions for substance abuse if there had been an earlier substance abuse treatment episode. Finally, the lack of data on patient characteristics means case mix adjustments may not be feasible and makes it difficult to assess biases in patterns of care and the need for culturally and gender-specific services.

Despite these limitations, administrative data sets are an efficient and important source of information for the assessment of quality of services. Program managers, program evaluators, and consumers, however, must be aware of the potential problems and biases and include an assessment of a data set's limitations in the analyses of services and the conclusions about quality. It is also critical to assess the potential for combining information from commercial and public administrative data systems so that the nature and extent of out-of-plan utilization can be assessed and added to the evaluation of the quality of care.

If you give information to providers and you work with information systems with the goal of providing information in real time, then quality assurance initiatives can be transformed from an external administrative burden into a powerful tool for improving clinical practice and increasing efficiency.

Geoffrey Reed
American Psychological Association
Public Workshop, April 18, 1996, Washington, DC

ROLE OF GOVERNMENT IN QUALITY ASSURANCE

Historically, the federal government's involvement in quality review and accreditation has been indirect. For example, in the area of hospital accreditation, the federal government has typically given an accreditation organization such as JCAHO deemed status. This means that the federal government makes use of the information collected by JCAHO and relies on JCAHO's judgments regarding the quality of hospitals in setting eligibility rules for reimbursement by Medicare.

States also are beginning to review and update traditional regulatory and contracting practices and to develop arrangements for deemed status. For example, COA holds deemed status in 22 states that recognize the COA accreditation process in lieu of Medicaid certification, state monitoring, or licensing (COA, 1996c).

Similar sets of arrangements already are in force in other markets. For example, the American Society for Testing and Materials holds deemed status in judging the quality of building materials. Table 6.3 displays a variety of consumer protection models for comparison.

Deeming can be a powerful tool, especially when the market for accreditation and measurement appears to be rather competitive. The federal or state government would grant deemed status to all organizations meeting standards of measurement and standard setting. For example, the federal or state government may decide that it will grant deemed status to any group that provides measures and standards across a specified range of domains. This would create an incentive for health plans and other organizations to develop quality measures and for accreditation organizations to measure a range of domains that extend beyond what any subset of interest groups might propose.

Achieving deemed status could also require that measurements be uniformly defined and collected by third parties. Under such arrangements, the federal government's influence would stem primarily from its role as a major purchaser through Medicare, Federal Employees Health Benefits Program, CHAMPUS, and other programs. The federal government would not be regulating the quality measurement and accreditation industry, nor would it choose among competing technologies, thereby allowing innovations to continue to emerge. As states continue to re-evaluate their contracting and regulatory mechanisms, more states may develop deemed status arrangements.

Under these conditions, government purchasing power would be used to promote approaches to measurement and accreditation that are consistent with concepts of efficient markets for insurance as well as consumer protection. Making use of deemed status in this manner may be particularly important in the behavioral health care arena if the market failures outlined above are significant.

This discussion suggests that the interests of enrollees and consumers of health care may be underrepresented in existing measurement and accreditation processes. The federal government could also serve to enhance the significance of consumer input. First, existing governmental efforts such as SAMHSA's sponsorship of a consumer-oriented report card can be used to increase consumer input to the development of health plan rating systems. This has been done with some success under the SAMHSA report card project.

A second approach would be for the government to make use of information based on consumer groups' ratings of the raters. That is, organizations such as American Association of Retired Persons, National Seniors Health Cooperative, Consumers Union, and the National Alliance for the Mentally Ill could be asked to rate accreditation and quality measurement systems. This information could be incorporated into the federal government's decision to give an accreditation organization deemed status. Again, this approach uses the federal government's purchasing power to advance representation of the interests that the market may fail to give adequate weight.

TABLE 6.3 Selected Regulatory and Consumer Protection Models

Name	Establishment	Duties	Structure	Industry Regulation
Better Business Bureaus	Established in 1912	Provide consumer reports on businesses, charity groups, and organizations; resolve consumer-business disputes; promote ethical and voluntary self-regulation of business	Community-based, private and nonprofit; supported mostly by membership dues paid by business and professional groups; coordinated by Better Business Bureaus Council, Inc.	No legal powers; dispute resolution through telephone conciliation, mediation, or nonbinding arbitration
Federal Aviation Administration	Air Commerce Act of May 20, 1926	Ensure the safety and efficiency of the air transportation system; maintain public confidence; regulate air navigation and air traffic control; minimize environmental impact of aviation; and conduct/ support aviation research and development	Operating arm of the U.S. Department of Transportation; the administrator is nominated by the President	Monitors operation of the nation's air traffic control system; certifies pilots, aircraft, and airports; establishes and enforces aviation and security rules
Federal Deposit Insurance Corporation	Banking Act of 1933 (Glass-Steagall Act)	Maintain stability and public confidence in the banking system	Board of directors and a chairman; one member is Comptroller of the Currency; one is Director of Office of Thrift Supervision; three are presidential appointees	Establishes criteria under which a bank is eligible for federal deposit insurance
Federal Reserve System	Federal Reserve Act of 1913	Conduct monetary policy; supervise and regulate banking institutions; maintain stability of financial system; protect consumers	Independent government agency; Board of Governors with chair and vice-chair appointed by President; 12 regional Federal Reserve Banks; 25 branches; advisory bodies include 30-member Consumer Advisory Council	Review member banks for compliance with banking regulations every 18 months on average, with poor performers reviewed more frequently and good performers reviewed every 24 months; investigate complaints; maintain national database to identify potential institutional or industrywide problems

Federal Trade Commission	Federal Trade Commission Act of 1914	Enforce federal antitrust and consumer protection laws; ensure fair and efficient operation of the market; safeguard informed choice of consumers	Independent government agency; five presidentially appointed commissioners	Rule-making; investigation of complaints or infractions with results of voluntary compliance (no guilt admitted but suspect practice halted), a "cease and desist" order to end the offending practice; facilitate consumer redress in civil courts
Financial Accounting Standards Board	Designated by the Securities and Exchange Commission (SEC) in 1973	Establish standards of financial accounting and reporting; keep standards in line with current industry practice and ensure international comparability of reporting methods; improve common understanding of information in financial reports	Private, nonprofit; operates under the Financial Accounting Foundation; seven members including a chair and vice-chair assisted by Financial Accounting Standards Advisory Council	Conduct a deliberative process that seeks to develop neutral standards; authority delegated by SEC
Food and Drug Administration	Food and Drugs Act of 1906; organized as the Food and Drug Administration in 1930	Ensure the safety of food, cosmetics, medicines, medical devices, radiation-emitting products, feed and drugs for pets and farm animals; provide for informed consumer choice through fair and open product labeling	Since 1988 an official agency of the U.S. Department of Health and Human Services with a Commissioner appointed by the President; 9,000 employees located in Washington, DC and 157 offices across the country	Regulation of approximately 95,000 U.S. businesses; investigations and inspections to verify manufacture and labeling; verification of producer product tests; approval of import safety; the Food and Drug Administration approves chemicals and products for use in the U.S.; enforcement capabilities include encouraging voluntary correction, recalls, court ordered recall and cessation of sales; fines and/or imprisonment
National Association of Insurance Commissioners	Established in 1871	Protect the interests of insurance consumers through coordination of regulations across multi-state insurers	Private, nonprofit organization encompassing all insurance regulators involved in life, accident, health, commercial, and special insurance from 50 states and District of Columbia	Require insurance departments to have adequate statutory and administrative authority to regulate an insurer's corporate and financial affairs through accreditation program; evaluations are conducted every 5 years; publish and

continues on next page

TABLE 6.3 Continued

Name	Establishment	Duties	Structure	Industry Regulation
				disseminate consumer guides; create models for legislation, regulation, and guidelines (e.g., Quality Assessment and Improvement Model Act and Health Care Assessment and Improvement Model Act)
Occupational Safety and Health Administration	Occupational Safety and Health Act of 1970	Save lives, prevent injuries, and protect the health of America's workers	Element of the Department of Labor under the Assistant Secretary for Occupational Safety and Health; three-person, presidentially appointed, Occupational Safety and Health Review Commission; advisory organs include National Advisory Committee on Occupational Safety and Health which includes participation by Department of Health and Human Services; over 200 regional offices nationwide	Establish regulations on employee health and safety; provide consultation and assistance with interpretation and applications of regulations; undertake inspections, investigate complaints, and issue citations to ensure compliance with regulations; provide training on occupational health and safety issues; the Commission may pursue penalties including cessation of hazardous activities, fines, and/or prison terms for violations
Securities and Exchange Commission	Securities and Exchange Act of 1934	Ensure fair competition and provision of services; ensure fair and free access to information; protect the interests of the consumer	Independent government agency; five presidentially appointed commissioners, with one serving as chair; 11 regional offices across United States	Provide interpretation and guidance on regulatory compliance; engage in rule-making or modification; conduct investigations and hold hearings; decisions may include suspension or revocation of registration and censure or ban from securities associations; work with criminal authorities in matters of mutual interest

SOURCES: Board of Governors of the Federal Reserve System (1994), Council of Better Business Bureaus Inc. (1996), FAA (1996), FASB (1996), FDA (1995), FDIC (1996), FTC (1996), GPO (1994), NAIC (1995, 1996a, b), OSHA (1996), and SEC (1996).

TABLE 6.4 Desirable Attributes of a Quality Assurance Program

---

- addresses overuse, underuse, and poor technical and interpersonal quality;
- intrudes minimally into the patient-provider relationship;
- is acceptable to professionals and providers;
- fosters improvement throughout the health care organization and system;
- deals with outlier practice and performance;
- uses both positive and negative incentives for change and improvement in performance;
- provides practitioners and providers with timely information to improve performance;
- has face validity for the public and for professionals (i.e., is understandable and relevant to patient and clinical decision-making);
- is scientifically rigorous;
- positive impact on patient outcomes can be demonstrated or inferred;
- can address both individual and population-based outcomes;
- documents improvement in quality and progress toward excellence;
- is easily implemented and administered;
- is affordable and is cost-effective; and
- includes patients and the public.

SOURCE: IOM (1990).

SUMMARY

As discussed in Chapters 1 to 3 of this report, quality measurement is complex and is evolving rapidly. This chapter has reviewed the existing means for quality assessment and has suggested some trends that may continue to develop in the future.

A previous IOM committee evaluated quality measurement activities for Medicare and developed a list of desirable attributes for a quality assurance program (IOM, 1990, p. 49). The present committee believes that the list is still appropriate and is a fitting closing for this chapter (see Table 6.4).

REFERENCES

AMBHA (American Managed Behavioral Healthcare Association, Quality Improvement and Clinical Services Committee). 1995. *Performance Measures for Managed Behavioral Healthcare Programs.* Washington, DC: American Managed Behavioral Healthcare Association.

Board of Governors of the Federal Reserve System. 1994. *The Federal Reserve System: Purposes and Functions.* Washington, DC: Board of Governors of the Federal Reserve System.

CARF (The Rehabilitation Accreditation Commission). 1996. *Standards Manual and Interpretive Guidelines for Behavioral Health.* Tucson, AZ: The Rehabilitation and Accreditation Commission.

CMHS (Center for Mental Health Services). 1995. *MHSIP Consumer-Oriented Mental Health Report Card: Phase II Task Force.* Washington, DC: Center for Mental Health Services.

COA (Council on Accreditation of Services for Families and Children). 1996a. *Standards for Agency Management and Service Delivery.* New York, NY: Council on Accreditation of Services for Families and Children.

COA. 1996b. *Council on Accreditation Profile.* New York: Council on Accreditation of Services for Families and Children.

COA. 1996c. *Council on Accreditation Recognition Report.* New York: Council on Accreditation of Services for Families and Children.

Cody P. 1996. CMHS offers states grants to test performance indicators. *Mental Health Report* 20(13): 114.

Council of Better Business Bureaus, Inc. 1996. *The Better Business Bureaus World Wide Web Homepage.* [http://www.igc.org/cbbb]. September.

DHHS (U.S. Department of Health and Human Services). 1990. *Healthy People 2000.* Washington, DC: Public Health Service, U.S. Department of Health and Human Services.

DHHS. 1992. *Prevention 91/92.* Washington, DC: Public Health Service, U.S. Department of Health and Human Services.

DHHS. 1995. *Healthy People 2000: Midcourse Review.* Washington, DC: Public Health Service, U.S. Department of Health and Human Services.

Digital Equipment Corporation. 1995. *HMO Performance Standards.* Maynard, MA: Digital Equipment Corporation.

Donabedian A. 1982. *Explorations in Quality Assessment and Monitoring: The Criteria and Standards of Quality.* Vol. 2. Ann Arbor, MI: Health Administration Press.

Ellwood PM. 1988. Outcomes management: A technology of patient experience. *The New England Journal of Medicine* 318(23):1549-1556.

FAA (Federal Aviation Administration). 1996. *The Federal Aviation Administration World Wide Web Homepage.* [http://www.faa.gov]. September.

FACCT (Foundation for Accountability). 1995. *Guidebook for Performance Measurement Prototype.* Portland, OR: Foundation for Accountability.

FASB (Financial Accounting Standards Board). 1996. *The Financial Accounting Standards Board World Wide Web Homepage.* [http://www.rutgers.edu/Accounting/raw/fasb/home.htm]. September.

FDA (Food and Drug Administration). 1995. *The Food and Drug Administration World Wide Web Homepage.* [http://www.fda.gov]. September.

FDIC (Federal Deposit Insurance Corporation). 1996. *The Federal Deposit Insurance Corporation World Wide Web Homepage.* [http://www.fdic.gov]. Septmeber.

FTC (Federal Trade Commission). 1996. *The Federal Trade Commission World Wide Web Homepage.* [http://www.ftc.gov]. September.

Garnick DW, Hendricks AM, Comstock CB. 1994. Measuring quality of care: Fundamental information from administrative datasets. *International Journal for Quality in Health Care* 6:163-177.

GPO (U.S. Government Printing Office). 1994. *United States Code.* Washington, DC: U.S. Government Printing Office.

HIAA (Health Insurance Association of America). 1996. *Sourcebook of Health Insurance Data, 1995.* Washington, DC: Health Insurance Association of America.

IOM (Institute of Medicine). 1989a. *Controlling Costs and Changing Patient Care? The Role of Managed Care.* Washington, DC: National Academy Press.

IOM. 1989b. *The Future of Public Health.* Washington, DC: National Academy Press.

IOM. 1990. *Medicare: A Strategy for Quality Assurance.* Vol. 1. Washington, DC: National Academy Press.

JCAHO (Joint Commission on Accreditation of Healthcare Organizations). 1995. *Accreditation Manual for Mental Health, Chemical Dependency and Mental Retardation/Developmental Disabilities Services—Standards.* Vol. 1. Oakbrook Terrace, IL: Joint Commission on Accreditation of Healthcare Organizations.

JCAHO. 1996. *Comprehensive Accreditation Manual for Health Care Networks.* Oakbrook Terrace, IL: Joint Commission on Accreditation of Healthcare Organizations.

Mattson MR, ed. 1992. *Manual of Psychiatric Quality Assurance.* Washington, DC: American Psychiatric Association.

NAIC (National Association of Insurance Commissioners). 1995. *A Tradition of Consumer Protection.* Washington, DC: National Association of Insurance Commissioners.

NAIC. 1996a. *Health Care Professional Credentialing Verification Model Act.* Washington, DC: National Association of Insurance Commissioners, Adopted June 1996.

NAIC. 1996b. *Quality Assessment and Improvement Model Act.* Washington, DC: National Association of Insurance Commissioners, Adopted June 1996.

NCQA (National Committee for Quality Assurance). 1996a. *HEDIS 3.0 Draft for Public Comment.* Washington, DC: National Committee for Quality Assurance.

NCQA. 1996b. *Accreditation Standards For Managed Behavioral Healthcare Organizations.* Washington, DC: National Committee for Quality Assurance.

OSHA (Occupational Safety and Health Administration). 1996. *The Occupational Safety and Health World Wide Web Homepage.* [http://www.osha.gov]. September.

Rodriguez AR. 1985. *The CHAMPUS Psychiatric and Psychological Review Project. Psychiatric Peer review: Preclude and Promise.* Washington, DC: American Psychiatric Press.

Rodriguez AR. 1988. An introduction to quality assurance in mental health. In: Stricker G, Rodriguez AR, eds. *Handbook of Quality Assurance in Mental Health.* New York: Plenum Press.

SAIC (Science Applications International Corporation). 1995. *A Comparison of JCAHO and NCQA Quality Oversight Programs.* National Quality Monitoring Project, Task 1b, Submitted to the Office of the Assistant Secretary of Defense, Health Affairs. Beaverton, OR: Science Applications International Corporation.

SAMHSA (Substance Abuse and Mental Health Services Administration). 1996. *Mental Health Measures in Medicaid HEDIS.* Washington, DC: Center for Mental Health Services, U.S. Department of Health and Human Services.

SEC (Securities and Exchange Commission). 1996. *The Securities and Exchange Commission World Wide Web Homepage.* [http://www.sec.gov]. September.

Slaven T. 1996. Personal communication to the Committee on Quality Assurance and Accreditation Guidelines for Managed Behavioral Health Care. Rehabilitation Accreditation Commission. May.

Slee V. 1974. PSRO and the hospital's quality control. *Annals of Internal Medicine* 81:97-106.

URAC (Utilization Review Accreditation Commission). 1996. *National Network Accreditation Standards.* Washington, DC: Utilization Review Accreditation Commission.

Valdez RO. 1996. Presentation at the Public Workshop of the Committee on Quality Assurance and Accreditation Guidelines for Managed Behavioral Health Care. Washington, DC. April 18.

7

Outcomes

DEFINITIONS OF SUCCESS

Evidence about treatment outcomes has become increasingly important in the health field in general and has become especially important in the behavioral health care field. A wide range of effective treatments are available for individuals with mental health and substance abuse problems, including psychosocial, pharmacological, and educational interventions. By now a large body of research demonstrates that treatment for these problems can be effective (Hubbard et al., 1989; McLellan et al., 1996; Polich et al., 1981; Simpson and Sells, 1990; Tims et al., 1991).

Defining outcomes for behavioral health problems is difficult. First, there are important differences among mental health and alcohol or other drug problems. For example, the same outcomes should not necessarily be expected for each drug of abuse, for example, heroin versus alcohol, or for every person with a substance abuse problem, for example, a pregnant woman, an adolescent, and a person with a dual diagnosis of mental health and substance abuse problems. The same is the case for mental health problems; outcomes differ by diagnoses (e.g., mild or major depression, chronic schizophrenia vs. adjustment disorder) and depend on individual characteristics (e.g., children vs. adults). It is appropriate to expect different outcomes at different stages of treatment, as the review of McLellan et al. in Appendix B points out. Differences in types of problems, the severities of problems, stages of illness and recovery, and other patient characteristics require a range of services and a multidimensional approach to measuring outcomes (Burnam, in press; Miller et al., 1995).

A second issue affecting the selection of outcomes measures has to do with the actual goals of treatment and the lack of consensus about what is considered successful treatment. For mental health problems, the goals of treatment differ according to the diagnosis, the severity of the illness, and past responses to treatment. Treatment generally begins with a comprehensive assessment that results in an individualized treatment plan. In many cases, full recovery from a mental health problem can be expected, with an individual returning to his or her former preillness level of functioning. Treatment also may have the goal of controlling symptoms or preventing relapses among those with recurring episodes of a disorder, such as depression. Improvements in functioning, rather than a complete return to preillness functioning, may be the goal for those with severe and chronic disorders such as schizophrenia. Improving quality of life by facilitating access to social services (e.g., through case management) may also be a goal, particularly for patients with severe debilitating and chronic mental disorders. Finally, the avoidance of violence may be a goal, such as when persons with suicidal or homicidal tendencies are restrained in a heavily supervised setting such as a hospital or locked nursing facility. Additional goals could include an improved ability to live independently in the community, or an ability to maintain employment in a supervised setting.

In the substance abuse field, a fundamental and sometimes controversial issue is whether treatment goals should be directed toward abstinence versus improvement. On the whole, alcohol treatment programs are oriented to an abstinence model rather than one of controlled drinking or improvement. Political considerations related to the management of illicit substances have played a large part in shaping treatment goals for chronic substance abusers (IOM, 1990a; Marlatt, 1983; Roizen, 1987). As a consequence of these strong ideological stances, some of the treatment interventions with proven efficacy (e.g., methadone maintenance with heroin addicts and controlled drinking strategies with carefully selected populations) are not often found in managed care treatment systems and therefore cannot be included in current managed care outcomes studies.

An additional issue affecting the definitions of outcomes for mental health and substance abuse treatment has to do with the public and policy expectations of treatment. Although some mental health and substance problems are chronic relapsing conditions like other medical problems, they also raise issues concerning individual and community responsibility that are not usually associated with other medical problems. Concerned stakeholders include individual clients, treatment programs, reimbursers, regulatory agencies or monitors, family members, agencies that have legal (the criminal justice system) or contractual relationships (employers), and the public. The goals of these groups are often conflicting, and the group whose interests are primary changes over time. These goals result in broad expectations of treatment, including reduced crime, improved health status, prevention of human immunodeficiency virus infection, reduction of unsafe sexual practices, improved employment, and improved family functioning. Reduced levels of alcohol or drug use or improved mental health symptoms are not necessarily the predominant expectations by these groups (McLellan and Weisner, 1996).

Thus, measurement of treatment outcomes for behavioral health treatment is complex. In its 1990 study of alcohol treatment, the Institute of Medicine (IOM) approached treatment effectiveness with the following question: "Which kinds of individuals, with what kinds of alcohol problems, are likely to respond to what kinds of treatments by achieving what kinds of goals when delivered by which kinds of practitioners?" (IOM, 1990b, p. 7). This perspective is appropriate for addressing treatment outcomes for drug and mental health problems as well.

We believe that the full evaluation of an organization has to combine knowledge of current outcomes with the standards-based information that lets you know and predict future outcomes.

Paul Schyve
Joint Commission on Accreditation of Healthcare
  Organizations
Public Workshop, April 18, 1996, Washington, DC

In approaching these multidimensional questions, the committee takes an evidence-based approach to defining outcomes in populations with substance abuse and mental health problems. This approach recognizes some fundamental commonalities across conditions and levels of severity. In the next section, the committee considers the general outcomes indicators of improvements in health and social functioning, such as improved quality of life and fewer family, employment, legal, and medical problems, that are applicable for each of these conditions. However, the committee also recognizes the value of condition-specific indicators, such as reduced alcohol and drug use and reductions in the symptoms of mental health problems (such as sleep and appetite disturbances as depressive symptoms, or hyperventilation for anxiety).

GENERAL AND SPECIFIC MEASURES OF OUTCOMES

It is important to identify the outcomes that treatment can be expected to bring about (see Table 7.1), including drawing a distinction between short-term and long-term goals. For example, the short-term goals of substance abuse treatment include detoxification, which is the reduction or elimination of alcohol use; the concomitant reduction of the signs, symptoms, and consequences of alcohol use; and a modification in attitude toward drinking behavior leading to a commit-

TABLE 7.1   Substance Abuse-Specific Outcomes Objectives by Level of Treatment

Level of Treatment	Outcomes Measures
Detoxification	Reduction in physiological and emotional instability; lack of serious medical or psychiatric complications; integration and engagement in rehabilitation phase of treatment
Rehabilitation	Maintain changes initiated during detoxification; prevent relapse; develop and practice changes in alcohol and drug use behaviors showing improvements in personal health (medical and psychiatric); improved social functioning (family, friends, employment, and legal areas); engagement in ongoing aftercare
Aftercare and recovery	Maintain changes developed in rehabilitation; continued abstinence and/or levels of use that are nonproblematic; continued improvement in personal health and social functioning

ment to resolution of the problem in the future. The attainment of these goals is a major therapeutic achievement (see Appendix B).

The longer-term outcomes of treatment have to do with the maintenance of these goals over time, for example, whether improvements in drinking or drug use behavior, as well as social functioning, have been accomplished. It is also important to distinguish between outcomes measures that are broadly relevant to mental health-, alcohol-, and drug-related conditions and those that are specific to the different disorders and conditions, characteristics of patients with the disease, and particular levels of treatment. This chapter provides a general framework for the development of performance measures in the context of outcomes research. Appendixes B and C provide more detailed discussions on substance abuse outcomes and mental health outcomes.

Many outcomes studies examining different facets of treatment have been conducted over the past 20 years. However, only recently have managed care organizations been the subject of such studies. The review by McLellan et al. (see Appendix B) indicates that those listed in Table 7.1 are the best supported.

New Approaches in Outcomes Measurement

Outcomes measurement can improve accountability and lead to an improved understanding of which practices are most effective in producing positive outcomes with different kinds of patients (Kane et al., 1995; Appendix C). Basic forms of outcomes assessment include patient satisfaction surveys, ratings by clinicians, and reviews of clinical charts. To standardize the assessment of mental

TABLE 7.2   General Outcome Measures for Substance Abuse and Mental Health Populations

---

- Improvement in employment or vocational status (e.g., return to work or school)
- Improvement in medical status (including morbidity and mortality)
- Improvement in family and social functioning
- Improvement in legal problem status
- Improvement in cognitive functioning
- Improvement in quality of life

---

health outcomes and improve the collection of outcome data, two new approaches show promise.

One approach is the development of clinical outcomes information systems, with most of the information coming directly from patients and clients through questionnaires or other forms of self-report (Ellwood, 1988; Kane et al., 1995). The information can easily be analyzed and assessed in standard formats. Another development in outcomes assessment is the design of modules or standardized sets of validated instruments that combine information from the patient and the clinician to assess the outcomes of treatment (Rost et al., 1992). The emphasis in the development of these modules has been the systematic approach to validating the instruments through field testing, primarily with routine clinical interventions (Smith et al., in press). (See Appendix C for a discussion of research priorities in the measurement of mental health outcomes.)

General Measures of Outcome in Behavioral Health

Many variables are common to substance abuse and mental health treatment (see Table 7.2). Some of the newly developed outcomes information management systems may make outcomes assessment more feasible to achieve (Kane et al., 1995), but the systems can be expensive to implement and to support and currently are more common in the private sector. Still, in behavioral health, it is important to identify and use measures that can be monitored fairly easily, such as functional outcomes of returning to work or school. Organizations that lack the capacity to implement a computerized outcomes information system can develop their own ways to build this basic information into their existing monitoring systems.

There is no evidence that a particular treatment setting (an inpatient, outpatient, or community-based setting, or a hospital) or even treatment modality (group vs. individual counseling) produces better outcomes across all patient groups (see Appendix B). The types of treatment settings (e.g., inpatient, outpatient, medical, and nonmedical settings) do not seem to be as important as the services received (DHHS and NIAAA, 1996; McLellan et al., 1996).

The committee notes that the evidence base across types of disorders and types of treatment approaches is very uneven. For example, for some treatment approaches, the research base is very strong (e.g., cognitive behavioral therapy for depression and methadone maintenance for heroin addiction), whereas for other treatments and types of mental and substance use disorders, research is lacking or equivocal (e.g., 28-day hospital programs for cocaine addiction and medication for childhood depression). Thus, Figure 7.1 provides an analytical framework for the development of an outcomes research base.

One application of this type of framework has been developed using the format of a psychiatric outcomes module (Rost et al., 1992). The module consists of

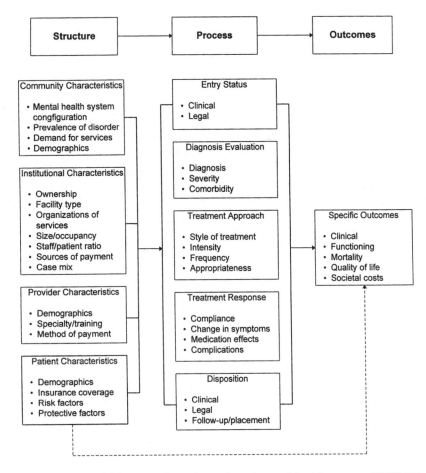

FIGURE 7.1   Model for research on the quality of mental health services. SOURCE: McGlynn et al. (1988). Reprinted by permission of the Blue Cross and Blue Shield Association. Copyright 1988. All rights reserved.

four different forms that are used to assess the types of care, outcomes of care, and patient characteristics associated with different outcomes and types of care. The forms include baseline assessments made by patient and clinician; a follow-up assessment; and a medical record review form. These tools can be used to inform administrative decisions about the quality of care and potentially can influence the decisions made by clinicians, patients, and payers of care (Smith et al., in press).

LINKS AMONG STRUCTURE, PROCESS, AND OUTCOMES

The committee uses a conceptual framework of structure, process, and outcome as characterized in the work of A. Donabedian (1992). The framework provides a multidimensional assessment of quality. From this perspective, outcome can be seen as emanating from important structural and process characteristics.

Within this framework, structure refers to the larger environment—the delivery system, the health care organization and system of delivery, interorganizational networks, communications, lines of authority, and the individual provider agency and staff. It is argued that organizational characteristics have differential effects on outcome (and access and utilization as well) and should be taken into consideration in outcomes research. These variables have not often been examined, especially in the context of managed care organizations. Studies by D'Aunno and Vaughn (1995) and others address the importance of examining the organizational characteristics within managed care organizations as part of outcomes monitoring.

Measuring process is an important part of assessing outcomes. It is necessary to determine which treatment characteristics and modalities have been applied and how they interact with patient characteristics to affect the outcomes. Once the indicators of the process of treatment are associated with outcomes, performance indicators can be more easily monitored by the field.

Within this framework an outcome is defined as the expected achievement. Donabedian (1992) describes outcomes measures as being integrative and reflecting the contributions of all those who provide care, including the contributions of patients to their own care. This includes examining the contributions of organizational and treatment characteristics. Currently, less is known about indicators of outcomes than about structural and process indicators.

Thus, examining outcomes is extremely important at this stage in quality improvement efforts since so little is known about the factors that influence treatment. The relative effectiveness of different approaches needs to be known, and routine monitoring of outcomes in a treatment setting or system of care can be a basis for continuous quality improvement within a treatment delivery organization (Berwick, 1989). A 1990 IOM study argued, "In a larger sense, outcome data provide an ethical justification for purveying treatment and a means of improving its effectiveness. From an ethical standpoint the provision of treatment in the absence of knowledge of results is a questionable procedure" (IOM, 1990b, p. 323).

TABLE 7.3 Performance Indicators Based on Outcomes Research

Performance indicators based on outcomes research require individual client-level data in addition to aggregated, agency-level data. Examples include the following:

1. percentage of individuals who show reductions in symptoms;
2. percentage of patients who show improved functioning;
3. number of patients who return to work;
4. after return to work, average number of consecutive days worked without absences
5. for children and adolescents, number who return to school;
6. for children and adolescents, average number of consecutive days in attendance at school;
7. number of clients returning to earlier levels of treatment;
8. number who are able to live independently in the community;
9. number whose substance-free status is validated through regular breath and urine testing; and
10. number who increase participation in community activities.

PERFORMANCE INDICATORS AS OUTCOMES MEASURES

Table 7.3 lists potential performance indicators as outcomes measures that emerge from the outcomes literature.

In addition to recognizing the importance of these treatment characteristics, studies have demonstrated the efficacies of particular treatment methods, such as coping skills training, cognitive behavioral therapies, methadone treatments at particular dosage levels, naltrexone therapy (naltrexone is a narcotic antagonist), along with counseling or psychotherapy, disulfiram therapy (more commonly known as Antabuse), relapse prevention, community reinforcement approaches, motivational enhancement, and marital or family therapy (DHHS and NIAAA, 1996). Studies have also indicated that treatment intensity, length of stay, and therapist characteristics affect outcomes (Gotheil et al., in press) (see Appendix B).

This is a complex literature based on clinical trials rather than studies conducted in real-world settings. These studies are also often conducted on narrow sets of patient characteristics. Many strategies have not been evaluated across types and severities of substances and patient characteristics, particularly severity, comorbidity, age, ethnicity, and so forth. Clinical management information systems in managed care organizations can be designed to identify the practices that tend to be associated with better outcomes with particular types of patients (Kane et al., 1995).

Differences in outcomes have not been compared for carved-out programs versus treatment integrated with medical services, particularly among populations receiving care in the public and private sectors. Information on such differences is particularly crucial considering the trend toward the use of managed care organizations for public populations across states, as discussed in Chapter 2, Trends in Managed Care. The range of treatment strategies, such as the provision of brief interventions for their prevention role, as well as treatment, should be examined within managed care organizations.

It is better to have a 10-item scale that works reasonably well than a 450-item scale that works perfectly that nobody will use.

Ron Manderscheid
Center for Mental Health Services
Public Workshop, April 18, 1996, Washington, DC

EFFICACY AND EFFECTIVENESS

Donabedian (1990a, b) and others (DHHS and NIAAA, 1996; IOM, 1990c) distinguish between efficacy and effectiveness. *Efficacy* is the assessment of treatment characteristics under ideal clinical conditions. The committee is concerned here with effectiveness as measured in the real world across different types of organizations. *Effectiveness* is improvement in health that is achieved, or that can be expected to be achieved, under the ordinary circumstances of everyday practice. In defining and assessing quality, effectiveness can be more precisely specified as the degree to which the care whose quality is to be assessed attains the level of health improvement that studies of efficacy have established (Donabedian, 1990a, b; Lohr, 1988).

A goal of integration between efficacy and effectiveness research is to conduct basic clinical research on structure, process, and outcomes to provide information on the characteristics associated with particular outcomes for particular client groups. Then, ongoing performance outcomes linked research can assess how well programs are doing, given what should be expected in terms of treatment characteristics and case mix.

For a variety of practical and ethical reasons, however, it is not always possible to conduct highly controlled research to evaluate the impacts of various structural and process components of treatment on outcomes. For this reason, it is desirable for quality assessment systems to begin to incorporate direct measures of client outcomes, in addition to treatment characteristics and client case mix.

OUTCOMES AND QUALITY IMPROVEMENT

The treatment field has been internally and externally motivated to assess performance. Data such as provider ratings and consumer satisfaction report cards are most often used to assess performance. However, some managed care organizations (such as Kaiser Permanente and Group Health Cooperative of Puget Sound) are initiating the use of routine outcomes monitoring systems; for example, they are establishing internal research divisions that perform research on their own internal standards and outcomes or contract with outside entities to conduct evaluations. These are important efforts; of concern is standardization and the comparability of measures and methodologies and the development of performance indicators related to the main predictors of good outcomes.

We encourage programs to use structured instruments. If they don't use structured instruments, we encourage them not to use dichotomous measures, like were you sober or were you not. If they have a measure like that, they don't have anything they can do in terms of program planning.

Tim Slaven
Rehabilitation Accreditation Commission
Public Workshop, May 17, 1996, Irvine, CA

The IOM and Agency for Health Care Policy Research approach to practice guidelines is one in which guidelines based on outcomes research provide the basis of performance measures and accreditation when possible (IOM, 1990c). In the behavioral health field, relatively few practice guidelines have been developed, and they tend not to have a direct relationship to the practice of accreditation. As accreditation organizations begin to focus more on outcomes research, the opportunities and need for further guideline development will increase.

The difficulties in conducting outcomes research within behavioral health care programs are well recognized. Such research is costly and imposes a burden on the programs; it also requires expertise not always available in smaller organizations. To make these efforts truly worthwhile, regardless of whether the research is done internally or externally, what is called for is the use of standardized instruments (with good reliability and validity) by all providers to assess outcomes, standardized instruments measuring content and process of treatment, instruments and methods that are not burdensome (require short response times) or costly, and instruments that are easily interpretable.

CRITERIA FOR EVALUATING OUTCOMES MEASURES

Many of the current indicators assess client satisfaction, which is a reflection of what is easy to measure given the constraints and costs of measuring outcomes.

Although this is an important area, additional emphasis should be placed on improvements in symptoms and functioning. To move the field forward and to begin to develop a process that injects data into a continually improving system, instruments and methods need to be standardized. Comparable, reliable, and valid instruments need to be used, and a system that does not put unreasonable burdens on programs needs to be developed. The existing indicators do not live up to these ideals.

Potential Data Sources for Outcomes Research

The only data source that can truly assess outcomes is client-level outcome information. This usually involves sample surveys of clients, often combined with other indicators assessing the validity of self-reports, such as breath analysis and urinalysis in substance abuse studies. This is the highest standard; however, its high cost and the expertise that is required to carry out the work are limitations to its use (see Appendix B).

Claims data are useful for examining utilization of care, appropriateness of treatment, retreatment rates, costs of treatment, and the cost offsets of care (e.g., money spent on mental health or substance abuse treatment that reduces the costs of treatment in primary care or other specialty care). The strength of claims data is their availability and low cost. Their limitations include a lack of direct measurement of outcomes. That is, claims data include diagnoses, clinical procedures, and numbers of visits, but do not include clinical information such as symptom reductions or behavioral changes experienced by the client or patient.

We need to provide outcome information to purchasers, especially medical cost offset findings, that clarifies it is in the best financial interests of their companies to care about quality because in the long run it will lower costs.

Tom Trabin
Institute for Behavioral Healthcare
Public Workshop, May 17, 1996, Irvine, CA

Admission or discharge forms (and medical records) can be used to assess the severity of a behavioral problem at intake and the provider's assessment of the patient's status at discharge. They also should be available for all programs. Their limitations include a lack of standardization across agencies and among staff within agencies with regard to the data collected and the time frames and definitions that are used. They also do not provide data following treatment discharge; thus, information on the posttreatment retention of the improvement is not available.

Retreatment rates can often be determined through analysis of claims data or admission data collected by managed care organizations. These rates do not reflect outcomes well because they are confounded, for example, by issues related to access and by the dropping of clients from insurance plans.

Accountability for Outcomes

The outcomes field would be improved significantly by developing standardized data that are publicly available. To accomplish this, it is necessary to move away from the focus on client satisfaction-based indicators of outcome to clinically-based indicators of outcome. This is not an easy transition to make. Client satisfaction indicators are easier to develop and to collect than are clinical indicators of outcomes, for reasons that are discussed throughout this chapter. Ideally, the steps should include clinical efficacy trials and then health services effectiveness trials, followed by comparisons of different practice settings, case mix adjustments, and so forth, for the assessment of outcomes in managed care settings. The assessments of outcomes could then become public information, through report cards or through other means.

As the treatment field moves in the direction of accountability for outcomes within programs, several difficult issues need to be addressed. The first has to do with external versus internal monitoring of treatment outcomes. External monitoring brings with it a higher potential for standardization across programs, the input of those with expertise in methodologies, and the credibility that comes from independent evaluations. Internal monitoring lacks those particular strengths, but offers the ability to collect the precise kinds of data most useful to managed care organizations in improving their particular programs.

All of our purchasers, including government and private purchasers, are looking at setting up outcomes and performance measures. Everybody has their own idea about what's a good outcome. Unless there can be some sort of consensus about what that means, I think increasingly we're going to see plans that are going to be ineffective at measuring outcomes.

Michael Jeffrey
William R. Mercer, Inc.
Public Workshop, May 17, 1996, Irvine, CA

A second issue has to do with finding valid measures for outcomes and requiring their collection by programs. Ongoing collaboration between outcomes researchers and clinicians can promote the further development of such measures by combining what is learned from outcomes research and clinical consensus to select those particular indicators that predict good outcomes. Until valid and reliable measures are available, it may be appropriate to accept proxies—indirect measures—of outcomes.

The development of a system of programs that perform their own follow-ups with standardized instruments would complement and strengthen outcomes research. Programs could gauge themselves against the findings related to outcomes and could use the information to develop a means of continual improvement for their systems. Using the standardized information generated by these programs, researchers could isolate the treatment elements that are associated with good treatment outcomes and those elements that become the indicators for improvements in quality.

This can result in the development of a real partnership between research and practice, one that is geared to moving the outcomes measurement field forward and also to generating useful information for program improvement. Anonymity would be provided for programs and organizations in outcomes studies and would provide programs and consumers with applied evaluation information. This information also would be valuable for assessing the cost-effectiveness of various treatment strategies.

It is only by speaking with a single voice, and, more importantly, by talking with data rather than with promises, that the cause of quality will be advanced in the ongoing policy debate about behavioral health care and the role that it is going to play in the health care delivery system in this country.

John Bartlett
American Managed Behavioral Healthcare Association
Public Workshop, April 18, 1996, Washington, DC

SUMMARY

Outcomes research does not yet explicitly identify those performance indicators associated with good outcomes across patient characteristics and types of programs. Furthermore, few outcomes studies are under way that will provide this specific information, especially across types of managed care organizations and patient characteristics, in the near future. At the same time, existing performance indicators do not yet attempt to specify particular treatment characteristics (organizational and clinical) that can be argued to represent a consensus of clinical judgment with regard to their relation to outcomes.

In the committee's view, outcomes research is vitally important to improving the evidence base for treatment effectiveness. However, much needs to be done to standardize outcomes information and to link findings from outcomes research with the development of practice guidelines, performance measures, and accreditation approaches.

REFERENCES

Berwick DM, 1989. Health services research and quality of care: Assignments for the 1990s. *Medical Care* 27(8):763-71.

Burnam MA. In press. Measuring outcomes of care for substance abuse and mental disorders. In: Steinwachs DM, Flynn L, eds. *New Directions for Mental Health Services: Using Outcomes to Improve Care.* San Francisco: Jossey-Bass.

D'Aunno T, Vaughn TE. 1995. An organizational analysis of service patterns in outpatient drug abuse treatment units. *Journal of Substance Abuse* 7(1):27-42.

DHHS (U.S. Department of Health and Human Services) and NIAAA (National Institute on Alcoholism and Alcohol Abuse). 1996. *Final Report: Panel on Effectiveness and Outcome.* Washington, DC: National Advisory Council on Alcohol Abuse and Alcoholism, August.

Donabedian A. 1990a. The seven pillars of quality. *Archives of Pathology and Laboratory Medicine* 114(11):1115-1118.

Donabedian A. 1990b. Quality and cost: Choices and responsibilities. *Journal of Occupational Medicine* 32(12):1167-1172.

Donabedian A. 1992. The role of outcomes in quality assessment and assurance. *Quality Review Bulletin* 18(11):356-360.

Ellwood PM. 1988. Outcomes management: A technology of patient experience. *The New England Journal of Medicine* 318(23):1549-1556.

Gotheil E, McLellan AT, Druley KA. In press. Length of stay, patient severity and treatment outcome: An example from the field of alcoholism. *Journal of Studies on Alcohol.*

Hubbard RL, Marsden ME, Rachal JV, Harwood HJ, Cavanaugh ER, Ginzburg HM. 1989. *Drug Abuse Treatment: A National Study of Treatment Effectiveness.* Chapel Hill, NC: University of North Carolina Press.

IOM (Institute of Medicine). 1990a. *Treating Drug Problems.* Vol. 1. Washington, DC: National Academy Press.

IOM. 1990b. *Broadening the Base of Treatment for Alcohol Problems.* Washington, DC: National Academy Press.

IOM. 1990c. *Clinical Practice Guidelines: Directions for a New Program.* Washington, DC: National Academy Press.

Kane RL, Bartlett J, Potthoff S. 1995. Building an empirically based outcomes information system for managed mental health care. *Psychiatric Services* 46(5):459-462.

Lohr KN. 1988. Outcome measurement: Concepts and questions. *Inquiry* 25:37-50.

Marlatt GA. 1983. The controlled-drinking controversy: A commentary. *American Psychologist* 38:1097-1110.

McGlynn EA, Norquist GS, Wells KB, Sullivan G, Liberman R. 1988. Quality of Care research in mental health: Responding to the challenge. *Inquiry* 25:157-170.

McLellan AT, Weisner C. 1996. Achieving the public health potential of substance abuse treatment: Implications for patient referral, treatment "matching" and outcome evaluation. In: Bickel W, DeGrandpre R, eds. *Drug Policy and Human Nature*. Philadelphia: Wilkins and Wilkins.

McLellan AT, Woody GE, Metzger DS, McKay J, Durell J, Alterman AI, O'Brien CP. 1996. Evaluating the effectiveness of addictions treatments: Reasonable expectations, appropriate comparisons. *The Milbank Quarterly* 74(1):51-85.

Miller WR, Westerberg VS, Waldron HB. 1995. Evaluating alcohol problems. In: Hester RK, Miller WR, eds. *Handbook of Alcoholism Treatment Approaches: Effective Alternatives, Second Edition*. New York, NY: Allyn and Bacon. Pp. 61-88.

Polich JM, Armor DJ, Braiker HB. 1981. *The Course of Alcoholism: Four Years After Treatment*. New York: John Wiley and Sons.

Roizen R. 1987. The great controlled drinking controversy. In: Galanter M, ed. *Recent Developments in Alcoholism*. New York: Plenum. Pp. 245-279.

Rost KM, Smith GR, Burnam MA, Burns BJ. 1992. Measuring the outcomes of care for mental health problems: The case of depressive disorders. *Medical Care* 31:189-200.

Simpson DD, Sells SB, eds. 1990. *Opioid Addiction and Treatment: A 12-Year Follow-up*. Malabar, FL: Robert E. Krieger Publishing Company.

Smith GR, Rost KM, Fischer EP, Burnam MA, Burns BJ. In press. Assessing the effectiveness of mental health care in routine clinical practice: Characteristics, development, and uses of patient outcomes modules. *Evaluation and the Health Professions*.

Tims FM, Fletcher BW, Hubbard RL. 1991. Treatment outcomes for drug abuse clients. In: Pickens RW, Leukefeld CG, Schuster R, eds. *Improving Drug Abuse Treatment*. Washington, DC: U.S. Government Printing Office. Pp. 93-113.

8

Findings and Recommendations

M anaged care is increasingly being used throughout the health care system, and the variability in approaches to managed care is also increasing. Managed care methods are growing at a faster rate in the behavioral health care sector than in the rest of the health care system because of their demonstrated ability to control costs in private health plans and because states are turning to managed care as a strategy to control Medicaid costs. Furthermore, because of this rate of change and because of the unique structure of mental health and substance abuse care (e.g., the existence of substantial publicly paid systems at the state and local levels), ensuring consumer protection and quality improvement are important challenges.

The increased use of managed care approaches in behavioral health care presents both opportunities and risks. For example, the use of case management to coordinate care for individuals with complex conditions and conditions that are costly to treat can improve care and control costs, making it more feasible to improve insurance coverage and to integrate private and public systems. Conversely, managed care approaches that emphasize cost control over quality of care can reduce access to care and can shift the costs of care for needier individuals to an overburdened public system.

Many interested parties are using a variety of methods to protect consumers and improve the quality of care in this environment of rapid change. The charge and focus of this committee are on managed care, although the committee recognizes that other issues such as licensure of practitioners and state inspection and certification of provider agencies play critical roles in consumer protection. Furthermore, in its focus on managed care, the committee has been particularly concerned with two prominent strategies: the accreditation of managed care entities and the use of performance measurement systems. At the same time, it has considered complementary strategies that can aid in consumer protection and quality improvement, such as consumer choice of health plans and better integration of research and practice.

This comprehensive approach is required, in the committee's view, given the interrelated, significant, and complex changes that are under way and the vulnerability of individuals who suffer from serious mental illness and addictions to alcohol and other drugs. The committee believes that there is increasing evidence that treatment for mental health and substance abuse problems is effective and that its effectiveness is generally comparable to that of treatment provided in other areas of medicine. The committee also believes that robust steps to address consumer protection and quality improvements are essential, particularly through improved accreditation and performance measurement systems.

This chapter sets out the committee's recommendations in 12 areas. Each set of recommendations is preceded by the findings that led the committee to make the recommendations. In many cases, the findings build on cross-cutting themes from testimony, research, and the committee's deliberations.

1. STRUCTURE AND FINANCING

Findings

•   Historically, the structure and financing of treatment for mental health and substance abuse problems have been inherently problematic. Insurance coverage for mental health and substance abuse care has been limited and frequently has not covered the prolonged treatment that consumers and families need to address complex problems.

•   The separate publicly-financed health care system creates incentives for the private sector to limit benefits and thus to undermine the basic purpose of insurance; that is, to provide protection for large losses. Costly care is often shifted to the underfinanced public system, a process that is sometimes called "dumping."

•   Traditionally, the health care system inhibits access to care and tolerates poor quality of care, and thus contributes to poor outcomes.

•   The problems of reduced access and increased cost shifting may be aggravated by the use of managed care approaches that focus exclusively on reducing costs.

•   High-quality managed care, however, can provide tools to control costs in an integrated system. For example, case management for high-cost treatment can improve access to appropriate treatment while controlling costs.

•   Existing measures and indicators are inadequate for use as evidence of dumping, skimming, and cost-shifting.

•   Historically, the categorical and fragmented nature of public funding has contributed to fragmentation in service delivery.

- A recent trend is to combine Medicaid funds with other state and local public funds in the financing of public systems.
- The fundamental problems in mental health and substance abuse care cannot be fully addressed without changing the structure and financing of the system and attending to the problem of the separate public and private sectors of care.

Recommendations

1.1   The reform of systems of care financed by states and counties must: (1) recognize current aspects of private health care in those states and counties and (2) consider the design and development of mechanisms to inhibit cost-shifting.

1.2   Payment arrangements that reduce incentives to underserve individuals with behavioral health conditions should be encouraged.

1.3   The reform of state and local systems through the use of managed care should incorporate a recognition of and responsiveness to the unique needs of consumers served by public systems.

1.4   Accreditation organizations, when appropriate, and purchasers should develop criteria and guidelines that: (1) recognize and measure dumping, skimming, and cost-shifting; and (2) specify rewards for organizations, groups, and individuals that provide appropriate care and penalties for those that do not.

1.5   Purchasers should ensure continuity of care for consumers when managed care contracts are awarded to different provider organizations.

2. ACCREDITATION

Findings

- The wide array of consumer and quality protections includes accreditation, performance measurement, clinical practice guidelines, state licensure, and contract requirements. Some of these functions overlap.
- Accreditation of managed care plans by independent national bodies is an important and powerful tool of consumer protection and quality improvement in health care and behavioral health care.
- Accreditation of service delivery organizations, such as hospitals, is well developed, but accreditation of managed care plans is in its infancy.
- In the field of managed behavioral health care, accreditation alone is not sufficient to guarantee high-quality care.
- Currently, multiple competing organizations perform measurement, reporting, and accreditation functions in the health and behavioral health care sectors. In the behavioral health care area, the Rehabilitation Accreditation Commission (CARF), Council on Accreditation of Services for Families and Children (COA), Joint Commission on Accreditation of Healthcare Organizations (JCAHO), National Committee for Quality Assurance (NCQA), and Utilization

Review Accreditation Commission (URAC) all play roles in accrediting managed care plans that cover mental health and substance abuse care. The American Managed Behavioral Healthcare Association, NCQA, the Substance Abuse and Mental Health Services Administration (SAMHSA), and a number of corporate buyers (e.g., Digital Equipment Corporation) have also developed performance rating systems.

- Accreditation organizations compete for accreditation business on the basis of their credibility with payers, providers, and consumers.
- Benefits consultants and other consultants are advising corporate purchasers and state agencies on procurement, contracting, and other aspects of accountability. This is a significant new industry.
- Data collection is an intricate part of the assessment of quality of care. Many of the data currently collected are internal, not validated by external sources, and may not be relevant to outcomes of care.
- Accreditation tends to focus on measures of the structure and process of care rather than on measures of clinical outcomes. However, examples of movement in the direction of outcome measurement can be found, such as consumer satisfaction surveys and measures of clinical appropriateness.
- Variability exists in utilization review (a formal assessment of the necessity for services and their appropriateness and efficiency), which can be done on a prospective (precertification), concurrent, or retrospective basis.
- In public systems of mental health and substance abuse care, uninsured and publicly insured individuals can often access a greater selection and intensity of benefits for behavioral health care than are available to individuals with private insurance.
- Federal and state government agencies sometimes require accreditation and specify which accreditation organization's standards will be accepted. This process is known as granting an accreditation organization "deemed status." Thus, the organization is "deemed" to act in the public interest. Deeming is not done extensively in health care but is common in other sectors, such as in the construction industry.
- Quality improvement methods have great potential but are still in preliminary stages for mental health and substance abuse services. Existing behavioral health performance measurement systems have used different strategies in their development, with varying degrees of consumer involvement.

Recommendations

Monitoring Quality of Care

2.1   Public and private purchasers, consumers, providers, practitioners, behavioral health care plans, and accreditation organizations should continue to monitor and assess the quality of care in the following ways:

2.1.1   Quality improvement should be a priority, and principles and methods of improving quality should be adopted.

2.1.2   Accreditation and review processes must be reliable and valid and must be continuously reviewed and improved.

2.1.3   Domains relevant to the effective treatment and prevention of behavioral health problems must be emphasized in accreditation processes. These include practitioner training, consumer education, improvements in consumer self-care, and the presence of a continuum of services, including wraparound services such as housing assistance, child care, and transportation.

2.1.4   Accreditation processes must focus on areas of managed care in which there may be a risk of quality problems: (1) variability in utilization review; (2) inconsistent or inappropriate precertification processes; (3) vulnerable groups and those who are unfamiliar with managed care processes; and (4) conditions that occur frequently and are treated by many practitioners, giving opportunities for variation in treatment practices.

2.1.5   Performance measures must be relevant to treatment processes and outcomes.

2.1.6   Data must have demonstrable integrity. External, independent audits can help to validate data quality.

2.1.7   Stakeholder consensus and consumer satisfaction measures must be included in the tools used to monitor quality of care.

2.1.8   Outcomes measures should increasingly be based on evidence from research.

Contracting

2.2   Quality of care should be clearly addressed in contracts between purchasers and providers.

2.2.1   When plans contract or subcontract for the management and delivery of behavioral health care services (e.g., health maintenance organizations contracting with carved-out managed behavioral health care firms), purchasers can benefit from independent audits of the contractor regarding the level of adherence to prespecified standards of performance with respect to quality.

2.2.2   Purchasers can benefit from carefully constructed contract language to ensure the quality, accessibility, and effectiveness of behavioral health plans. Contracts should also specify the ways in which the quality and effectiveness standards will be monitored and enforced, including conditions for applying positive incentives for meeting or exceeding the standards and penalties for substandard performance.

Role of the Federal Government

2.3   The federal government should play a role in consumer protection in managed care by:

2.3.1   Promoting the improvement and use of performance measures for managed care.

2.3.2   Monitoring and studying the use and effectiveness of quality assurance, accreditation, performance measures, and outcomes measurements.

2.3.3   Establishing minimum standards for accreditation organizations to achieve deemed status (i.e., when the government, in its role as purchaser of managed care services, accepts accreditation as a measure of adequate quality and consumer protection).

Role of State Governments

2.4   The role of state governments in consumer protection should include the following:

2.4.1   Support the development of consumer protection standards for managed behavioral health care by state mental health and substance abuse agencies, state Medicaid agencies, state insurance departments, state licensing boards, state hospitals, and state child welfare agencies. State consumer groups, such as the chapters of the National Mental Health Association (NMHA), National Depressive and Manic Depressive Association (NDMDA), National Association for Research on Schizophrenia and Depression (NARSD), and National Alliance for the Mentally Ill (NAMI), should be included in the development of standards.

2.4.2   Maintain the minimum necessary regulatory standards, including the use of accreditation, to assure consumer protection while encouraging innovations in the delivery of care.

2.4.3   Consider offering deemed status to specific accreditation organizations that meet state-defined standards for quality of managed behavioral health care services.

Roles of All Levels of Government

2.5   Both federal and state governments should:

2.5.1   Encourage the development of report cards or other similar materials to help inform consumers and families about specific plans and the quality of care.

2.5.2   Include all stakeholders (accreditation organizations, employers, state agencies, consumers, families, providers, and practitioners) in the development, implementation, and use of standards.

Provider Inclusion

2.6   Because managed care methods are increasingly applied to public systems, accreditation bodies and managed care plans should evaluate the inclusion of a variety of types of practitioners, including substance abuse counselors and mental health workers, in provider panels; collect information on practitioner effectiveness; and remove any practitioners from networks only for performance reasons (e.g., poor outcomes and poor consumer satisfaction).

2.6.1 The Substance Abuse and Mental Health Services Administration (SAMHSA), Agency for Health Care Policy and Research (AHCPR), Health Resources and Services Administration (HRSA), and National Institutes of Health (NIH) (National Institute on Alcohol Abuse and Alcoholism [NIAAA], National Institute on Drug Abuse [NIDA], and National Institute of Mental Health [NIMH]) should cosponsor research to evaluate the components of treatment that are most effective in providing behavioral health care, including strategies used by psychiatrists, psychologists, social workers, counselors, and primary care practitioners.

2.6.2 The Substance Abuse and Mental Health Services Administration (SAMHSA), Agency for Health Care Policy and Research (AHCPR), Health Resources and Services Administration (HRSA), and National Institutes of Health (NIH) (National Institute on Alcohol Abuse and Alcoholism [NIAAA], National Institute of Drug Abuse [NIDA], and National Institute of Mental Health [NIMH]) should cosponsor research to evaluate the cost-effectiveness of using different practitioner types to provide behavioral health care, including individual psychiatrists, psychologists, social workers, counselors, primary care practitioners, and teams with different practitioner combinations.

3. CONSUMER INVOLVEMENT

Findings

- Individuals who have been treated for severe mental health problems are most often referred to as "consumers," both by the individuals themselves and by the organizations that represent them.
- Consumers and families strongly desire to participate fully in decision-making in treatment, setting behavioral health care standards, and developing performance measures.
- Public behavioral health service systems make use of self-help groups, consumer-operated services, and experientially trained counselors (e.g., mental health workers and substance abuse counselors) as service providers. These practices are both valuable and highly valued in these systems because they help to support consumers and, for example, to assist with medication compliance.
- Quality measures are being developed by organizations with various degrees of involvement by consumers and consumer groups. Among consumers, the report card developed by the Center for Mental Health Services (CMHS) is viewed as having the most consumer involvement.

Recommendations

3.1   Health care purchasers must be responsive to consumers and families and should develop means of ensuring their meaningful participation in treatment decisions, measurement of satisfaction, and measurement of treatment effectiveness.

3.2   Accreditation bodies should evaluate the extent of inclusion of consumers and families in treatment decisions and program planning.

3.3   The activities that are used to develop and review quality measures should include all stakeholders, including consumers, families, practitioners, and researchers.

4. CULTURAL COMPETENCE

Findings

•   Racial and ethnic minorities frequently lack access to culturally appropriate care.

•   In the effort to create smaller and more efficient provider networks, there is a risk of eliminating providers and groups who have special expertise with different cultures and different healing practices (e.g., Afrocentric counseling and Spanish-speaking services, sweat lodges for Native Americans, and American Sign Language services for individuals who are deaf).

•   Often, the reason given for exclusion of cultural practices is that accepted evidence of effectiveness does not exist. The committee observes, however, that controlled trials or other outcomes assessments have not been done for many, if not most, medical treatments.

Recommendations

4.1   Health plans and programs should be responsive to community demographics and to the cultural needs of the populations that they serve.

4.2   Practitioners of alternative and innovative treatments without an accepted research base should not arbitrarily be excluded from health plans. If these treatments are used, their effectiveness should be studied so that standards of quality improvement can be developed.

4.3   Health plans should have an explicit mechanism for evaluating new and innovative techniques and types of practitioners.

5. SPECIAL POPULATIONS

Findings

- People with disabilities, such as individuals who are deaf, hard of hearing, or blind, who use wheelchairs, or who have had traumatic brain injury, frequently lack access to care that is appropriate.
- Individuals who have child care responsibilities, most of whom are women, often have barriers to participating in treatment.
- Individuals who have co-occurring substance abuse and mental health problems need coordinated care to maintain their recovery.

Recommendations

5.1   Research is needed to identify incentives for plans to serve vulnerable populations. The Substance Abuse and Mental Health Services Administration (SAMHSA) should work with other federal agencies to develop a plan to conduct such research.

5.2   Plans that serve distinct populations should measure and evaluate the needs of those groups through reviews of research literature, consumer surveys, and other appropriate mechanisms.

5.3   All plans should meet the same core standards. Supplemental standards can be developed for special populations, whether they are in stand-alone programs or in mainstream plans, for example, for a child of an employed person with family coverage.

6. RESEARCH

Findings

- Health services research stimulates collaboration among providers, researchers, and managed care organizations and can facilitate the development of valid and useful measures of treatment processes and outcomes through such collaborations.
- Research and practice interact too infrequently, and few incentives exist for collaboration among researchers, practitioners, and policymakers.
- Outcomes research is often unresponsive to emerging problems in clinical practice and also rarely provides direction for accreditation and quality improvement efforts.
- The federal government plays a key role in the support of health services research and thus in the development of the necessary knowledge base for improving the quality of behavioral health care.

Recommendations

6.1 The committee recommends continued development of collaborative health services research in substance abuse and mental health, and encourages the Agency for Health Care Policy and Research (AHCPR), Centers for Disease Control and Prevention (CDC), Health Resources and Services Administration (HRSA), National Institutes of Health (NIH) (National Institute on Alcohol Abuse and Alcoholism [NIAAA], National Institute on Drug Abuse [NIDA], and the National Institute of Mental Health [NIMH]), and Substance Abuse and Mental Health Services Administration (SAMHSA) to maintain, to evaluate, and, where necessary, to expand programs and initiatives that support collaborative health services research.

6.2 The agencies mentioned above should support further research on the effectiveness of different treatment strategies for a variety of practitioner types and for consumers with different needs.

6.3 Researchers should become more involved in studies carried out in managed care organizations and community-based settings and in other clinical outcomes research used to develop standards and performance measures.

7. WORKPLACE

Findings

- Society and individual workers need safe and supportive work environments.
- The federal government has responded through the passage of legislation (e.g., the Family and Medical Leave Act and the Americans with Disabilities Act) and regulations concerning safety and other standards.
- The workplace environment provides an excellent arena in which to address behavioral health problems.

Recommendations

7.1 Employers should investigate the benefits of wellness activities, employee assistance programs, and health risk reduction initiatives that enhance prevention, early intervention, access, and treatment adherence for health and behavioral health problems.

7.2 The Substance Abuse and Mental Health Services Administration (SAMHSA) should identify models of successful behavioral health programs in the workplace and increase public awareness of these models.

8. WRAPAROUND SERVICES

Findings

- For long-term recovery to be sustained, the social aspects of consumers' lives must be addressed as part of the behavioral health care provided.
- Medical and managed care models often do not take these rehabilitative and support services into account. In the substance abuse field, these are known as wraparound services and in the mental health field they are also known as enabling services.
- Some symptoms of mental illness and substance abuse—such as severe anxiety and depression, active psychosis, and substance abuse withdrawal—interfere with social judgment and functioning.

Recommendations

8.1 Further research is needed to prioritize the essential components of a treatment regimen that can address adequately the complex behavioral aspects of recovery from alcoholism and other drug addictions.

8.2 To maximize full functioning for individuals with severe and persistent mental illness, and to optimize conditions supporting recovery for individuals with chronic substance abuse problems, wraparound services such as social welfare, housing, vocational, and rehabilitative services should be available and should be coordinated.

8.3 For children and adolescents with severe emotional disturbances, educational and home environment-family support services should be coordinated and integrated with mental health care.

8.4 Accreditation systems must address the social and rehabilitative aspects as well as the medical aspects of comprehensive treatment for addiction and severe and persistent mental illness.

9. CHILDREN AND ADOLESCENTS

Findings

- Services for children and adolescents are fragmented across many different agencies, such as mental health, child abuse and neglect, and juvenile justice.
- Many treatment models focus on a high-risk child or adolescent and do not involve the family or other caretakers.
- Developmentally appropriate, comprehensive models for intervention and treatment for adolescents are not well-defined or applied in the current public and private systems.

- The needs of many high-risk youth are unmet because traditional systems do not focus on this population.
- Prevention and treatment programs for mental health and substance abuse problems are not adequately linked.

Recommendations

9.1   The Substance Abuse and Mental Health Services Administration (SAMHSA), National Institutes of Health (NIH) (National Institute on Alcoholism and Alcohol Abuse [NIAAA], National Institute on Drug Abuse [NIDA], and National Institute of Mental Health [NIMH]), and the Health Resources and Services Administration (HRSA) should identify exemplary models of coordinated systems of care for children and adolescents.

9.2   The Substance Abuse and Mental Health Services Administration (SAMHSA), National Institutes of Health (NIH) (National Institute on Alcoholism and Alcohol Abuse [NIAAA], National Institute on Drug Abuse [NIDA], and National Institute of Mental Health [NIMH]), and the Health Research and Services Administration (HRSA) should identify exemplary models of linking behavioral health treatment and prevention programs for children and adolescents to address suicide, substance abuse, and other areas.

9.3   The Substance Abuse and Mental Health Services Administration (SAMHSA), National Institutes of Health (NIH) (National Institute on Alcoholism and Alcohol Abuse [NIAAA], National Institute on Drug Abuse [NIDA], and National Institute of Mental Health [NIMH]), and the Health Resources and Services Administration (HRSA) should support research to identify the elements of developmentally appropriate treatment that should be available to adolescents who are abusing alcohol or drugs or who have mental health problems.

9.4   The public and private systems must make efforts to develop service capabilities to meet the needs of adolescents who are abusing alcohol or drugs and adolescents who have mental health problems.

10. CLINICAL PRACTICE GUIDELINES

Findings

- Practice guidelines are developed by professional organizations, managed care organizations, and other groups. The development of guidelines is not always systematic, and guidelines are not always linked to empirical findings. Little or no information is available on successful strategies for implementing guidelines.
- Accreditation tends to measure whether plans or managed care organizations have guidelines in place and does not address the quality of the guidelines

used by plans or organizations, or the extent to which care is actually monitored and changed according to those guidelines.

Recommendations

10.1 The development of clinical practice guidelines should be linked to outcomes research, performance standards, and accreditation.

10.2 The Agency for Health Care Policy and Research (AHCPR), Substance Abuse and Mental Health Services Administration (SAMHSA), and other agencies and organizations that develop guidelines should sponsor additional research that examines the successful implementation of guidelines and identifies successful implementation models.

10.3 Practitioners and consumers should be included in the development of practice guidelines.

11. PRIMARY CARE

Findings

- Many individuals (10 to 20 percent of the population) consult primary care physicians for behavioral health problems.
- Responsibility for behavioral health care is frequently divided between primary and specialty settings, which are not well integrated, and this division of responsibility results in poor coordination of care.
- Few guidelines exist for behavioral health treatment in primary care.
- Some individuals may be treated more successfully in specialty settings than in primary care settings.

Recommendations

11.1 This committee endorses the view of the Institute of Medicine (IOM) Committee on the Future of Primary Care, which recommended "the reduction of financial and organizational disincentives for the expanded role of primary care in the provision of mental health services" and "the development and evaluation of collaborative care models that integrate primary care and mental health services more effectively. These models should involve both primary care clinicians and mental health professionals" (IOM, 1996, p. 137).

11.2 This committee recommends that the above recommendation include alcohol and other drug abuse problems as a defined area of expertise.

12. ETHICAL CONCERNS

Findings

- The field of health care ethics embodies ethical principles that address risks in the areas of autonomy, access, informed consent, practitioner-patient relationships, and confidentiality.
- Ethical challenges and problems exist in both the traditional fee-for-service system and in the rapidly developing managed care system, although the incentives, risks, and oversight strategies differ in the two settings.
- Cultural competence and sensitivity are ethical issues.

Recommendations

12.1 Managed care organizations should be able to demonstrate that they recognize and have concern for the ethical risks created by managed care systems. Additionally, they should substantiate the use of safeguards that protect and maintain ethical standards and practices. These would include the following:

- a clear description of a plan, its benefits, and grievance procedures,
- accessible and responsive grievance, complaint, and appeals procedures,
- effective strategies to maintain confidentiality while meeting the needs of practitioners to coordinate care,
- culturally appropriate and gender-specific service practitioners in the network,
- consumer surveys and measures of consumer satisfaction,
- consumer representation on policy development and grievance resolution,
- continuous improvement protocols to promote better outcomes, and
- no contractual or other limitations for physicians and other practitioners concerning the discussion of clinically appropriate treatment options with patients and families.

12.2 A careful review of ethical issues in various settings, for example, managed care organizations, networks, and fee-for-service settings, is needed. The Substance Abuse and Mental Health Services Administration (SAMHSA), Health Care Financing Agency (HCFA), and Agency for Health Care Policy and Research (AHCPR) should develop a plan to examine ethical issues.

REFERENCE

IOM (Institute of Medicine). 1996. *Primary Care: America's Health in a New Era.* Washington, DC: National Academy Press.

Glossary

Access   The extent to which an individual who needs care and services is able to receive them. Ease of access depends on several factors, including insurance coverage, availability and location of appropriate care and services, transportation, hours of operation, and cultural factors, including languages and cultural appropriateness.

Accreditation   An official decision made by a recognized organization that a health care plan, network, or other delivery system complies with applicable standards.

Adverse selection   Individuals enrolling in health plans tend to select plans that will best suit their expected health care needs, and individuals with a greater chance of needing particular kinds of care will select health care plans with generous benefits for those services. Health plans do not know who those individuals are, so the plans have an incentive to strictly limit coverage and access to those services and thus avoid drawing an adverse selection of the enrolled population.

Appropriateness   The extent to which a particular procedure, treatment, test, or service is clearly indicated, is not excessive, is adequate in quantity, and is provided in the setting best suited to a patient's or member's needs (NCQA, 1995, p. 45).

Autonomy   A principle in biomedical ethics that refers to having respect for every individual's independence and freedom of choice. This is usually expressed as the need to obtain informed consent from an individual or his or her representatives before undertaking treatment.

Behavioral health   Managed care term that applies to the assessment and treatment of problems related to mental health and substance abuse. Substance abuse includes abuse of alcohol and other drugs.

Benchmark   For a particular indicator or performance goal, the industry measure of best performance. The benchmarking process identifies the best performance in the industry (health care or non-health care) for a particular process or outcome, determines how that performance is achieved, and applies the lessons learned to improve performance (NCQA, 1995, p. 45).

Capitation   A fixed rate of payment to cover a specified set of health services. The rate is usually provided on a per-member per-month basis (IOM, 1989, p. 288).

Carve-out   A decision to purchase separately a service that is typically a part of an indemnity or health maintenance organization plan. For example, a health maintenance organization may "carve out" the behavioral health benefit and select a specialized vendor to supply these services on a standalone basis (United HealthCare Corporation, 1994, p. 16).

Consumer   Any individual who does or could receive health care or services. Includes other more specialized terms, such as beneficiary, client, customer, eligible member, recipient, or patient.

Co-occurring disorders   Individuals who have more than one disorder, for example, a depressed person who also is an alcoholic. Usually, the term is used to refer to a combination of mental health and substance abuse problems, but it can also refer to individuals who have a behavioral health diagnosis as well as a medical diagnosis or disability.

Cost-sharing   The part of health expenses that are paid by the person who receives services, including deductibles and copayments.

Credentialing   The process of assessing and validating the qualifications of a licensed independent practitioner to provide member services in a health care network or its components. The determination is based on an evaluation of the individual's current license, education, training, experience, current competence, and ability to perform privileges requested. The credentialing process is the basis for making appointments to the panel or staff of the health care network and its components. It also provides information for the process of granting clinical privileges to licensed independent practitioners (based on JCAHO, 1996, p. 406).

Cultural comptence   Actions that indicate an awareness and acceptance of the importance of addressing cultural factors while providing care; ability to meet the needs of clients and patients from diverse backgrounds.

Deemed status   A method of quality assurance in which public agencies hold an organization accountable to standards developed by, for example, a nonprofit accreditation organization. For example, Health Care Financing Administration requires hospitals to conform to the Joint Commission on Accreditation of Healthcare Organizations standards to receive Medicare reimbursement.

Dual diagnosis   *See Co-occurring disorder.*

Indicator   A defined, measurable variable used to monitor the quality or appropriateness of an important aspect of patient care. Indicators can be activities, events, occurrences, or outcomes for which data can be collected to allow comparison with a threshold, a benchmark, or prior performance (NCQA, 1995, p. 47, from the JCAHO *Managed Care Standards Manual,* 1989, p. 56).

Integrated delivery system   System of providers and diverse organizations working collaboratively to coordinate a full range of care and services within a community.

Managed behavioral health care   Any of a variety of strategies to control behavioral health (i.e., mental health and substance abuse) costs while ensuring quality care and appropriate utilization. Cost-containment and quality assurance methods include the formation of preferred provider networks, gatekeeping (or precertification), case management, relapse prevention, retrospective review, claims payment, and others. In many health plans, behavioral health care is separated from care available in the rest of the health plan for the separate management of costs and quality of care (EAPA, 1996, p. 19).

Managed care   Arrangements for health care delivery and financing that are designed to provide appropriate, effective, and efficient health care through organized relationships with providers. Includes formal programs for ongoing quality assurance and utilization review, financial incentives for covered members to use the plan's providers, and financial incentives for providers to contain costs.

Outcome   Results or effects achieved through a given service or procedure.

Outcomes research   Studies that measure the effects of care or services.

Performance goals   The desired level of achievement of standards of care or service. These may be expressed as desired minimum performance levels (thresholds), industry best performance (benchmarks), or the permitted variance from the standard. Performance goals usually are not static but change as performance improves and/or the standard of care is refined (NCQA, 1995, p. 47).

Performance measure(s)   Methods or instruments to estimate or monitor the extent to which the actions of a health care practitioner or provider conform to practice guidelines, medical review criteria, or standards of quality (IOM, 1990a, p. 50).

Practice guidelines   Systematically developed statements to standardize care and to assist practitioner and patient decisions about the appropriate health care for specific circumstances. Practice guidelines are usually developed through a process that combines scientific evidence of effectiveness with expert opinion. Practice guidelines are also referred to as clinical criteria, practice parameters, protocols, algorithms, review criteria, preferred practice patterns, and guidelines.

Privileging   The process of authorizing by an appropriate authority (e.g., a governing body, where one exists) in a component of a health care network or by the network itself a practitioner to provide specific patient care services in the component or the network, as appropriate, within defined limits, on the basis of an individual practitioner's license, education, training, experience, competence, ability to perform assigned tasks, and judgment (JCAHO, 1996, p. 411).

Quality assessment   The measurement of the technical and interpersonal aspects of health care and the outcomes of that care (IOM,1990b, p. 45, based on IOM, 1989, p. 291).

Quality assurance   A systematic and objective approach to improving the quality and appropriateness of medical care and other services. Includes a formal set of activities to review, assess, and monitor care and to ensure that identified problems are addressed appropriately.

Quality improvement A set of techniques for continuous study and improvement of the processes of delivering health care services and products to meet the needs and expectations of the customers of those services and products. It has three basic elements: customer knowledge, a focus on processes of health care delivery, and statistical approaches that aim to reduce variations in those processes (IOM, 1990b, p. 46).

Quality of care The degree to which health services for individuals and populations increase the likelihood of desired health outcomes and are consistent with current professional knowledge (IOM, 1990b, p. 4). NOTE: Adopted by National Committee for Quality Assurance and Joint Commission on Accreditation of Healthcare Organizations.

Recovery A term used by some individuals and groups to refer to the process of making a commitment to change personal behaviors in order to overcome addiction. Thus, an individual who has chosen to make changes is "in recovery."

Report card on health care An emerging tool that can be used by policy makers and health health care purchasers, such as employers, government bodies, employer coalitions, and consumers, to compare and understand the actual performance of health plans. The tool provides health plan performance data in major areas of accountability, such as health care quality and utilization, consumer satisfaction, administrative efficiencies and financial stability, and cost control (United HealthCare Corporation, 1994, p. 64).

Risk sharing The process of establishing financial arrangements that share the financial risk of providing care among providers, payers, and those who use the services.

Standard(s) Authoritative statements of (1) minimum level of acceptable performance or results, (2) excellent levels of performance or results, or (3) the range of acceptable performance or results (IOM, 1990a).

Utilization The extent to which eligible individuals use a program or receive a service or group of services over a specified period of time.

Utilization management A set of techniques used by or on behalf of purchasers of health benefits to manage health care costs by influencing the decisions about patient care made by providers, payers, and patients themselves. Includes techniques such as prior authorization, concurrent review, retrospective review, and case management.

Utilization review   A formal assessment of the medical necessity, efficiency, or appropriateness of health care services and treatment plans on a prospective, concurrent, or retrospective basis (United HealthCare Corporation, 1994, p. 74).

REFERENCES

EAPA (Employee Assistance Professional Association). 1995. *Glossary of Employee Assistance Terminology*. Arlington, VA: Employee Assistance Professional Association, Inc.

IOM (Institute of Medicine). 1989. *Controlling Costs and Changing Patient Care: The Role of Utilization Management*. Washington, DC: National Academy Press.

IOM. 1990a. *Clinical Practice Guidelines: Directions for a New Program*. Washington, DC: National Academy Press.

IOM. 1990b. *Medicare: A Strategy for Quality Assurance*. Washington, DC: National Academy Press.

JCAHO (Joint Commission on Accreditation of Healthcare Organizations). 1989. *Managed Care Standards Manual*. Chicago, IL: Joint Commission on Accreditation of Healthcare Organizations.

JCAHO. 1996. *1996 Comprehensive Accreditation Manual for Health Care Networks*. Chicago, IL: Joint Commission on Accreditation of Healthcare Organizations.

NCQA. (National Committee for Quality Assurance). 1995. *Standards for Accreditation, 1995*. Washington, DC: National Committee for Quality Assurance.

United HealthCare Corporation. 1994. *The Managed Care Resource: The Language of Managed Health Care and Organized Health Care Systems*. Minneapolis, MN: United HealthCare Corporation.

Appendixes

A

Committee Biographies

JEROME H. GROSSMAN, MD, *Chair* (IOM), is the President and Chief Executive Officer of Health Quality LLC, a medical information management company in Boston, and a Scholar-in-Residence at the Institute of Medicine. He is the former Chairman and Chief Executive Officer of the New England Medical Center and Professor of Medicine at Tufts University, School of Medicine. Dr. Grossman has been active in the HMO movement, as an original staff member of Harvard Community Health Plan and a founder of the Tufts Associated Health Plan. Nationally Dr. Grossman has held several leadership positions in the Association of American Medical Colleges, the Council of Teaching Hospitals, the Academic Medical Center Consortium, and the Institute of Medicine. In 1988 he founded the Health Institute at New England Medical Center to pursue research and development of initiatives to improve the organization and financing of medical care to achieve better health outcomes. Dr. Grossman serves as Trustee/Director for several corporations and institutions, including Massachusetts Institute of Technology, Massachusetts Business Roundtable, and Arthur D. Little, Inc. In 1989, he chaired the IOM Committee on Utilization Management by Third Parties, and in 1990, he chaired the IOM Committee to Advise the Public Health Service on Clinical Practice Guidelines.

ROBERT BOORSTIN has served as Senior Advisor to Secretary of State Warren Christopher since November 1995. From 1994 to 1995, Mr. Boorstin served as Senior Director for Speechwriting at the National Security Council, was responsible for writing and editing President Clinton's remarks on foreign policy, and accompanied the President on international trips. Prior to that position, he served as Special Assistant to the President for Policy Coordination and helped develop communications strategy for the Clinton Administration's health care reform efforts. As Deputy Communications Director for the Clinton/Gore campaign, Mr. Boorstin oversaw the policy and research staffs and the production of campaign documents, including the candidates' agenda, *Putting People First*. Mr. Boorstin has worked with several national consumer groups and has been active in speaking about mental health consumer issues since 1987, when he was diagnosed with manic depressive illness. He received his undergraduate degree in history from Harvard and did graduate work at King's College, Cambridge. Subsequently, he worked as a journalist for *The New York Times* and contributed to *Newsweek, The Washington Post*, and WBGH public television. Mr. Boorstin also founded and directed a New York City branch of the National Manic Depressive Association, which counsels people with mental illness and their families.

JOHN J. BURKE is Executive Vice President for Workplace Services at Value Behavioral Health, in Falls Church, Virginia. Mr. Burke is the former President of Burke-Taylor Associates, the largest EAP in the Southeast. He has experience in Employee Assistance Programs (EAP) delivery, management and credentialing and has served as National Chair of the Employee Assistance Certification Commission. Mr. Burke has been a member of several committees for the National Employee Assistance Professionals Association and was a Co-Chairman of the Mental Health and Substance Abuse Committee for the North Carolina Health Planning Commission. Mr. Burke is a Certified Employee Assistance Professional (CEAP).

M. AUDREY BURNAM, PhD, is Senior Behavioral Scientist for the RAND Corporation in Santa Monica, California. She has been actively involved in mental health and substance abuse research for over 15 years, directing studies on the epidemiology of mental health and substance abuse problems, and on delivery of services for persons with these problems. She is a Co-Director of the Drug Policy Research Center at RAND, and a Visiting Researcher to the Department of Psychiatry at the University of Arkansas for Medical Sciences. Her doctoral degree is in social psychology, and she completed post-doctoral training in mental health epidemiology and evaluation methods.

BARBARA CIMAGLIO is Director of the Illinois Department of Alcoholism and Substance Abuse, and a member of the Board of Directors for the National Association of State Alcohol and Drug Abuse Directors (NASADAD). Her expertise is in state administration of substance abuse services and community-based care. She is a former board member of the National Prevention Network and the Illinois Women's Substance Abuse Coalition and several other organizations. Ms. Cimaglio is a clinically certified substance abuse counselor.

MOLLY JOEL COYE, MD, MPH (IOM), is Executive Vice President for Strategic Development at Healthdesk Corporation in Berkeley, California. Previously, she was Senior Vice President of Clinical Operations for the Good Samaritan Health System, Health Dimensions Incorporated, in San Jose, California. From 1991-93, Dr. Coye was the Director of the California Department of Health Services, where she directed MediCal's transition to managed care. She also was the Commissioner of Health in New Jersey and has served on the Board of Directors of the Association of State and Territorial Health Officials (ASTHO). Currently, Dr. Coye is on the Board of Directors for UMQC, which certifies managed care providers. Her past academic appointments include professor on the clinical faculty in the Department of Community Health at the University of California at Davis, Head of the Division of Public Health at the Johns Hopkins University of School of Hygiene and Public Health, and visiting professor at the UCLA School of Public Health. Dr. Coye is a former Medical Investigative Officer (Commissioned Corps) for the National Institute for Occupational Safety and Health.

LYNNE DeGRANDE, ACSW, CEAP, is Senior Consultant to the Salaried Employee Assistance Program at General Motors Corporation. She was involved in the development and implementation of General Motors' EAP, where she interacts with managed care firms providing services to GM enrollees. Ms. DeGrande has more than 20 years administrative and clinical experience developing and managing behavioral health programs in corporate, industrial and health care settings. She is a member of the Corporate Advisory Board for the Washington Business Group on Health and serves on the Bio-Ethics Committee of St. John's Hospital in Detroit. Ms. DeGrande is a member of the Academy of Certified Social Workers, a Certified Employee Assistance Professional, and a Substance Abuse Professional with the Employee Assistance Professional Association (EAPA).

RICHARD FRANK, PhD, is Professor of Health Economics at the Department of Health Care Policy at Harvard Medical School, and a Research Associate with the National Bureau of Economic Research in Cambridge, Massachusetts. Dr. Frank is a former professor with the Department of Health Policy at the Johns Hopkins University School of Hygiene and Public Health. He has published extensively on cost-effectiveness and costs of mental health/ substance abuse treatment, the design of mental health benefits plans, health care financing, and the organization and delivery of health services. Dr. Frank was a staff member of the President's Task Force on Health Care Reform and a Commissioner for the Maryland Health Services Cost Review Commission.

JOHN E. FRANKLIN, MD, is an Associate Professor in the Department of Psychiatry and Behavioral Sciences at Northwestern University Medical School, and the Medical Director for the Consultation Liaison Service at Northwestern's Stone Institute of Psychiatry. He is a member of the Executive Committee and the Utilization Review Committee of the Department of Psychiatry and has many teaching responsibilities for medical students and residents. Dr. Franklin received an award for teaching excellence in 1986-87 when he was on the faculty of the New Jersey Medical School. He has served as a consultant to the National Institute of Drug Abuse and currently is Principal Investigator for an grant on homelessness. Dr. Franklin is a member of the American Academy on Addiction Psychiatry.

MICHAEL F. HOGAN, PhD, has been the Director of the Ohio Department of Mental Health since March of 1991. The Department operates 14 accredited hospitals, funds and monitors services through 53 local/county boards, and serves over 150,000 citizens annually. Previously, he was the Commissioner of the Connecticut Department of Mental Health, the Deputy Commissioner in the same Department, and also held a variety of positions with the Massachusetts Department of Mental Health. Dr. Hogan has published many articles and book chapters on mental health services and policy, and he is a frequent speaker in national conferences on managed behavioral health care. Dr. Hogan received his doctoral degree in administration of special education from Syracuse University.

DENNIS McCARTY, PhD, is a Research Professor at the Heller School at Brandeis University and director of the substance abuse group in the Institute for Health Policy. He is the Principal Investigator for Brandeis/Harvard Research Center on Managed Care and Drug Abuse Treatment, a health services research center funded by NIDA. The Center examines the effects of managed care on the organization and financing of services for the treatment of dependency on alcohol and other drugs. Previously, Dr. McCarty served as the director of the Massachusetts state authority for drug and alcohol abuse treatment and prevention services. He collaborated with Massachusetts Medicaid to facilitate the introduction of a managed care carve-out for mental health and substance abuse services. Dr. McCarty designed and implemented the current Massachusetts substance abuse management information system and also initiated a Quality Improvement Collaborative for substance abuse treatment programs throughout Massachusetts.

J. MICHAEL McGINNIS, MD, MPP, is currently a Senior Policy Advisor and Team Leader for the World Health Organization's Health Reform and Reconstruction Programme in Bosnia, and a Scholar-in-Residence for the Commission on Behavioral and Social Sciences and Education at the National Academy of Sciences. As Deputy Assistant Secretary of Health from 1977-1995, Dr. McGinnis pioneered the development of public health objectives through directing the Healthy People 2000 initiative. Under his leadership, the year 2000 framework involved more than 10,000 individuals from national, state, and local public health agencies and organizations. Dr. McGinnis also directed the development of national guidelines for clinical preventive services, including screening and evaluation for substance abuse. He has published many articles on health policy, health objectives, health economics, clinical preventive medicine, and other areas, and served as the editor of many reports for the U.S. Department of Health and Human Services. Dr. McGinnis is a fellow of the American College of Preventive Medicine and the American College of Epidemiology and has served on several boards and committees for the World Health Organization. Dr. McGinnis resigned from the committee in August 1996 because of his WHO commitments overseas.

RHONDA ROBINSON-BEALE, MD, is the Senior Associate Medical Director for Behavioral Medicine at Health Alliance Plan/Henry Ford Health System. Dr. Robinson-Beale has been an administrative lead in the development of the behavioral medicine delivery system for HAP, a mixed model HMO, PPO, and POS. She has experience developing and implementing utilization and quality management activities within the HMO setting. As a provider, Dr. Robinson-Beale has managed a capitated behavioral medicine population which included private and public patients for ten years. Dr. Robinson-Beale has been one of the lead HMO representatives in Michigan during an initiative on the part of the State Department of Mental Health and Medical Services Administration to integrate the behavioral medicine care of Medicaid recipients between the HMOs and Community Mental Health. She has extensive experience in addiction medicine. She has worked in conjunction with the Detroit Department of Substance Abuse in the development of specialized addiction day treatment programs for pregnant addicts and their children and cocaine-addicted males. Dr. Robinson-Beale has served as a reviewer for the National Committee on Quality Assurance (NCQA), and has performed committee activities for NCQA. She has also served on the Committee on Standards for the American Society on Addiction Medicine and on the Quality Assurance Committee for the American Psychiatric Association.

ALEX RODRIGUEZ, MD, is Vice President and Medical Director, National Account Consortium, Inc., a service company of Blue Cross/Blue Shield Plans that are committed to acquiring and retaining national accounts. For ten years, Dr. Rodriguez was the Chief Medical Officer of two national managed care companies, Preferred Health Care, Ltd. and subsequently Preferred Works/Value Health, Inc. Previously, Dr. Rodriguez was the National Medical Director and Director, Office of Quality Assurance of the Office of Civilian Health and Medical Program of the Uniformed Services (CHAMPUS). He also served as Special Assistant to two Secretaries of the Department of Health and Human Services while he was a White House Fellow. Dr. Rodriguez is currently President-Elect of the American College of Medical Quality, and holds a faculty appointment at Yale University School of Medicine. He maintains an active medical practice in the Naval Reserve as a staff physician with primary care and psychiatric privileges at the Naval Hospital, Groton, Connecticut, and at the National Naval Medical Center, Bethesda, Maryland.

STEVEN S. SHARFSTEIN, MD, MPA, is currently President, Medical Director, and Chief Executive Officer at the Sheppard Pratt Health System and Clinical Professor of Psychiatry at the University of Maryland. A practicing clinician for over 20 years, he specializes in psychotherapy and psychopharmacology, especially for patients with long-term mental illness. He spent 13 years with the National Institute of Mental Health, where he was Director of Mental Health Service Programs and also held positions in consultation/liaison psychiatry and research in behavioral medicine on the campus of the National Institutes of Health. He has written on a wide variety of clinical and economic topics and has published more than 140 professional papers, 40 book chapters, and 10 books, including (as co-author) Madness and Government: Who Cares for the Mentally Ill?, a history of the federal community mental health centers program. A graduate of Dartmouth College and the Albert Einstein College of Medicine, he trained in psychiatry at the Massachusetts Mental Health Center in Boston from 1969 to 1972. Dr. Sharfstein also received a Master's degree in Public Administration from the Kennedy School of Government in 1973 and a certificate from the Advanced Management Program at the Harvard Business School in 1991. He was Secretary of the American Psychiatric Association from 1991-95, and is a member of the Board on Neuroscience and Behavioral Health at the Institute of Medicine.

DONALD L. SHUMWAY, MSS, is Co-director of Self-Determination for Persons with Developmental Disabilities, Institute on Disability at the University of New Hampshire. Mr. Shumway is the former Director of the Division of Mental Health for the New Hampshire Department of Health and Human Services, where he directed the development of New Hampshire's Medicaid 1115 Waiver for comprehensive health care reform. Mr. Shumway also was responsible for leading a legislatively mandated reengineering of the department and the reduction of the budget by $32,000,000. He restructured the state's mental health system and managed the first closing nationally, of all institutional services for persons with developmental disabilities. Mr. Shumway is a former member of the National Advisory Mental Health Council at the National Institute of Mental Health, and a former Board President of the National Association of State Mental Health Program Directors.

CONSTANCE WEISNER, DrPH, MSW, is Senior Scientist for the Alcohol Research Group, a member of the faculty of the School of Public Health at the University of California at Berkeley, and an Adjunct Investigator for Kaiser Permanente Division of Research, Northern California Region. She directs the Community Epidemiology Laboratory, a large study of the epidemiology of alcohol and drug problems across populations of health and human services agencies and the general population. Dr. Weisner is Principal Investigator of NIAAA and NIDA research grants that study the cost and effectiveness of alcohol and drug treatment interventions in Kaiser. Other current studies examine access, utilization, and outcome across public and private sector programs. Dr. Weisner has been an advisor to the World Health Organization, the Robert Wood Johnson Foundation, the John D. and Catherine T. MacArthur Foundation, and state governments. She is a member of the World Health Organization Expert Advisory Panel on Drug Dependence and Alcohol Problems and was a member of the IOM committee that produced the report *Broadening the Base of Treatment for Alcohol Problems.*

Committee Staff

MARGARET EDMUNDS, PhD, joined the IOM in October 1995 as Study Director for Quality Assurance and Accreditation Guidelines for Managed Behavioral Health Care. From 1992 to 1995, she was an Assistant Research Psychologist at the Institute for Health Policy Studies, University of California, San Francisco, and the project director for a multisite clinical evaluation conducted for the California Department of Health Services. In 1991-92, she was the project director for the Primary Care-Substance Abuse Linkage Initiative, a national initiative on health care reform sponsored by the Public Health Service. From 1986-92, Dr. Edmunds was with the Johns Hopkins Behavioral Medicine Clinic, where she was a member of the affiliate staff of the Johns Hopkins Hospital, a clinical and research fellow (1986-89), an Instructor of Medical Psychology at the Johns Hopkins School of Medicine (1989-92), and a frequent lecturer with the Preventive Medicine Residency Program. Dr. Edmunds is a member of the Board of Directors and a Fellow of the Society of Behavioral Medicine. She has published articles on integrated health care delivery systems; financing and payment reform for primary care and substance abuse; clinical practice guidelines; smoking cessation; multidisciplinary treatment of chronic pain; and policy research.

CONSTANCE PECHURA, PhD, Director of the IOM Division of Neuroscience and Behavioral Health, has a B.S. degree in psychology and a Ph.D. in anatomy and neuroscience. Following a post-doctoral fellowship at the National Institute of Neurological Disorders and Stroke, she joined the Institute of Medicine staff in 1988. She has directed projects and edited reports on a variety of topics including chemical weapons exposures to World War II veterans, integrating computer technologies to map the human brain, scientific and ethical issues of fetal and embryo research, mental and addictive disorders in women, ethical and science policy issues related to cross-species organ transplantation, and health and human rights. Dr. Pechura is a recipient of a National Science Foundation Graduate Fellowship, Uniformed Services University of the Health Sciences Outstanding Teaching Award, and National Academy of Sciences/National Research Council Special Achievement Award. Dr. Pechura holds an adjunct faculty position at the George Washington University School of Medicine, teaches a health policy tutorial in the Stanford in Washington program, and chairs the Board of Directors of Student Pugwash USA.

MOLLA S. DONALDSON, MS, is Senior Staff Officer at the Institute of Medicine and adjunct professor at the George Washington University School of Medicine and Health Sciences (GWU). Currently she is project director the IOM's National Roundtable on Health Care Quality and its associated Managed Care Panel. She has been at the Institute of Medicine (IOM) since 1988 when she joined the staff as an Associate Study Director to develop a strategy for quality assurance in the Medicare Program. Since then she has directed studies on conflict of interest in patients outcomes research teams (PORTs), on development of a model process for setting priorities for health technology assessment, on clinical uses of antiprogestins (including RU 486), and on a study of regional health data networks that examined public disclosure of health information and protections for privacy and confidentiality. She co-directed a recently published report, *Primary Care: America's Health in a New Era.* Before coming to the IOM, she was Associate Professor at GWU in its primary care department. She directed the HMO's quality assurance program and taught in various medical school, health administration, and public health programs on issues of quality assurance, survey research, health services research in ambulatory care, and bioethics. Ms. Donaldson received a Masters of Science degree from the University of Virginia. She currently holds a Pew Doctoral Fellowship in Health Policy at the University of Michigan.

CARRIE INGALLS, MPH, is a Research Associate in the Institute of Medicine's Division of Neuroscience and Behavioral Health. Since 1993, Ms. Ingalls has worked on several projects at the Institute of Medicine focusing on behavioral health care, substance abuse, genetics, fetal alcohol syndrome, environmental and occupational health, toxicology and environmental health information resources, and risk communication. Ms. Ingalls received her M.P.H. from George Washington University in 1995 with a concentration in health policy and programs. Her interests and research activities include epidemiology, health policy, and environmental and behavioral health.

THOMAS J. WETTERHAN, MA, is a Project/Research Assistant with the Institute of Medicine (IOM). He received his MA in European Studies in 1994 from George Washington University's Elliott School of International Affairs. Since joining the IOM in 1995, he has worked on projects on behavioral health care, raising the profile of substance abuse research, genetics, toxicology and environmental health information resources, and the health of military women for the Division of Neuroscience and Behavioral Health and the Food and Nutrition Board.

B

Can the Outcomes Research Literature Inform the Search for Quality Indicators in Substance Abuse Treatment?

A. Thomas McLellan, Mark Belding, James R. McKay,
David Zanis, and Arthur I. Alterman

Penn-Veterans Affairs Center for Studies of Addiction, Philadelphia

Over the past 20 years, treatment researchers within the field of substance abuse have focused on questions of whether treatment is effective and which type of substance abuse treatment is most effective (Bale, 1979; Gerstein et al., 1994; Hubbard and Marsden, 1986; McLellan et al., 1992, 1994; Sells and Simpson, 1980). The data on these questions have been quite consistent, with well-substantiated evidence available from both controlled clinical trials and field studies, suggesting four important conclusions.

1.   Many of the traditional forms of substance abuse treatment (e.g., methadone maintenance, therapeutic communities, outpatient drug-free treatment) have been evaluated multiple times and have been shown to be effective (Ball and Ross, 1991; Gerstein et al., 1994; Hubbard and Marsden, 1986; IOM, 1990a, b; McLellan et al., 1980; Simpson and Sells, 1982).

2.   The benefits obtained from these treatments typically extend beyond the reduction of substance use to areas that are important to society, such as reduced crime, reduced risk of infectious diseases, and improved social function (Ball and Ross, 1991; Gerstein et al., 1994; IOM 1990a, b; McLellan et al., 1980).

3.   Individuals who complete treatment or receive more days of treatment typically show more improvements than those who leave care prematurely (DeLeon, 1984; Gerstein et al., 1994; Hubbard et al., 1989; Sells and Simpson, 1980).

4.   The costs associated with the provision of substance abuse treatment provide three- to sevenfold returns to employers, the health insurers, and society within

3 years following treatment (French et al., 1991; Gerstein et al., 1994; Holder and Blose, 1992).

HOW DO THESE RESULTS TRANSLATE INTO RECOMMENDATIONS FOR PROVIDING QUALITY TREATMENT?

Although the conclusions from this line of research are important and gratifying, they are not adequate to inform important clinical, economic, or health and social policy questions regarding the delivery of substance abuse treatment services. Knowledge that some of these treatments can work and that better outcomes are associated with longer treatment does not help to determine (1) which of the multiple elements in these multicomponent treatments are causally related to the favorable outcomes (i.e., the so-called active ingredients of treatment), (2) how long or at what level of intensity these ingredients should be delivered, or (3) the point at which the additional provision of these ingredients is no longer associated with increased benefits.

If the field of substance abuse treatment research is to help guide and inform the search for better, faster, less expensive treatments, it will be necessary to develop better, faster, less expensive means of evaluating the specific effects of substance abuse treatments. To respond to this need, the treatment field has begun to look for markers of or proxies for true outcomes that can be easily measured during the course of treatment (ideally as part of a management information system) and that have been associated with favorable outcomes following treatment. These early indicators of subsequent favorable outcomes have been called "quality indicators."

Until now, these indicators have typically been developed by groups of clinicians and administrators who have simply selected indicators that have a clear, "face-valid" or intuitive link with longer-term outcomes. This common sense approach has had great appeal because the results have been measures that can be collected, analyzed, and reported rapidly and inexpensively, with the results being clear to patients, clinicians, and administrators alike.

Furthermore, because these indicators could be measured for individual patients and during the early course of an individual's treatment, they have the potential for use as early warning signs to correct inappropriate treatments. Because of their potential clinical and administrative value, systems of quality indicators have already been widely adopted by treatment providers, and there is a widespread effort to build the reporting of these measures into existing clinical or management information systems.

The existing and proposed quality indicators for the substance abuse field (e.g., American Managed Behavioral Healthcare Association and the National Committee for Quality Assurance) have been useful in identifying obvious problems in the conduct of treatment, in bringing the consumer perspective into the treatment setting, and in stimulating the treatment field toward greater self-examination and self-evaluation. At the same time, there is some concern that these initial indicators may only identify extremely poor outcomes, bordering on malpractice (e.g., prescribing antipsychotic medications to patients without psychosis diagnoses). Furthermore, although the indicators have been developed to encourage improved clinical practices, some of them can be made to show *apparent* improvement through administrative action without actually changing treatment practices (e.g., an administrative decision not to readmit discharged patients within 1 month posttreatment to give the impression of a low 1-month relapse rate). Thus, the current indicators may be insufficient to differentiate subtler levels of treatment quality or to offer guidance for providers searching for more effective treatment methods.

WHAT QUALITIES ARE NECESSARY FOR AN IDEAL QUALITY INDICATOR?

Some of the problems with the existing quality indicators result from the lack of a clear rationale or conceptual basis for what would and would not constitute an indicator that is valid and useful. In our view, such an indicator would be a **measure of a treatment process or a patient characteristic that can be recorded easily during treatment and that has been clearly associated with a favorable outcome.**

It is important to examine the rationale for and subtleties of each of the components of this definition of an ideal quality indicator. First, the definition includes both treatment process factors and patient changes during treatment. Although the majority of current quality indicators focus on treatment practices, policies, and processes, it is potentially more practical and more informative to focus upon interim patient changes brought about during the course of treatment. The distinctions between these two types of potential indicators are important and are discussed at the end of this paper.

The definition also suggests that the measures that will ultimately serve as these indicators must be easily, inexpensively, and reliably made during the course of treatment at the individual patient level. Ease of measurement is essential if these indicators are to be used widely in standard clinical settings. Furthermore, these measures should be recorded at the individual patient level because early indications of favorable or unfavorable treatment progress could be extremely useful for clinical management of individual patients, again increasing the likelihood that they will be adopted and used regularly in the clinical setting. Moreover, indicators that are recorded at the individual patient level can always be aggregated through sampling to permit reporting at the program level. However, indicators that are based on the aggregate data from a treatment program can rarely be reduced to provide clinically significant information at the individual patient level.

Finally and most importantly, the true value of potential quality indicators rests ultimately upon the relationship of those indicators to treatment outcomes.

Although this may seem apparent, there has been, in fact, a lack of agreement about how to define and measure outcomes, which in turn makes it difficult to identify useful indicators. One way to approach this issue is to identify two separate and distinct stages of substance abuse treatment: detoxification-stabilization and rehabilitation. Each of these stages has distinct therapeutic goals, different treatment processes, and markedly different expectations with regard to outcome.

Thus, this paper will review the available outcomes research for the detoxification-stabilization stage and the rehabilitation stage of treatment. Each section will include a description of processes and therapeutic goals for the treatment stage, define outcomes on the basis of these therapeutic goals, discuss a strategy for reviewing the literature based on the outcomes definitions, and finally, present research findings pertinent to the identification of quality indicators within that stage of treatment.

The review includes only data from clinical trials, treatment matching program studies, or health services studies where the patients were adults who were clearly alcohol or drug (excluding tobacco) dependent by contemporary criteria, where the treatment provided was a conventional form of either detoxification or rehabilitation (any setting or modality), and where there were measures of either treatment processes or patient change during the course of treatment as well as posttreatment measures of outcome as defined later in the paper.

THE DETOXIFICATION OR ACUTE STABILIZATION STAGE

Before the advent of managed care strategies in the United States, the acute stage of substance dependence treatment was synonymous with hospitalization, regardless of whether the focus of the treatment was the medical detoxification of a true withdrawal syndrome (i.e., neuroadaptation, withdrawal symptoms, etc.) or simply the stabilization of physiological and emotional symptoms associated with the cessation of drug use that might not produce a bona fide withdrawal syndrome. Currently, detoxification from alcohol, opiate, barbiturate, or benzodiazepine use is generally the only type of treatment for which hospital admission may be warranted, and even the majority of these "true detoxifications" now occur in outpatient or nonmedical settings.

However, this review includes both true detoxification as well as initial stabilization from the acute effects of drugs in which tolerance and withdrawal are less clearly documented (e.g., phencyclidine, LSD, marijuana, and even cocaine). The therapeutic settings, procedures, and goals are quite similar for both forms of these acute treatments, which seek to stabilize the patient medically and psychologically and to develop an effective discharge plan that includes continued rehabilitative care, almost always in an outpatient setting.

The acute stage of treatment is associated with lasting improvements only when there is continued rehabilitative treatment (IOM, 1990a, b). This association is quite important in the development of indicators of treatment effectiveness and quality for this stage of treatment.

Goals of Detoxification and Stabilization

Patients and Treatment Settings

The detoxification and stabilization phase of treatment is designed for patients who have been actively abusing alcohol or street drugs, or both, and who are suffering physiological or emotional instability, or both. In cases of severe withdrawal potential or extreme physiological or emotional instability, detoxification-stabilization helps to prevent serious medical consequences of abrupt withdrawal, to reduce the physiological and emotional signs of instability, and to motivate necessary behavioral change strategies that will be the focus of rehabilitation. This stage of treatment may take place in inpatient settings, either a hospital or a nonhospital, residential setting, or in outpatient settings, such as in a hospital-based clinic or a residential or social setting.

Treatment Elements and Methods

Medications are available for both physiological withdrawal signs and for the temporary relief of acute medical problems associated with physiological instability (e.g., sleep medications, antidiarrheal medications, vitamins, and nutritional supplements). Motivational counseling is widely used to address shame and ambivalence, as well as to increase adherence with recommendations for continued rehabilitation.

Duration

Regardless of the setting, stabilization of acute problems is typically completed within 2 to 10 days, with the average being 3 to 5 days (Fleming and Barry, 1992). True detoxification is necessary only for cases of severe alcohol, opiate, benzodiazepine, or barbiturate use, although many cocaine-dependent and other drug-dependent patients suffer from significant physiological and emotional instability that precludes immediate participation in rehabilitation. The duration of the detoxification-stabilization process depends on the presence and severity of the patient's dependence symptoms as well as concurrent medical and psychiatric problems. Stays longer than 5 days are unusual and typically are due to conjoint medical or psychiatric problems or physiological dependence upon some forms of sedatives (e.g., alprazolam).

Key Findings for Detoxification and Stabilization Treatment

This section reviews research on treatment processes or patient changes during the course of detoxification and stabilization that have been associated with sustained reductions in physiological and emotional instability and, particularly, with continued engagement in the rehabilitation stage of treatment. As suggested earlier, there are recognized tolerance and withdrawal syndromes following the heavy use of alcohol, opiates, benzodiazepines, and barbiturates.

The standard detoxification strategy for barbiturate withdrawal was described more than a decade ago by Robinson and colleagues (Robinson et al., 1981). The majority of published work on detoxification strategies for alcohol and opiates has been reviewed in two former Institute of Medicine publications (IOM, 1990a, b). Much less has been written regarding detoxification procedures for benzodiazepine dependence, perhaps because dependence upon this group of drugs is much less prevalent.

Although cocaine "withdrawal" has been recognized in the *Diagnostic and Statistical Manual*, Fourth Edition (DSM IV), there is continued debate regarding the treatment and even the existence of a bona fide withdrawal syndrome following cocaine use (Satel et al., 1991; Weddington, 1992). At the same time, there is clear agreement that patients who have used cocaine or crack continuously over sustained periods, suffer two to five day periods of measurable physiological and psychiatric instability (Gawin and Ellinwood, 1988; Gawin and Kleber, 1986). For this reason, stabilization is included along with detoxification in this treatment category and was included with detoxification in the few available studies that have investigated factors associated with the acute stabilization of cocaine cessation.

Setting of Care: Medical or Nonmedical and Inpatient or Outpatient

Debate regarding the appropriate setting of care in which to detoxify alcohol-dependent patients has been substantial. Since the mid-1970s, medical settings such as residential treatment facilities or even outpatient treatment centers have conducted detoxification or stabilization treatments for alcohol, opiates, and more recently, cocaine. Although studies have not systematically compared social settings with medical settings for detoxification from alcohol dependence, there are reports of favorable outcomes in both (Naranjo et al., 1983; Whitfield et al., 1978).

In the presence of significant physiological signs of alcohol, opiate, benzodiazepine, or barbiturate withdrawal, however, the standard treatment includes medical supervision in either a hospital or an outpatient medical clinic (Fleming and Barry, 1992; IOM, 1990b). Although research is not extensive, medical settings are generally viewed as being more appropriate for detoxifications involving medical problems (particularly those with a history of seizures) and psychiatric problems (particularly for individuals with depression and at risk of suicide) and also when patients have concurrent cocaine dependence. This last group of patients now makes up the majority of many clinical populations (DATOS, 1992; ONDCP, 1995).

Alcohol Detoxification. Within the framework of medically supervised alcohol detoxification, the relative effectiveness and costs of inpatient versus outpatient alcohol detoxification have been examined (Hayashida et al., 1989; Stockwell et al., 1986). In a study by Hayashida et al. (1989), chronic alcohol-dependent patients without histories of serious psychiatric or medical complications were randomly assigned to receive medically supervised alcohol withdrawal in either an inpatient or a day-hospital setting. On two of the outcome domains considered important for detoxification treatments (safe elimination of withdrawal signs and engagement in ongoing rehabilitation), the inpatient group showed significantly better performance, but the readdiction rates were less than 12 percent for both groups. Despite this statistically significant advantage for the inpatient setting, it was 10 times more costly than outpatient detoxification in an outpatient setting.

There may be some advantage to inpatient detoxification when a patient does not have the social or personal supports necessary to comply with the outpatient attendance requirements. However, despite somewhat lower retention rates for outpatient than for inpatient alcohol detoxification (Hayashida et al., 1989; Stockwell et al., 1991), outpatient detoxification may be more acceptable to a wider range of drinkers who wish to avoid the stigma of treatment in a designated detoxification (Stockwell et al., 1990).

Opiate Detoxification. Available evidence suggests that opiate detoxification with methadone can generally be accomplished in an outpatient setting under medical supervision with gradually reduced doses of methadone (Cushman and Dole, 1973; IOM, 1995a). However, completion rates for treatment of opioid dependence may be higher in inpatient than in outpatient detoxification programs (Gossop et al., 1986; Lipton and Maranda, 1983).

Cocaine and Crack Detoxification. Few studies have examined the appropriate setting for the stabilization of physiological and psychiatric signs and symptoms associated with extended cocaine or crack use. The prevailing practice has been to attempt to stabilize all but the most severely affected patients through outpatient care (Higgins et al., 1994). Patients who are in the acute stages of cocaine cessation and who are more severely affected (medically or psychiatrically) are placed into a hospital if they have significant cardiac problems or significant psychiatric symptomatology or are at least placed in inpatient social settings for the first 3 to 5 days of treatment (Fleming and Barry, 1992).

The available literature is replete with accounts of early dropouts during the first 2 to 3 weeks of outpatient cocaine treatment (Alterman et al., 1994; Carroll et al., 1994; Higgins et al., 1993; Kang et al., 1991), with attrition rates ranging from a low of 27 percent to a high of 47 percent in the first few weeks of care. As discussed below, it is reasonable to conclude that the patients with the most severe medical and psychiatric problems are most susceptible to drop out of treatment early.

Length of Stay and Criterion for Completion

Alcohol and Opiates. Several detoxification studies (Cushman and Dole, 1973; Hayashida et al., 1989; Senay et al., 1981) have measured detoxification as 3 consecutive days of abstinence from observable withdrawal signs or symptoms (opiate or alcohol), using standardized inventories of these physical measures. Lengths of stay for alcohol detoxifications vary from about 3 days to as long as 1 month. However, the great majority of detoxifications can be accomplished in 3 to 5 days (Fleming and Barry, 1992), and there is no evidence of greater effectiveness from extended stays.

In an early study by Cushman and Dole (1973), only 3 percent of 525 opiate-dependent patients who failed to provide an opiate-negative urine specimen following the outpatient detoxification (signifying at least 3 days of abstinence) were able to engage in the suggested abstinence-oriented rehabilitation program following detoxification. One hundred percent of these patients were readdicted to opiates at the 6-month follow-up.

Cocaine. A recent study of cocaine-dependent patients entering outpatient rehabilitation also offers some relevant information on the clinical importance of developing a criterion of successful completion. In a study of cocaine-dependent veterans, Alterman et al. (1996) found that the single best predictor of engagement in the rehabilitation process, and ultimately program completion (elimination of cocaine use verified by urinalysis), was the presence or absence of cocaine metabolites in the urine sample submitted upon admission to the program, signifying recent cocaine use. Of those patients without cocaine metabolites present in their urine on admission, 79 percent engaged in and completed the outpatient treatment, whereas only 39 percent of those with a positive urine sample on admission engaged and completed the outpatient treatment.

Potential Quality Indicators for Detoxification and Stabilization

The therapeutic goals of detoxification and stabilization are focused primarily on the amelioration and stabilization of the acute medical, psychiatric, or substance use symptoms that were out of control and thus responsible for preventing the patient from entering directly into rehabilitation. Thus, the goal of detoxification-stabilization is removal of the physiological and emotional instability that has impeded direct entry to rehabilitative treatment. Readiness for the rehabilitation stage of treatment should be assessed separately.

Patient-Level Indicators

Detoxification can be said to have succeeded if shortly after discharge (i.e., 1 week to 1 month) the patient has:

1.   shown significant reductions in physiological and emotional instability (at least to levels appropriate for rehabilitation entry),
2.   has not had serious medical or psychiatric complications, and
3.   has been integrated into and engaged in an appropriate rehabilitation program.

Program-Level Indicators

As summarized above, serious consequences can result from not addressing medical complications from alcohol detoxification, such as seizure history. Thus, a potential indicator for nonmedical or social detoxification settings could be the number of patients admitted with a history of medical complications, such as seizures or cardiac arrhythmias.

Given that alcohol-dependent and perhaps cocaine-dependent patients may not have the requisite personal or social resources to comply with the daily attendance requirements associated with outpatient detoxification regimens, one potential negative indicator could be the number of individuals in outpatient treatment who are homeless or who have previously failed outpatient detoxification.

Evidence suggests that it may be possible to set measurable thresholds for determining whether the detoxification has at least reduced the physiological and emotional symptoms that were the foci of treatment. This threshold may be importantly related to subsequent performance in rehabilitation treatment, at least for outpatient rehabilitation. Thus, a potential positive indicator of detoxification performance could be the number of patients who are discharged or transferred from acute care (detoxification or stabilization) who have had 3 consecutive days without withdrawal signs or symptoms. This might be measured by standard inventories of symptoms and signs or at least by breathalyzer and urinalysis measures.

REHABILITATION

Goals of Rehabilitation

Patients and Treatment Settings

Rehabilitation is appropriate for patients who are no longer suffering from the acute physiological or emotional effects of recent substance use and who need behavioral change strategies to regain control of their urges to use substances.

Rehabilitation can take place in inpatient settings, such as a hospital (which is very rare) or a residential setting (which is increasingly rare). More frequently, however, rehabilitation takes place in a hospital-based clinic or a residential or social setting.

Treatment Elements and Methods

The purposes of this stage of treatment are to prevent a return to active substance use that would require detoxification-stabilization; to assist the patient in developing control over urges to use alcohol or drugs, or both, usually through sustaining total abstinence from all drugs and alcohol; and to assist the patient in regaining or attaining improved personal health and social function, both as a secondary part of the rehabilitation function and because these improvements in lifestyle are important for maintaining sustained control over substance use.

Professional opinions vary widely regarding the underlying reasons for the loss of control over alcohol and drug abuse, for example, genetic predispositions, acquired metabolic abnormalities, learned, negative behavioral patterns, deeply ingrained feelings of low self-worth, self-medication of underlying psychiatric or physical medical problems, character flaws, and lack of family and community support for positive function. Thus, there is an equally wide range of treatment strategies and treatments that can be used to correct or ameliorate these underlying problems and to provide continuing support for the targeted patient changes.

Strategies have included such diverse elements as psychotropic medications to relieve "underlying psychiatric problems"; medications to relieve alcohol and drug cravings; acupuncture to correct acquired metabolic imbalances; educational seminars, films, and group sessions to correct false impressions about alcohol and drug use; group and individual counseling and therapy sessions to provide insight, guidance, and support for behavioral changes; and peer help groups (e.g., Alcoholics Anonymous [AA] and Narcotics Anonymous [NA]) to provide continued support for the behavioral changes thought to be important for sustaining improvement.

Duration

Typically, inpatient hospital-based forms of treatment last 7 to 11 days (ONDCP, 1995; White Paper, 1995). Nonhospital forms of residential rehabilitation are typically longer, ranging from 30 to 90 days; therapeutic community modalities typically range from 6 months to 2 years in. Outpatient forms of treatment (at least abstinence-oriented treatments) range from 30 to 120 days (ONDCP, 1995; White Paper, 1995).

Many of the more intensive forms of outpatient treatment (intensive outpatient and day hospital) begin with full or half-day sessions five or more times per week for approximately 1 month. As the rehabilitation progresses, the intensity of the treatment reduces to shorter-duration sessions of 1 to 2 hours delivered twice weekly to semimonthly. The final part of outpatient treatment is typically called "continuing care" or "aftercare," with biweekly to monthly group support meetings continuing (in association with parallel activities in self-help groups) for as long as 2 years. Maintenance forms of treatment are designed with an indeterminate length, with some intended to continue throughout the patient's life.

Maintenance Medications

Although the majority of rehabilitation treatment programs in the United States are abstinence oriented, a significant number of rehabilitation programs maintain patients on a medication that is designed to either block the effects of the abusable drugs (e.g., disulfiram and naltrexone) or, in the case of opiates and nicotine, a medication that is designed to override the effects of the abusable drugs through the development of tolerance to a safer, more potent, and longer-acting form of the drug (nicotine patch, methadone, buprenorphine, levo-alpha-acetylmethadol [LAAM]). These maintenance approaches are quite similar to current strategies for ameliorating the physiological or emotional problems in individuals with other chronic medical conditions, such as long-term maintenance on antidepressant, antipsychotic, or other psychotropic medications for psychiatric patients; maintenance on beta-blockers and other normotensive agents for patients with hypertension; antiasthmatics for asthma sufferers; and insulin for diabetics.

The use of medications in general and maintenance medications in particular has been controversial because this general medical approach has often conflicted with the broader view that it is important to teach substance-dependent patients to live without a reliance on *any* type of medication. At the same time, a substantial amount of research has shown that these medications can be very effective in the rehabilitation of several forms of addiction (IOM, 1995a; O'Malley et al., 1992; Transdermal Nicotine Study Group, 1991; Volpicelli et al., 1992).

Among the most widely and thoroughly studied medications in the pharmacopoeia is methadone. Despite this fact, methadone, at least as a maintenance medication in the rehabilitation of opiate dependence, remains a controversial medication (IOM, 1995a). Compared with the medications used to treat other types of addiction, the medication is among the most tightly controlled and regulated, the chronicity and the severity of the patients' treatment problems are different from those of patients addicted to other drugs, and maintenance on methadone is often for 10 or more years, compared with 1 to 3 months maintenance for any other form of addiction medication.

This review, however, includes methadone maintenance, as well as maintenance with its long-acting form, LAAM, as part of the general category of rehabilitation treatments, because the psychosocial elements of methadone treatment and the overall rehabilitative goals of methadone treatment are quite similar to those for other forms of rehabilitation. Many of the same patient and treatment variables that have been predictive of outcomes from other forms of rehabilitation are also predictive of the same outcomes from methadone maintenance treatments (McLellan et al., 1994).

Key Findings in the Rehabilitation Stage of Treatment

Defining Outcomes

A variety of outcomes have been proposed from several perspectives, for example, cost offset, patient satisfaction, and abstinence. However, regardless of the specific setting, modality, philosophy, or methods of rehabilitation, the goals of all forms of rehabilitation are to:

1.   maintain the physiological and emotional improvements that were to be initiated during detoxification, preventing relapse to redetoxification,

2.   enhance and sustain reductions in or elimination of alcohol and drug use (most rehabilitation programs suggest a goal of complete abstinence), and

3.   provide services and encourage behaviors that lead to improved personal health, improved social function, and reduced threats to public health and public safety.

Defining Outcomes

For substance abuse treatment, particularly rehabilitative forms of treatment, to be worthwhile to society, **outcomes must be lasting improvements in those problems that led to the treatment admission and that are important to the patient and to society.** Each component of the definition will be explained below.

This definition of outcomes is restricted to improvements that can be shown to have an enduring or lasting quality (McLellan and Durell, 1995; McLellan et al., 1995; McLellan and Weisner, 1996). Because these disorders are chronic and relapsing, a "cure" for substance use disorders is not now achievable in most cases. In the case of extended outpatient abstinence-oriented treatments or maintenance treatments in which the patient is expected to remain in treatment for many months to many years, the expected improvements should be in evidence by at least the third month and should remain in evidence throughout the course of the maintenance period. The literature is replete with evaluation studies showing sustained improvements in important outcome domains at periods of 6 months to 1 year following treatment (Anglin et al.,1989; DeLeon, 1984, 1994; Finney et al., 1981; IOM 1990a, b; McLellan and Ball, 1995; Simpson and Savage, 1980).

The definition also is restricted to those improvements in problems that led to the treatment admission and that are important to the patient and to society. For the patient, and particularly for the many stakeholders, the effectiveness of treatment will be measured in some significant part by the extended effects of treatment on the addiction-related problems that have limited personal health and social function in the patient and that may have become public health and public safety concerns, such as the risk of acquiring or transmitting infectious diseases or committing personal and property crimes. These are generally the precipitating factors leading to the treatment admission.

In this regard, achievement of the primary goal of reducing alcohol and drug use is necessary, but not always sufficient, to improve the addiction-related problems that are typically so prominent among individuals seeking treatment. Furthermore, without additional improvements in these associated problems, addiction treatment is not worthwhile either to the patient who undergoes it or to the society that supports it (McLellan and Ball, 1995; McLellan and Durell, 1995; McLellan and Weisner, 1996; McLellan et al., 1995).

Outcome Domains

Three domains are relevant to the rehabilitative goals of the patient and to the public health and safety goals of society. The first two domains are quite consistent with the primary and secondary measures of effectiveness typically used by the Food and Drug Administration (FDA) to evaluate new drug or device applications in controlled clinical trials and are quite consistent with the mainstream of thought regarding the evaluation of other forms of health care (Stewart and Ware, 1989). The final outcome dimension is more specific to the treatment of substance use disorders, because it acknowledges the significant public health and public safety concerns associated with addiction.

Sustained Reduction of Alcohol and Drug Use. Sustained reduction of drug and alcohol use is the foremost goal of treatment for substance dependence and is the primary outcome domain in this review, consistent with the FDA view. In this review, operational evidence for improvement in this domain includes both objective data from urinalysis and breathalyzer readings as well as patients' self reports of alcohol and drug use, when those reports were recorded by independent interviewers under conditions of privacy and impartiality.

Sustained Improvements in Personal Health and Social Function. Improvements in the patients' medical and psychiatric health and social function are important from a societal perspective, because these improvements reduce the problems produced by the disorders and thereby the expenses associated with their treatment. In addition, improvements in these areas are clearly related to maintenance of gains in the primary outcome area of reduced substance use. Within this review, evidence is included from measures such as general health status inventories, psychological symptom inventories, family function measures, and simple measures of days worked and dollars earned, collected either directly from the patient via confidential self report or from independent medical or psychiatric evaluations and employment records.

Sustained Reductions in Threats to Public Health and Public Safety. The threats to public health from substance abusing individuals come from behaviors that spread infectious diseases, such as human immunodeficiency virus infection and AIDS. Specifically, the sharing of needles, unprotected sex, and trading sex for drugs are serious behaviors that have clearly been linked to addiction and are significant threats to public health. Within the review, sources of evidence include confidential self-reporting techniques or objective measures of the acquisition of AIDS, sexually transmitted diseases, tuberculosis, and hepatitis from laboratory tests, although the latter are rarely available.

Major threats to public safety include personal and property crimes committed by an individual under the influence of alcohol and drugs or for the purpose of obtaining alcohol or drugs and the irresponsible or dangerous use of automobiles or equipment by an individual under the influence of alcohol or drugs. In the studies reviewed, these behaviors were measured either by confidential interviews and questionnaires or by objective records of arrests and incarcerations.

Key Findings for Rehabilitation Treatment Outcomes

Studies are included in this review only if they measured one or more of the above three domains at 6 or more months following discharge from any form of rehabilitation treatment or 6 months or more following the initiation of a maintenance form of rehabilitation. This necessarily excludes results such as increased treatment retention, short-term improvements in symptom reduction, and patient satisfaction, because these do not represent lasting behavioral changes in any of the problem areas that are typically responsible for treatment initiation (McLellan and Weisner, 1996). Patient satisfaction has been found to be almost completely independent from most of the commonly accepted behavioral outcomes (e.g., reduced drug use, unemployment, and health care service utilization) (McLellan and Hunkeler, in press).

Summarized below are the most robust and well-replicated variables from two general categories: patient factors and treatment factors. Although a number of patient factors have been reliably related to posttreatment outcomes, very few of these, by themselves, are directly translatable into potential quality or performance indicators. However, any review of potential quality indicators should include variables that might be important as case mix adjusters, or factors that could be used to adjust two or more groups of patients in a comparative evaluation of factors that would likely affect outcome, independent of the treatment process.

Patient Factors

Demographic Factors. Demographic factors are typically important predictors of the development of drug abuse problems (IOM, 1990b; Johnston et al., 1996; Wilsnack and Wilsnack, 1991). However, there is not much compelling evidence that race, gender, age, or educational level are consistent predictors of treatment outcome. A wide range of treatment outcome studies in the substance abuse rehabilitation field have found that demographic factors such as age, education, race, and even treatment history are relatively poorly related to outcome (as defined above) across the major rehabilitation modalities (Ball and Ross, 1991; Finney and Moos, 1992; McLellan et al., 1994; Rounsaville et al., 1987).

There may be some important exceptions. Pregnant and parenting women are an important subgroup of the larger patient population. For these individuals different features of treatment programs are required to allow them to gain access to treatment, as are different constellations of treatment services needed to address their often significant treatment problems (Gomberg and Nirenberg, 1993; Wilsnack and Wilsnack, 1993). More specifically, many of these women have been reluctant to get into standard treatments because of stigma and because of the absence of services for their children (Gomberg, 1989; Hagan et al., 1994; Weisner, 1993; Weisner et al., 1995).

Experimental programs have been created to meet these needs but there have been very few long-term outcome studies of specialized treatments for these women. The limited evidence suggests that the following may be valuable:

1.   An inpatient or residential setting. This would offer protection from potentially aggressive spouses, because a large proportion of the women come from abusive relationships and because there may be few community resources and few opportunities for self support (Finnegan, 1991; Hagan et al., 1994).

2.   The availability of general medical, obstetric-gynecologic, and psychiatric services. These women have been shown to have medical and psychiatric problems that are of much greater severity than those of their male counterparts (Gomberg, 1989; Hagan et al., 1994).

3.   The availability of quarters and care for children are likely to be necessary for these women to be able to enter treatment (Finnegan, 1991).

Severity of Substance Abuse

Patients who have more serious drug dependence problems at the outset of treatment have been found to benefit less from standard treatment [Carroll et al., 1991, 1994, 1995; McKay et al., in press(a)]. This has been true of alcohol-dependent patients (Babor et al., 1988; Finney and Moos, 1992), opiate-dependent patients in therapeutic communities and in patients on methadone maintenance (Ball and Ross, 1991; DeLeon, 1994; Simpson et al., 1986), and cocaine-dependent patients treated in outpatient and inpatient settings (Alterman et al., 1994; Carroll et al., 1991, 1994; McLellan et al., 1994). In all studies, a professional therapy (relapse prevention therapy) condition seemed to result in better outcomes than those from standard forms of peer counseling for highly cocaine-dependent patients.

Although the level of severity of substance use at the time of treatment admission predicts posttreatment substance use, it does not predict changes in the other domains of personal health and social function or public health and safety (Kosten et al., 1987; McLellan et al., 1984, 1994). Furthermore, the predictive relationship of level of severity of substance use to treatment response is not particularly robust, because it generally accounts for less than 10 percent of the total outcome variance (Babor et al., 1988; McLellan et al., 1994), even in the substance abuse domain.

Severity of Psychiatric Problems

Another general patient variable predicting treatment response and posttreatment outcome has been the chronicity and severity of the psychiatric problems presented by the patient at the start of treatment. Psychiatric problems have been measured by using many scales and interviews, and all have attempted to distinguish more enduring or chronic psychiatric symptoms from the acute and temporary effects of alcohol and drug withdrawal (Carroll et al., 1991, 1994, 1995; Kadden et al., 1990; McLellan et al., 1982,1983a, b; Powell et al., 1982; Project MATCH Research Group, in press; Rounsaville et al., 1987; Woody et al., 1983, 1984, 1987).

For opiate-dependent patients on methadone maintenance, the psychiatric severity scale from the Addiction Severity Index (ASI), a general measure of the number and severity of psychiatric symptoms, has been found to be among the best predictors of 6-month substance use, personal health, and social adjustment in studies by McLellan and colleagues (1983a, b). Similar findings have been shown by Ball and Ross (1991) in their study of 6 methadone maintenance treatment programs and by studies of Kosten et al. (1987) and Rounsaville et al. (1982, 1983) of patients on methadone maintenance.

Measures of psychiatric severity have also been shown to be predictive of dropout and posttreatment substance use in studies of opiate-dependent and multiple-drug-dependent patients entering an inpatient therapeutic community setting (DeLeon, 1984, 1994). In a study by McLellan and colleagues (1984), the patients with high-severity psychiatric problems who stayed in therapeutic community treatment the longest actually showed the worst posttreatment status, suggesting that the therapeutic environment that had been demonstrably effective for the patients with problems that were not psychiatrically severe was actually countertherapeutic for the patients with high severity problems.

Poorer outcomes have been found for cocaine-dependent patients with greater psychiatric pathologies. Similar results have been found for outpatient treatment (Carroll et al., 1991) as well as for treatment in a day-hospital and an inpatient rehabilitation setting (Alterman et al., 1994).

Among alcohol-dependent patients, there has been a great deal of evidence for the predictive power of general psychiatric symptomatology (Rounsaville et al., 1987). The severity of depression and anxiety (Powell et al., 1982; Schuckit et al., 1985, 1988, 1990) have been predictive of posttreatment drinking and posttreatment social adjustment among various samples of alcohol-dependent patients. More recently, findings from a multisite study of patient treatment matching sponsored by the National Institute on Alcohol Abuse and Alcoholism (NIAAA) (Project MATCH Research Group, in press) showed that the psychiatric severity scale from the ASI was a significant general predictor of posttreatment drinking and posttreatment social adjustment in a sample of more than 1,200 alcohol-dependent patients and three types of outpatient rehabilitation treatment.

Although the data relating the severity of psychopathology and posttreatment outcome are consistent, Schuckit and colleagues have argued cogently against overdiagnosing psychiatric symptoms, on the grounds that much of the serious psychopathology seen among alcohol-dependent patients at the time of admission for treatment is reduced following even 4 weeks of abstinence (Brown et al., 1991; Schuckit et al., 1990). There is evidence for this position among opiate-dependent patients and for patients following abstinence from cocaine.

Potential Quality Indicators

In summary, almost any general measure of severity of psychiatric symptomatology (i.e., the psychiatric severity scale from the ASI, total score on the Symptom Checklist 90, general pathology scale on the Minnesota Multiphasic Personality Inventory, number of diagnostic symptoms, etc.) can predict scores for almost all pertinent outcomes measures following standard rehabilitation treatments for alcohol, cocaine, or opiate dependence. In general, as the severity of psychiatric symptomatology increases, the likelihood of a successful outcome decreases.

This relationship appears to be attenuated by more professional forms of treatment, such as the addition of psychotropic medications to relieve depression symptoms or the provision of professional forms of family or individual psychotherapy. That is, there appears to be general evidence that previously detoxified and stabilized patients suffering from significant psychiatric symptoms such as depression, thought disorder, or anxiety perform better during treatment and have substantially better posttreatment outcomes when they receive psychotropic medications or professional therapies that would generally be prescribed to nondependent patients with these conditions.

Thus, a potential quality indicator of treatment might be the percentage of patients who are in rehabilitation for alcohol, cocaine, or opiate dependence, who have been diagnosed with major or intermittent depression, generalized anxiety disorder, or other psychiatric condition, and who have been provided adjunctive pharmacotherapy (an appropriate antidepressant or anxiolytic) or professional psychotherapy during the course of their treatment.

Patient Motivation or Stage of Change

Motivation for treatment has traditionally been conceptualized and measured as the extent to which patients had entered treatment under their own free will, without external pressure from legal, family, or employment sources. Many studies have measured motivation in this way, with results that are generally quite consistent: performance during treatment and posttreatment outcomes are comparable for patients who are seemingly forced to enter a substance abuse treatment against their will, based on legal or work-related pressure (Anglin and Hser, 1990; Inciardi, 1988; Lawental et al., 1996; Roman, 1988) and for internally motivated patients (see IOM [1990a] for additional information on the history of coerced treatments). When motivation is conceptualized and measured in terms of the degree to which the patient has been coerced into treatment, it has not been an important predictor of treatment response.

However, motivation, as defined as "readiness for change" and conceptualized and measured in stages as suggested by Prochaska and DiClemente and associates (Prochaska et al., 1992), may be an important predictor of treatment response and treatment outcome. According to the model, behavior change occurs in a progression through five distinct stages, each of which is characterized by a different constellation of attitudes and behaviors. An individual in the precontemplation stage has no awareness of a problem and no desire to change. An individual in the preparation stage has made the decision to change and is already taking steps to do so. An individual in the maintenance stage has successfully made the desired change and is working to maintain that change.

Evidence supports the stages-of-change model. Stage of change may be measured by a brief questionnaire such as the University of Rhode Island Change Assessment (URICA) (McConnaughy et al., 1983) or by the use of an algorithm based on an individual's stated intentions regarding behavior change (DiClemente et al., 1991). Several studies have shown that stage classification can predict change in substance use behaviors for individuals both in and out of treatment across a variety of populations including smokers (DiClemente et al., 1991), heavy drinkers (Heather et al., 1993; Marlatt, 1988), and opiate users (Belding et al., in press).

The model postulates that progression through the stages is mediated by different types of activities or processes of change. The activities most conducive to behavior change vary according to stage. Thus, the model provides a way of identifying patients with different levels of motivation and outlines a way of tailoring interventions to match their stage of change. For example, different types of motivational enhancement therapies (MET) (Miller et al., 1994) can prepare a patient in the early stages of change for subsequent interventions that are typically found in rehabilitation treatments.

Research concerning motivation or stage of change provides an important breakthrough in the treatment of substance-dependent patients. Specifically, if patients do not acknowledge that they have a problem needing treatment, they are likely not to respond to the type of interventions that are often the focus of rehabilitation treatments. However, for decades, precontemplators who are presumed to have an alcohol or drug problem have been forced into treatments and typically confronted about their denial (IOM, 1990a). Thus, the true contribution of this line of research appears to be evidence that forced acceptance can be not only inefficient but also counter therapeutic.

Potential Quality Indicators

A potential quality indicator could be the proportion of recently admitted patients shown to be precontemplators who have received a form of treatment (such as MET or at least a motivational interview) designed to change their motivational readiness. Evidence would suggest that individuals who are potential admissions to rehabilitation and who have *not* shown at least "preparation for change" status will not be good candidates for traditional forms of rehabilitation treatment. Accordingly, this indicator could be most reasonable for use in the initial detoxification-stabilization phase of treatment.

Employment

Employment, employability, and self-support skills often are a significant problem for rehabilitating substance abuse patients, and unemployed patients are more likely to drop out of treatment prematurely and to relapse to substance use early following treatment (Dennis et al., 1993; Platt, 1995). McLellan et al. (1981) found that patients who derived most of their income from employment showed more improvement and better 6-month outcomes in several outcomes domains, including not only employment but also drug use, legal and psychiatric problems, and employment, than similar patients who derived the majority of their income from unemployment or welfare.

Unemployment has been found to be a significant predictor of early relapse to opiate use among detoxified heroin-dependent males (Hall et al., 1981). Similarly, in a sample of primarily employed, multiple substance abusers entering private inpatient or outpatient, abstinence-oriented treatment programs, problems with employment (not getting along with the supervisor, dissatisfaction with present job and salary, etc.) were one of the most significant predictors of both posttreatment substance use as well as posttreatment personal health and social function, measured at the 6-month follow-up (McLellan et al., 1993).

Similar to the findings from studies of the severity of the pretreatment alcohol and drug use, findings from studies of pretreatment employment problems also indicate that those patients (opiate, cocaine, and mixed drug abusers) who have more severe employment and self-support problems also have poorer outcomes following treatment, as measured by a return to substance use and posttreatment self support. In summary, employment problems appear to be a general predictor of poor outcome across most treatment modalities and patient subgroups.

Family and Social Supports

Social support has been conceptualized in a wide variety of ways. These include participation in peer-supported treatments such as AA and NA, the availability of relationships that are not conflict-producing (McLellan et al., 1980, 1985), the level of patient investment in relationships, the level of psychological support from those relationships, and the level of support from those relationships for abstinence from the alcohol or drug use (Longabaugh et al., 1993, 1995).

Among alcohol-dependent patients, those who are members of families with significant dysfunction are more likely to drop out of outpatient treatment programs earlier (McLellan et al., 1983a, b, 1994), to relapse to drinking earlier following treatment (Finney and Moos, 1992), and generally to function poorly after treatment (McCrady et al., 1986; McKay et al., 1993; Moos and Moos, 1984). Patients on methadone maintenance typically return to their families after treatment, and those families have been found to show significant instability and social pathology. The level of social pathology in the family of origin is associated with the use of heroin during methadone treatment (Stanton, 1979; Stanton and Todd, 1982). The family relationship scale on the ASI predicts posttreatment drug use and general personal and social function among opiate-dependent patients in either inpatient therapeutic communities or outpatient methadone maintenance treatment programs (McLellan et al., 1983a, b).

A paradoxically negative relationship has been found between the reported number of available family and friends of the patient and relapse to cocaine use following treatment. For primarily African-American cocaine-dependent patients, the return to cocaine use was earlier if more friends and family had contact with the patient (Havassy et al., 1991, 1994). Many interactive variables may combine in important ways to define the nature and strength of the effect between a particular family and social constellation and a specific treatment (Longabaugh et al., 1995; Moos et al., 1990).

Treatment Factors

Overview. Comparatively few treatment variables have been shown to be predictive of outcome; only those for which evidence for their predictive value has been replicated are presented here. In contrast to the number of studies of patient factors, there are few studies of treatment setting, modality, process, and service factors as predictors of outcome from substance abuse treatments. Perhaps this is because there have been many reliable and valid measures of various patient characteristics but still very few measures of treatment setting (Allison and Hubbard, 1982; Moos, 1974, 1987) or treatment services (McLellan et al., 1992). Developments such as the multisite NIAAA study of patient treatment matching (Project MATCH Research Group, in press) may begin to change this.

Treatment Setting. In the field of rehabilitation from alcohol dependence, several important studies have examined the role of treatment setting, generally showing that the setting of care might not be an important contributor to outcome (Alterman et al., 1994; McCrady et al., 1986). Reviews of the literature on inpatient and outpatient alcohol rehabilitation by Miller and Hester (1986) concluded that across a range of study designs and patient populations there was no significant advantage provided by inpatient care over that provided by outpatient care in the rehabilitation of alcohol dependence, despite the substantial difference in costs. One exception was a study of employed alcohol-dependent patients, which found that an inpatient program produced better outcomes than a very nonintensive form of outpatient treatment, largely Alcoholics Anonymous meetings (Chapman-Walsh et al., 1991).

In treatment of cocaine dependence differences in completion rates for inpatient and outpatient treatments do not appear to be related to longer-term outcome. Alterman et al. (1994) found that 89 percent of inpatients completed treatment, compared with a completion rate of 54 percent for day-hospital treatment. However, at 7 months posttreatment, both groups had made considerable improvements in their drug and alcohol use, family and social, legal, employment, and psychiatric problems. Abstinence rates for both groups were of 50 to 60 percent.

Similar findings have been reported in field studies of private substance abuse treatment programs treating primarily cocaine-dependent and cocaine-plus alcohol-dependent patients (McLellan et al., 1993; Pettinati et al., in press). In all of these studies, patients in outpatient treatment programs were less likely to complete treatment than those in inpatient programs, but those who did complete treatment showed equal levels of improvement and the outcomes in the two settings were comparable.

Attempts to formalize clinical decision processes regarding who should and who should not be assigned to inpatient and outpatient settings of care have had mixed results [McKay et al., 1992, 1994, in press(b)]. Partial support has been found for the predictive validity of the patient placement criteria of the American Society on Addiction Medicine (ASAM) [McKay et al., in press(b)], but research is in progress to evaluate whether the criteria can be effectively used to make decisions concerning placements to levels of care, defined by the amount and quality of medical supervision and monitoring.

Potential Quality Indicators

There may be an advantage for inpatient or residential forms of care for patients who may be less likely to complete treatment (e.g., homeless, more psychiatrically severe, and cocaine-dependent patients), but otherwise, there seem to be few differences in outcomes for inpatient and outpatient treatment. Thus, it would be useful to develop decision criteria that can effectively differentiate those patients who are not likely to show significant improvement from outpatient forms of treatment, such as the proportion of patients assigned to an outpatient treatment program who were found to meet ASAM criteria for placement in an inpatient or residential setting. Conversely, an indicator of clinical cost-effectiveness might be the proportion of patients assigned to inpatient hospitalization who were found to meet ASAM criteria for some form of outpatient treatment.

Length of Treatment and Adherence to Treatment

Virtually all studies of rehabilitation have shown that patients who stay in treatment longer or who attend the most treatment sessions have the best post-treatment outcomes (Armor et al., 1976; Ball and Ross, 1991; DeLeon, 1984, 1994; Simpson et al., 1986). Adherence with the suggestions of the health care provider (usually a physician for those with medical disorders or the counselor or treatment team for those with substance use disorders) has been found to be the single best predictor of continued favorable posttreatment function for substance abuse treatments as well as for other forms of chronic medical conditions, such as diabetes, hypertension, and asthma (McLellan and Durell, 1995; O'Brien and McLellan, 1996).

These relationships suggest that length of stay and patient adherence would appear to be exactly the type of measure that would be well suited to use as a quality indicator (e.g., the percentage of patients who have completed treatment or the percentage of patients who have attended 90 AA meetings in 90 days). However, such a measure would reflect an assumption that patients who enter treatment gradually acquire new motivation, skills, attitudes, knowledge, and supports over the course of their stay in treatment and that the gradual acquisition of these qualities or services is the reason for the favorable outcomes.

Patients who have been randomly assigned to receive a longer duration of treatment do not necessarily show better outcomes than those patients who have been randomly assigned to receive shorter treatments (Miller and Hester, 1986; Project MATCH Research Group, in press). Therefore, it is possible that better patients are likely to stay in treatment longer and to do more of what is recommended. If treatment gradually produces positive changes over time, it is clinically sound practice for patients to stay in treatment longer. On the other hand, if well-motivated, highly functioning, compliant patients enter treatment with the requisite skills and supports necessary to do well, they might also benefit from a shorter treatment regimen.

When a high proportion of patients in a program stay in treatment for the recommended duration and comply with all treatment requirements, does that mean that the treatment processes, policies, and therapists have been selected to instill motivation and engage patients into behavioral change strategies, or that the program has been successful in selecting motivated and compliant patients who are likely to do well regardless of the services that they receive? The distinction between adherence and length of treatment needs further exploration.

Potential Quality Indicators

Length of stay and adherence with treatment recommendations are perhaps the two most easily measured aspects of treatment and are both suitable for inclusion in contemporary clinical management information systems. However, the measures are more appropriately viewed as descriptive rather than as predictive indicators of quality, because there are still questions regarding the meaning of these two measures with regard to outcome (See McKay et al., 1991).

Participation in AA and NA

AA is recognized as a social organization and not a formal treatment. However, AA has become synonymous with the last part of rehabilitation, aftercare. Virtually all alcohol dependence rehabilitation programs and most cocaine dependence rehabilitation programs refer patients to AA and/or NA programs, with instructions to get a sponsor, to attend "share and chair" at meetings, and to attend 90 meetings in 90 days as a continued commitment to sobriety. There has always been consensual validation for the value of AA and other peer-support forms of treatment, but relatively few studies have evaluated the contributions of AA and NA because of the anonymous quality of the groups.

Evidence shows that patients who have participated in AA, NA, or some other form of peer-support group, who have a sponsor, or who have participated in the fellowship activities have much better abstinence records than patients who have received rehabilitation treatments but who have not continued in AA [McKay et al., 1994, in press(a); Timko et al., 1994].

Although studies have generally suggested that the peer-support component of rehabilitation is valuable, it is also difficult to sort out the extent to which AA attendance constitutes an active ingredient of successful treatment or is simply a marker of treatment adherence and motivation (Vaillant, 1996). Infrequent or irregular attendance of AA meetings following discharge from residential treatment was associated with a poorer prognosis than either regular attendance or no attendance (McLatchie and Lomp, 1988).

Potential Quality Indicators

There is no doubt that peer-support groups have made an important contribution for a significant minority of patients. Participation in AA during and following rehabilitation seems to be an excellent marker for sustained reductions in alcohol and drug use as well as improved personal and social function for a significant, if still inexact, proportion of alcohol-dependent patients.

Thus, quality indicators for rehabilitation treatment (at least for alcohol-dependent patients) could be the proportion of patients who have acquired an AA sponsor and the proportion of patients in aftercare who have attended more than three AA meetings in the first month of treatment.

Therapists and Counselors Who Provide Treatment

A drug or alcohol abuse counselor or therapist can make an important contribution to the engagement and participation of the patient in treatment and to the posttreatment outcome. One example of the role of individual counseling was in a study of methadone patients who were randomly assigned to receive individual counseling plus methadone or methadone alone. Fifty-three percent of patients who received counseling showed sustained elimination of opiate use and 41 percent showed sustained elimination of cocaine use over the 6 months of the trial. In contrast, 68 percent of patients assigned to the no counseling condition failed to reduce their level of drug use (confirmed by urinalysis), and 34 percent of these patients required at least one episode of emergency medical care.

However, different outcomes are found for different therapists, including professional psychotherapists with doctorate-level training (Luborsky et al., 1985, 1986), experiential substance abuse counselors (McLellan et al., 1988; Miller et al., 1980), and different individual counselors within an alcohol treatment program (McCaul and Svikis, 1991). What distinguishes more effective from less effective counselors is not clear. A client-centered approach emphasizing reflective listening has been found to be more effective for problem drinkers than a directive, confrontational approach (Miller et al., 1993). In a review of the literature on therapist differences in substance abuse treatment, Najavits and Weiss (1994) concluded, "The only consistent finding has been that therapists' in-session interpersonal functioning is positively associated with greater effectiveness" (p. 683). Among indicators of interpersonal functioning are the ability to form a helping alliance (Luborsky et al., 1985, 1986), measures of the level of accurate empathy (Miller et al., 1980; Valle, 1981), and a measure of "genuineness," "concreteness," and "respect" (Valle, 1981).

Counselor certification is available from several sources throughout the country. These include the Rehabilitation Accreditation Commission; Certified Addictions Counselor (CAC) program, as well as professional certification from the ASAM, American Academy of Addiction Psychiatry, and the American Psychological Association. Currently, there is no evidence to show whether patients treated by certified addictions counselors, physicians, or psychologists have better outcomes than patients treated by noncertified individuals. This is an important gap in the existing literature, and results from such studies would be quite important for the licensing efforts and health policy decisions of many states and health care organizations.

Medications

NIAAA and the National Institute on Drug Abuse have sponsored a great deal of research aimed at developing useful medications for the treatment of substance-dependent persons. Great progress has been made over the past 10 years in the development of new medications and in the application of existing medications for the treatment of particular conditions associated with substance dependence and for particular types of substance-dependent patients. Because of the vast amount of research, this review includes some of the clearest results from the use of medications in the treatment of substance dependence, as well as citations for more comprehensive reviews of medications for interested readers. Two types of medications are discussed: agonist and antagonist or blocking medications.

Agonist Medications. Two agonist medications are in use in the treatment of drug dependence. Both of these medications work by direct occupation of receptors within the body to mimic the effects produced by the target drug. The most prevalent agonist is nicotine replacement in the form of gum or a skin patch, which has recently been approved for over-the-counter sales. Nicotine replacement is typically prescribed and used for relatively brief periods (1 to 3 months) as part of an abstinence-oriented program for nicotine dependence.

For more than 25 years, methadone has been an approved agonist medication for the maintenance treatment of opiate dependence. The long-acting form of methadone (48 to 72 hours in duration), LAAM, has recently received FDA approval and has been accepted by 16 states for use in the same way as methadone; that is, it is available only at methadone maintenance programs. Buprenorphine is a partial opiate agonist that has been widely used in Europe and the United States. It is thought to have some advantages over methadone in that it produces many fewer withdrawal symptoms and often produces none. At the time of this writing, it is not approved for use, although approval is expected shortly.

Among the most robust findings in the treatment literature is the relationship between the dose of methadone and the general outcome of methadone treatment: higher doses are more effective than lower doses (Ball and Ross, 1991; D'Aunno and Vaughn, 1995; IOM, 1995a). In a well-controlled, double-blind, multisite study, Ling et al. (1976) found that 100 milligrams per day was superior to 50 milligrams per day, as indicated by staff ratings of global improvement and by a drug use index comprising weighted results of opiate urine tests.

In a more recent randomized, double-blind study, Strain et al. (1993) compared 50 milligrams and 20 milligrams with a 0 milligram placebo-only group. They found orderly dose-response effects on treatment retention, and they found that 50 milligrams was more effective than 20 milligrams or 0 milligrams at decreasing opiate and cocaine use, as measured by urinalysis results. In a randomized double-blind comparison of moderate (40 to 50 milligrams) and high (80 to 100 milligrams) doses of methadone, Strain et al. (1996) found a significantly lower rate of opiate-positive urine specimens among patients receiving the high dose of methadone (53 percent vs. 62 percent). They concluded that although the higher dose was more effective, substantial opiate use can persist even among patients treated with 80 to 100 milligrams of methadone per day. There are many other studies of opiate agonist medications, but space limitations do not permit more detail here (see IOM, 1995a for additional information).

Potential Quality Indicator

If methadone is prescribed for purposes of maintenance rehabilitation as opposed to detoxification, the dose should be high enough to block the euphoric effects of street opiates (heroin) and the craving for opiates. Thus, a potential quality indicator would be the proportion of patients on methadone maintenance who have continued regular opiate use (as evidenced by past two or three opiate-positive urine specimens) but who have not had increases in their methadone or LAAM dose. Because it is a federal requirement that urine samples be obtained from patients on methadone maintenance, the data should be readily available at the clinic level.

Antagonist and Abuse Blocking Agents. Naltrexone is an orally administered opiate antagonist that blocks the actions of externally administered opiates such as heroin by competitive binding to opiate receptors. Naltrexone under the trade name Trexan® has been used for more than 20 years in the treatment of opiate dependence. More recently, naltrexone (marketed under a different trade name: Revia®) has been found to be effective in the treatment of alcohol dependence (O'Malley et al., 1992; Volpicelli et al., 1992).

Naltrexone at 50 milligrams per day has been approved by the FDA for use with alcohol-dependent patients, because independent studies have shown that it is a safe, effective pharmacological adjunct for reducing heavy alcohol use among alcohol-dependent patients. Its mechanism of action appears to be the blocking of at least some of the high produced by alcohol consumption, again through competitive binding of the opiate receptors (O'Malley et al., 1992; Volpicelli et al., 1992).

With regard to other medications designed to block the effects of an abused drug, disulfiram (Antabuse®) has been used the longest and most pervasively in the treatment of alcohol dependence. Although both disulfiram and naltrexone can be used for extended periods, in practice they are generally prescribed for about 1 to 3 months as part of a more general rehabilitation program that includes behavioral change strategies (see the review by Anton, 1995). Many agents have been tried as blocking agents in the treatment of cocaine dependence, but there is still no convincing evidence that any of the various types of cocaine-blocking agents are truly effective for even brief periods of time or for even a significant minority of affected patients.

The use of opiate and alcohol antagonists or blocking agents is increasing as traditional addiction medicine physicians are becoming more comfortable with the prescription of adjunctive medications and as more substance dependence is treated by primary care physicians in office settings (Fleming and Barry, 1992). The past 10 years have witnessed innovation and discovery in this area, but the parameters that are most effective when using them are still not clear. Thus, some traditional addiction medicine physicians are reluctant to prescribe these medications unless therapy alone has been ineffective (IOM, 1995a, b).

The responsible and appropriate use of these antagonist or blocking medications in the treatment of substance dependence disorders may be among the most important topics for future research in the treatment field. Long-term studies are needed to evaluate the effects of these medications for various types of substance-dependent patients, as well as to determine the most appropriate and efficient mix of psychosocial and pharmacological services that will maximize the impact of rehabilitation.

Potential Quality Indicator

The available literature suggests that naltrexone can be very effective in the abstinence-oriented treatment of opiate dependence and that disulfiram and naltrexone can be effective as adjuncts in the treatment of alcohol dependence. A potential indicator of poor quality care for alcohol dependent patients could be the proportion of patients in abstinence-oriented rehabilitation for alcohol dependence who have continued to use alcohol (as evidenced by the past two or three positive breathalyzer readings) who have not been evaluated for naltrexone or disulfiram treatment.

Specialized Services

The majority of patients admitted to substance abuse treatment have significant addiction-related problems in one or more areas such as medical status, employment and self support, family relations, and psychiatric function (McLellan and Weisner, 1996). As indicated above, the severity of these problems is generally predictive of the response during treatment as well as posttreatment outcome.

Studies over more than a decade have documented that strategies designed to direct and focus specialized services to these addiction-related problems can be applied in standard clinical settings and can be effective in improving the results of substance abuse treatment (McLellan et al., in press). Adding professional marital counseling (O'Farrell et al., 1985; McCrady et al., 1986; Stanton and Todd, 1982), psychotherapy (Carroll et al., 1994; Woody et al., 1995), and medical care (Fleming and Barry, 1992; Schonberg, 1988) produces clinically significant better outcomes from substance abuse treatment. However, interventions that have been developed to improve employment and self support among substance-dependent patients have had mixed results (French et al., 1992; Hall et al., 1981; Zanis et al., 1994).

The majority of adjunctive forms of therapy and services have been most clearly associated with improved personal health and social function following treatment and have been less related to reduced alcohol and drug use. In addition, and not surprisingly, these treatments have only been shown to be effective with those patients having more severe problems in the target area (i.e., matching effect); that is, if there has been no indication of a relatively severe problem in the target area, there has typically been no evidence that the provision of the target therapy is effective or worthwhile (Woody et al., 1984).

Potential Quality Indicators

Significant problems in the areas of employment, medical and psychiatric health, and family relations are thought to be impediments to treatment for substance-dependent patients in two ways. First, the presence of these problems often complicates the provision of standard substance abuse treatment, and second, these problems, if left unattended, can provoke a relapse to substance use even among well-motivated, abstinent individuals. For these reasons, the provision of treatments for these problems is seen as important both for the immediate purpose of retaining patients in treatment and for reducing the risk of a relapse. If these specialized services are potent, it follows that they will have a direct effect on symptoms in the target problem area (e.g., reduction of symptoms of depression) but an indirect and possibly delayed effect on the substance use problems (e.g., longer latency until relapse).

Although many substance abuse treatment programs do not have the resources to provide specialized treatment services, it is at least possible for these programs to perform an active referral to an appropriate agency or practitioner to attempt to access these services. Thus, potential quality indicators would be the proportion of patients who showed evidence of a significant psychiatric problem (by the criteria of DSM IV) who received sessions of specialized psychiatric or psychological care, and the proportion of patients reporting significant family problems who receive sessions of specialized couples or family therapy.

SUMMARY AND DISCUSSION

The search for quality indicators in the research literature has revealed five major challenges. They are summarized in this section.

1.   The existing research on treatment outcomes has been disappointing with regard to informing the search for potential quality indicators.

Most of the outcomes studies in the current literature were conducted by clinical researchers, typically in controlled trials. The purpose of these studies was generally to determine whether the index treatment, when delivered under speci-fied conditions to rather highly selected samples of patients, could effect the ex-pected changes relative to standard or minimal treatment conditions.

However, most clinical trials reviewed here do not lend themselves to the identification of quality indicators. They often exclude important classes of pa-tients (e.g., users of multiple substances and psychotic patients) and focus on very specific outcomes (e.g., abstinence from a single substance). Under such condi-tions, it is difficult to flexibly tailor treatments to individual patients, because studies call for strict adherence to experimental protocols. In clinical practice, when a patient fails to respond to one type of intervention, the sensitive clinician will alter the approach. Thus, the interventions that are compared in experiments may not reflect what happens in practice.

Research has effectively established that treatment can be effective, but there are only preliminary indications at this time about why treatment is effective or what it is about or within treatment that makes it effective. Treatment research-ers are only now beginning to develop the measures and models that will be nec-essary for the exploration of questions regarding why treatment works. If the out-comes research field is really to inform the search for quality or performance indicators in substance abuse treatment, then it will be necessary to move beyond the question of *whether* treatment works to the question of *how* treatment works.

To accomplish this, researchers will need to make a methodology shift from the simple evaluation or comparison of treatment outcomes to the parametric study of the various types of treatment services and therapeutic processes deliv-ered within those treatments and their relationship to the target outcomes. The methodology will require measurement of more than just the target outcomes at a posttreatment follow-up point. Careful recording of the treatment services and processes provided during treatment will be necessary, as will the concurrent monitoring of during-treatment changes in patient attitude, cognition, motiva-tion, affect, and behavior that are the interim goals of these processes.

These types of dose-response or dose-ranging designs will ultimately permit the discovery of the important changes or therapeutic milestones that patients must achieve along their route to recovery and the active ingredients within a treatment that are responsible for those milestones and ultimately for lasting outcomes following treatment. This is a line of research that has been called for by several within the field, but the present review has uncovered very few studies to date that have pursued this line of research. Thus, one message from this paper is a call to the treatment research field for more systematic work along this line of investigation.

2.   Significant confusion and disagreement exist within the field on important and basic concepts that are essential for the identification of potential quality indicators. The most basic confusion has been on the definition of outcomes.

A reviewer of this field will get substantially different views about the outcomes of a substance abuse treatment depending on the perspective taken regarding what outcome is and when, how, and by whom it is measured. Consider three common perspectives on the evaluation of an outpatient treatment program. A quality assurance or service delivery evaluation of that treatment might conclude that the program had very good outcomes because there was no waiting for treatment entry and at discharge more than 80 percent of the patients were highly satisfied with their counselors and physicians. A clinical researcher, having interviewed a sample of patients at admission to the program and again 6 months following discharge, might conclude that the program had mixed outcomes because at the follow-up point only 50 percent of the patients were abstinent (the intended goal of the program) but there was a 70 percent reduction in the frequency of drinking and a 50 percent reduction in medical and psychiatric symptoms. Meanwhile, an economist or health policy analyst might have used Medicaid data tapes to compare the health services utilization rates of a sample of discharged patients 2 years prior to their treatment admission and 2 years following their discharge. The conclusion here might be that treatment had a very poor outcome because there had been no decrease in health care utilization from the pretreatment to the posttreatment period, and hence no cost offset to the public.

This example illustrates two points. First, these three common perspectives on outcomes have different purposes for their evaluations and different expectations regarding treatment. They measure different elements of the treatment process and the patient population and at different points in time. Second, these different measures of outcome are not well related to each other, and to the extent that quality indicators are expected to relate to outcomes, these different perspectives will suggest different quality indicators.

3.   Two stages of treatment exist for substance-dependent patients: the acute care, detoxification-stabilization stage and the subsequent rehabilitation stage. Each stage has different expected outcomes.

For the detoxification-stabilization stage, favorable outcomes include the elimination of the signs and symptoms of physical and emotional instability associated with the initial cessation of substance use and the motivation and engagement of the patient into continued rehabilitation. Treatment characteristics that were most closely associated with these outcomes were the inpatient setting of care (at least for patients likely to drop out prematurely) and treatment to the criterion of 3 consecutive days without withdrawal signs or symptoms.

For rehabilitative treatment to have an opportunity to succeed, the outcomes from the detoxification-stabilization stage would have to be achieved. An outcome from rehabilitative treatment should be lasting improvements in those problems that led to the treatment admission and that were important to the patient and to society. Three outcomes domains have been measured at least 6 months following treatment discharge: reduction in substance use, improvement in personal health and social function, and reduction in public health and safety problems.

Patient variables that had been reliably associated with better outcomes from rehabilitation included (1) low severity of dependence and psychiatric symptoms at admission, (2) "readiness for change" beyond the precontemplation stage of change, (3) being employed or self supporting, and (4) having family and social supports for sobriety. Treatment variables that have been reliably associated with better outcomes in rehabilitation included (1) staying longer in treatment and being more compliant with treatment recommendations, (2) having an individual counselor or therapist (particularly an effective one), (3) receiving proper medications, (4) participating in voucher-based, behavioral reinforcement interventions, (5) participating in AA or NA following treatment, and (6) having specialized services provided for adjunctive medical, psychiatric, or family problems.

Although none of these patient or treatment variables showed a completely unambiguous record of prediction outcomes, the findings have been replicated across more than one type of primary drug problem (alcohol, cocaine, or opiates) and in more than one evaluation. However, although some of the predictors identified (e.g., longer lengths of stay and greater adherence) are quite robust, there is no clear understanding of the basis for the predictive relationship.

No single rehabilitation modality or therapeutic process has yet been reliably associated with superior outcomes across all populations of patients. Furthermore, it was surprising that some of the treatment elements that are most widely provided in substance abuse treatment (e.g., group therapy) have not been associated with outcomes. Clearly, more research is needed to identify the "active ingredients" of treatment and the "minimal effective dose" of these ingredients.

4.   The ability to identify potentially useful quality indicators relies on a clear understanding of the ways in which these indicators will ultimately be used.

Quality indicators can be used in two ways: (1) at the individual patient level to provide clinicians with early warning signs for poor outcome and thus allow for modification of the treatment plan, and (2) in the aggregate, to provide evaluators and regulators with rapid, easily collected, and face-valid indications of treatment program performance, ultimately for purposes of interprogram comparisons and possibly for report cards.

Because a primary purpose for these indicators will be clinical decision support, they need to be measured at the individual patient level and to be collectable as early as possible in the course of treatment, using nonintrusive and rapid methods of data collection. These features are essential for the information to be relevant to clinical decision-making and, in turn, worthwhile for the clinicians who will ultimately be charged with recording these measures.

Not all variables identified as predictors of outcome will be useful in clinical decision-making, because many (e.g., gender and socioeconomic strata) cannot be modified in the course of treatment. At the same time, because a second purpose of these quality indicators will be to compare aggregated mean values between two treatment programs or among several patient subgroups, it will be important to have access to all variables that affect the outcomes of treatment independent of the treatment process. These "case mix adjusters" are important in any comparative study of outcomes or quality indicators to adjust the groups on variables that could have an independent effect on outcome, thus helping to provide a level playing field when the comparative evaluations are performed. Before any of the prospective quality indicators can be used in a comparative fashion, however, much more research comparing different case mix adjustment strategies and different combinations of predictor variables is needed.

5.   Although both treatment process and patient change variables can serve as quality indicators, patient change variables are conceptually and practically much better.

Only two types of measures meet the practical and conceptual needs of the clinical, management, and regulatory groups that are interested in identifying quality indicators. The first of these are treatment elements, processes and practices: interventions or services that are done to or for the patient during treatment. The second of these are interim changes in patient status: aspects of the patient's affect, knowledge, motivation, and behavior that are presumed to be problematic in the patient at the start of treatment and are thus the direct focus of the treatment elements within rehabilitation.

The great majority of the quality indicators used thus far in the evaluation of substance abuse and mental health treatments have been treatment process indicators (counseling provided to urge smokers to quit, referral to outpatient care following inpatient discharge, etc.). Typically, they have been measured by staff notations in treatment charts. There is justification for using these process measures. First, because costs or charges are typically associated with the provision of treatment processes, these measures are generally available and accessible in clinical management information systems. Second, and more importantly, there are clear indications from the outcomes literature that certain treatment processes and treatment elements are reliably related to outcomes.

This review has referred to these treatment process measures as *secondary indicators* of treatment quality for two reasons. The first reason is practical and based on the quality of available evidence. The simple notation in a chart that an activity, labeled as the appropriate or intended process, has been provided at some level of intensity, by someone with an unknown ability or training level, with no indication of its immediate effects, is not, by itself, the type of evidence that inspires confidence in the quality of that treatment.

The second reason for referring to even those treatment practices or treatment elements that have been reliably associated with outcomes as secondary indicators of quality relates to the level of inference that is available from such an association. No treatment element, service, or procedure produces a lasting outcome directly but, rather, produces an outcome through the production of at least one interim change in a patient's attitude, affect, knowledge, motivation, cognition, or behavior. For example, patients who attend rehabilitation following detoxification have better posttreatment outcomes than those who stop treatment following detoxification.

Thus, it can be said that the treatment process or the treatment practice of referring a patient to outpatient treatment is associated with a better posttreatment outcome. However, this association is only true when the referral has actually resulted in the patient's attendance and participation in the rehabilitation. Actually, it is this interim change in the patient's behavior (attendance) rather than the process of referral that is most directly associated with the ultimate outcome, and the treatment practice is only associated with that outcome through its ability to produce that interim result.

There is another reason to use measures of interim changes in patient status (symptoms, signs, behaviors, etc.) instead of treatment process measures as quality indicators. The majority of patient status measures can be measured in a more valid, unbiased, and verifiable way than most treatment process measures. Thus, although it would be possible to check a patient chart for a note indicating the current dose of methadone (a secondary indicator of treatment quality), greater confidence would come from primary indicators, such as interim results in the form of reductions in observed withdrawal signs and negative urine screens.

Although these measures of interim change in patient status may be slightly more difficult to collect, most are not burdensome and are, again, directly associated with the focus of the treatment elements or interventions being applied. Specifically, given a patient status variable that has been reliably associated with treatment outcome (e.g., a high-severity psychiatric problem at admission) and a treatment process variable that has also been reliably related to outcome (e.g., provision of professional psychotherapy), the responsible clinician and clinical regulator will be better informed regarding the quality of the care provided to the patient by measuring changes in psychiatric symptomatology over the course of treatment (e.g., a weekly change in Beck Depression Inventory) rather than measuring the number of therapy sessions provided during the course of treatment.

NEED FOR FURTHER RESEARCH

A new line of research is needed to address at least two central questions of effective and efficient treatment delivery.

1.   What types of interim changes in patients should be effected during treatment to provide the highest probability of lasting gains following treatment?

Not all of the changes in patients' attitudes, affects, motivation, knowledge, and behavior that are the interim goals of substance abuse treatments are important for attaining favorable posttreatment outcomes. An important role for future treatment research will be to identify those interim patient changes that are reliably predictive of lasting benefits following treatment. These ultimately will be the quality indicators that the field is searching for.

2.   Which treatment settings, modalities, and services provide the most potent and rapid ways of effecting the during-treatment changes that have been shown to be important predictors of lasting outcomes, and at what costs?

Not all of the treatment elements, services, or activities that are provided to patients in treatment will be appropriate or adequate to produce the interim patient changes that are desired. An important role for future treatment research will be to identify the active ingredients and the minimum effective dose of those ingredients that can effect the important interim changes in patients during the course of treatment.

Combinations of active ingredients will ultimately be translated into empirically derived clinical pathways and treatment guidelines. Because these combinations of proven effective treatment ingredients are compared for potency and duration of action as well as on the basis of their costs of delivery for both the provider and the patient, real estimates of the value and efficiency of treatments can be developed.

REFERENCES

Allison M, Hubbard RL. 1982. *Drug Abuse Treatment Process: A Review of the Literature.* TOPS Research Monograph. Raleigh, NC: Research Triangle Press.

Alterman AI, McLellan AT, O'Brien CP, August DS, Snider EC, Cornish JC, Droba M, Hall CP, Raphaelson A, Schrade F. 1994. Effectiveness and costs of inpatient versus day hospital cocaine rehabilitation. *Journal of Nervous and Mental Diseases* 182:157-163.

Alterman AI, McKay J, Mulvaney F, McLellan AT. 1996. Prediction of attrition from day hospital treatment in lower socioeconomic cocaine-dependent men. *Drug and Alchohol Dependence* 40:227-233.

Anglin MD, Speckart GR, Booth MW, Ryan TM. 1989. Consequences and costs of shutting off methadone. *Addictive Behaviors* 14:307-326.

Anglin MD, Hser Y. 1990. Legal coercion and drug abuse treatment. In: Inciardi J, ed. *Handbook on Drug Control in the United States*. Westport, CT: Greenwood Press.

Anton RF. 1995. New Directions in the pharmacotherapy of alcoholism. *Psychiatric Annals* 25:353-362.

Armor DJ, Polich JM, Stambul HB. 1976. *Alcoholism and Treatment*. Santa Monica, CA: The RAND Corporation Press.

Babor TF, Dolinsky Z, Rounsaville BJ, Jaffe JH. 1988. Unitary versus multidimensional models of alcoholism treatment outcome: An empirical study. *Journal of Studies on Alcohol* 49(2):167-177.

Bale RN. 1979. Outcome research in therapeutic communities for drug abusers: A critical review 1963-1975. *International Journal of the Addictions* 14:1053-1074.

Ball JC, Ross A. 1991. *The Effectiveness of Methadone Maintenance Treatment*. New York: Springer-Verlag.

Belding MA, Iguchi MY, Lamb RJ. In press. Stages and processes of change as predictors of drug use among methadone maintenance patients. *Experimental and Clinical Psychopharmacology*.

Brown SA, Irwin M, Schuckit MA. 1991. Changes in anxiety among abstinent male alcoholics. *Journal of Studies on Alcohol* 52:55-61.

Carroll KM, Rounsaville BJ, Gawin FH. 1991. A comparative trial of psychotherapies for ambulatory cocaine abusers: Relapse prevention and interpersonal psychotherapy. *American Journal of Drug and Alcohol Abuse* 17:229-247.

Carroll KM, Rounsaville BJ, Nich C, Gordon LT, Wirtz PW, Gawin F. 1994. One-year follow-up of psychotherapy and pharmacotherapy for cocaine dependence: Delayed emergence of psychotherapy effects. *Archives of General Psychiatry* 51(12):989-997.

Carroll KM, Nich C, Rounsaville BJ. 1995. Differential symptom reduction in depressed cocaine abusers treated with psychotherapy and pharmacotherapy. *Journal of Nervous and Mental Disease* 183:251-259.

Chapman-Walsh D, Hingson RW, Merrigan DM, Morelock Levenson S, Cupples,A, HeerenT, Coffman GA, Becker CA, Barker TA, Hamilton SK, McGuire TG, Kelly CA. 1991. A randomized trial of treatment options for alcohol-abusing workers. *The New England Journal of Medicine* 325:775-782.

Cushman P, Dole VP. 1973. Detoxification of rehabilitatied methadone-maintained patients. *Journal of the American Medical Association* 226:747-752.

D'Aunno TJ, Vaughn T. 1995. An organizational analysis of service patterns in drug abuse treatment. *Journal of Substance Abuse* 16:123-131.

DATOS (Drug Abuse Treatment Outcome Study). 1992. Drug abuse treatment outcome study. *NIDA Research Monograph No. 237*. Rockville, MD: National Institute on Drug Abuse.

DeLeon G. 1984. The therapeutic community: study of effectiveness treatment. *NIDA Research Monograph*. Publication No. 84-1286. Rockville, MD: National Institute on Drug Abuse.

DeLeon G. 1994. Therapeutic communities: Toward a general theory and model. In: Tims FM, De Leon G, Jainchill N, eds. *NIDA Research Monograph*. Washington, D.C.: National Institute on Drug Abuse.

Dennis ML, Karuntzos GT, McDougal GL, French MT. 1993. Developing training and employment programs to meet the needs of methadone treatment clients. *Evaluation Program Planning* 16:73-86.

DiClemente CC, Prochaska JO, Fairhurst SK, Velicer WF, Velasquez MM, Rossi JS. 1991. The process of smoking cessation: An analysis of precontemplation, contemplation, and preparation stages of change. *Journal of Consulting and Clinical Psychology* 59:295-304.

Finnegan LP. 1991. Treatment issues for opioid-dependent women during the perinatal period. *Journal of Psychoactive Drugs* 23:191-199.

Finney JW, Moos RH, Chan DA. 1981. Length of stay and program component effects in the treatment of alcoholism: A comparison of two techniques for process analyses. *Journal of Consulting and Clinical Psychology* 49:120-131.

Finney JW, Moos RH. 1992. The long-term course of treated alcoholism: II. Predictors and correlates of 10-year functioning and mortality. *Journal of Studies on Alcohol* 53:142-153.

Fleming MF, Barry KL, eds. 1992. *Addictive Disorders*. St. Louis: Mosby Yearbook Primary Care Series.

French MT, Rachal JV, Hubbard RL. 1991. Conceptual framework for estimating the social cost of drug abuse. *Journal of Health and Social Policy* 2:1-22.

French MT, Dennis ML, McDougal GL, Karuntzos GT, Hubbard RL. 1992. Training and employment programs in methadone treatment: Client needs and desires. *Journal of Substance Abuse Treatment* 9:293-303.

Gawin FH, Kleber HD. 1986. Abstinence symptomatology and psychiatric diagnoses in cocaine abusers. *Archives of General Psychiatry* 43:107-113.

Gawin FH, Ellinwood EH. 1988. Cocaine and other stimulants: Actions, abuse, and treatment. *The New England Journal of Medicine* 318:1173-1182.

Gerstein DR, Johnson RA, Harwood HJ, Fountain D, Suter N, Malloy K. 1994. *Evaluating Recovery Services: The California Drug and Alcohol Treatment Assessment (CALDATA)*. Fairfax, VA: Lewin-VHI and National Opinion Research Center at the University of Chicago.

Gomberg ESL. 1989. Alcoholic women in treatment: Early histories and early problem behaviors. *Advances in Alcoholism and Substance Abuse* 8:133-147.

Gomberg ESL, Nirenberg TD, eds. 1993. *Women and Substance Abuse*. Norwood, NJ: Ablex Publishing Corporation.

Gossop M, Johns A, Green L. 1986. Opiate withdrawal: Inpatient versus outpatient programmes and preferred versus random assignment. *British Medical Journal* 293:103-104.

Hagan TA, Finnegan LP, Nelson L. 1994. Impediments to comprehensive drug treatment models for substance abusing women: Treatment and research questions. *Journal of Psychoactive Drugs* 26:163-171.

Hall SM, Loeb P, LeVois P, Cooper J. 1981. Increasing employment in ex-heroin addicts. II: Methadone maintenance sample. *Behavioral Medicine* 12:453-460.

Havassy BE, Hall SM, Wasserman DA. 1991. Social support and relapse: Commonalities among alcoholics, opiate users, and cigarette smokers. *Addictive Behaviors* 16(5):235-246.

Havassy BE, Wasserman D, Hall SM. 1994. Social relationships and cocaine use in an American treatment sample. *Addiction* 18:145-161.

Hayshida M, Alterman AI, McLellan AT, O'Brien CP, Purtill JJ, Volpicelli JR, Raphaelson AH, Hall CP. 1989. Comparative effectiveness of inpatient and outpatient detoxification in patients with mild-to-moderate alcohol withdrawal syndrome. *The New England Journal of Medicine* 320(6):358-365.

Heather N, Rollnick S, Bell A. 1993. Predictive validity of the Readiness to Change Questionnaire. *Addiction* 88:1667-1677.

Higgins ST, Budney AJ, Bickel WK, Hughes JR, Foeg FE, Badger GJ. 1993. Achieving cocaine abstinence with a behavioral approach. *American Journal of Psychiatry* 150:763-769.

Higgins ST, Budney AJ, Bickel WK, Foerg FE, Donham R, Badger GJ. 1994. Incentives improve outcome in outpatient behavioral treatment of cocaine dependence. *Archives of General Psychiatry* 51:568-576.

Holder HD, Blose JO. 1992. The reduction of health care costs associated with alcoholism treatment: A 14-year longitudinal study. *Journal of Studies on Alcohol* 53(4):293-302.

Hubbard RL, Marsden ME. 1986. Relapse to use of heroin, cocaine and other drugs in the first year after treatment. In: *Relapse and Recovery in Drug Abuse*. NIDA Research Monograph No. 72. Rockville, MD: National Institute on Drug Abuse.

Hubbard RL, Marsden ME, Rachal JV, Harwood HJ, Cavanaugh ER, Ginzburg HM. 1989. *Drug Abuse Treatment: A National Study of Effectiveness.* Chapel Hill: University of North Carolina Press.

Inciardi JA. 1988. Some considerations on the clinical efficacy of compulsory treatment: Reviewing the New York experience. In: Leukefeld CG, Tims FM, eds. *Compulsory Treatment of Drug Abuse: Research and Clinical Practice.* NIDA Research Monograph No. 86. Rockville, MD: National Institute on Drug Abuse.

IOM (Institute of Medicine). 1990a. *Broadening the Base of Treatment for Alcohol Problems.* Washington, DC: National Academy Press.

IOM. 1990b. *Treating Drug Problems.* Vols. 1 and 2. Washington, DC: National Academy Press.

IOM. 1995a. *Federal Regulation of Methadone Treatment.* Washington, DC: National Academy Press.

IOM. 1995b. *Development of Medications for the Treatment of Opiate and Cocaine Addictions: Issues for the Government and Private Sector.* Washington, DC: National Academy Press.

Johnston LD, O'Malley PM, Bachman JG. 1996. *National Survey Results on Drug Use From the Monitoring the Future Study.* NIDA Publication No. 96-4027. Washington, DC: National Institute on Drug Abuse.

Kadden RM, Cooney NL, Getter H, Litt MD. 1990. Matching alcoholics to coping skills or interactional therapies: Post treatment results. *Journal of Consulting and Clinical Psychology* 57:698-704.

Kang SY, Kleinman PH, Woody GE, Millman RB, Todd TC, Kemp J, Lipton DS. 1991. Outcomes for cocaine abusers after once-a-week psychosocial therapy. *American Journal of Psychiatry* 148:630-635.

Kosten TR, Rounsaville BJ, Kleber HD. 1987. Multidimensionality and prediction and treatment outcome in opioid addicts: 2.5-year follow-up. *Comprehensive Psychiatry* 28:3-13.

Lawental E, McLellan AT, Grissom GR, Brill P, O'Brien CP. 1996. Coerced treatment for substance abuse problems detected through workplace urine surveillance: Is it effective? *Journal of Substance Abuse* 8(1):115-128.

Ling W, Charuvastra C, Kaim SC, Klett J. 1976. Methadyl acetate and methadone as maintenance treatments for heroin addicts. *Archives of General Psychiatry* 33:709-720.

Lipton DS, Maranda MJ. 1983. Detoxification from heroin dependency: An overview of method and effectiveness. *Advances in Alcohol and Substance Abuse* 2:31-55.

Longabaugh R, Beattie M, Noel N, Stout R, Malloy P. 1993. The effect of social investment on treatment outcome. *Journal of Studies on Alcohol* 54:465-478.

Longabaugh R, Wirtz PW, Beattie MC, Noel NE, Stout R. 1995. Matching treatment focus to patient social investment and support: 18-month follow-up results. *Journal of Consulting and Clinical Psychology* 63:296-307.

Luborsky L, McLellan AT, Woody GE, O'Brien CP. 1985. Therapist success and its determinants. *Archives of General Psychiatry* 42:602-611.

Luborsky L, Crits-Christoph P, McLellan AT, Woody GE. 1986. Do psychotherapists vary much in their effectiveness? The answer within four outcome studies. *American Journal of Orthopsychiatry* 56(4):501-512.

Marlatt GA. 1988. Matching clients to treatment: Treatment models and stages of change. In: Donovan DM, Marlatt A, eds. *Assessment of Addictive Behaviors.* New York: Guilford Press. Pp. 474-483.

McCaul M, Svikis D. 1991. Improving client compliance in outpatient treatment: Counselor-targeted interventions. *NIDA Research Monograph No. 106.* Rockville, MD: National Institute on Drug Abuse. Pp. 204-217.

McConnaughy EA, Prochaska JO, Velicer WF. 1983. Stages of change in psychotherapy: Measurement and sample profiles. *Psychotherapy: Theory, Research and Practice* 20:368-375.

McCrady BS, Noel NE, Abrams DB, Stout RL, Nelson HF, Hay WM. 1986. Comparative effectiveness of three types of spouse involvement in outpatient behavioral alcoholism treatment. *Journal of Studies on Alcohol* 47:459-467.

McKay JR, Alterman AI, McLellan AT. 1991. Does achieving goals of addiction treatment predict better outcomes? *Alcoholism: Clinical and Experimental Research* 15:383.

McKay JR, McLellan AT, Alterman AI. 1992. An evaluation of the Cleveland Criteria for inpatient treatment of substance abuse. *American Journal of Psychiatry* 149:1212-1218.

McKay JR, Longabaugh RC, Beattie M, Maisto S, Noel N. 1993. Changes in family functioning during treatment and drinking outcomes for high and low autonomy alcoholics. *Addictive Behaviors* 18:355-363.

McKay JR, Alterman AI, McLellan AT, Snider EC. 1994. Treatment goals, continuity of care, and outcome in a day hospital substance abuse rehabilitation program. *American Journal of Psychiatry* 151:254-259.

McKay JR, McLellan AT, Alterman AI, Cacciola J, Rutherford M, O'Brien CP. In press(a). Predictors of participation in aftercare sessions and self-help groups following completion of intensive outpatient treatment for substance abuse. *Journal of Studies on Alcohol.*

McKay JR, Cacciola J, Alterman A, McLellan AT, Wirtz P. In press(b). An initial evaluation of the psychosocial dimensions of the Americant Society on Addiction Medicine criteria for inpatient versus intensive outpatient substance abuse rehabilitation. *Journal of Studies on Alcohol.*

McLatchie BH, Lomp KG. 1988. Alcoholics Anonymous affiliation and treatment outcome among a clinical sample of problem drinkers. *American Journal of Drug and Alcohol Abuse* 14:309-324.

McLellan AT, Ball JC. 1995. Is methadone treatment effective? Background Paper prepared for IOM Committee on Federal Regulation of Methadone Treatment. In: IOM. *Federal Regulation of Methadone Treatment.* Washington, DC: National Academy Press.

McLellan AT, Durell J. 1995. Evaluating substance abuse and psychiatric treatments: Conceptual and methodological considerations. In: Sederer L, ed. *Outcomes Assessment in Clinical Practice.* New York: Williams and Wilkins.

McLellan AT, Weisner C. 1996. Achieving the public health potential of substance abuse treatment: Implications for patient referral, treatment "matching" and outcome evaluation. In: Bickel W, DeGrandpre R, eds. *Drug Policy and Human Nature.* Philadelphia: Wilkins and Wilkins.

McLellan AT, Hunkeler E. In press. Relationships between patient satisfaction and patient performance in addiction treatment. *American Journal of Psychiatry.*

McLellan AT, Luborsky L, O'Brien CP, Woody GE. 1980. An improved diagnostic instrument for substance abuse patients: The Addiction Severity Index. *Journal of Nervous and Mental Diseases* 168:26-33.

McLellan AT, O'Brien CP, Luborsky L, Woody GE, Kron R. 1981. Are the addiction-related problems of substance abusers really related? *Journal of Nervous and Mental Diseases* 169(4):232-239.

McLellan AT, Woody GE, Luborsky L, O'Brien CP, Druley KA. 1982. Is treatment for substance abuse effective? *Journal of the American Medical Association* 247:1423-1427.

McLellan AT, Luborsky L, Woody GE, Druley KA, O'Brien CP. 1983a. Predicting response to alcohol and drug abuse treatments: Role of psychiatric severity. *Archives of General Psychiatry* 40:620-625.

McLellan AT, Luborsky L, Woody GE, O'Brien CP, Druley KA. 1983b. Increased effectiveness of substance abuse treatment: A prospective study of patient-treatment "matching". *Journal of Nervous and Mental Diseases* 171(10):597-605.

McLellan AT, Griffith J, Childress AR, Woody GE. 1984. The psychiatrically severe drug abuse patient: Methadone maintenance or TC. *American Journal of Drug and Alcohol Abuse* 10(1):77-95.

McLellan AT, Luborsky L, Cacciola J, Griffith J. 1985. New data from the Addiction Severity Index: Reliability and validity in three centers. *Journal of Nervous and Mental Disease* 173:412-423.

McLellan AT, Woody GE, Luborsky L, Goehl L. 1988. Is the counselor an "active ingredient" in substance abuse rehabilitation? *Journal of Nervous and Mental Disease* 176:423-430.

McLellan AT, Alterman AI, Woody GE, Metzger D. 1992. A quantitative measure of substance abuse treatments: The treatment services review. *Journal of Nervous and Mental Disease* 180:100-109.

McLellan A, Grissom G, Durell J, Alterman AI, Brill P, O'Brien CP. 1993. Substance abuse treatment in the private setting: Are some programs more effective than others? *Journal of Substance Abuse Treatment* 10:243-254.

McLellan AT, Alterman A, Metzger DS, Grissom GR, Woody GE, Luborsky L, O'Brien CP. 1994. Similarity of outcome predictors across opiate, cocaine, and alcohol treatments: Role of treatment services. *Journal of Consulting and Clinical Psychology* 62(6):1141-1158.

McLellan AT, Alterman AI, Woody GE, Metzger D, McKay JR, O'Brien CP. 1995. Great Expectations: A review of the concepts and empirical findings regarding substance abuse treatment. In: *Alcohol and Substance Dependence.* London, England: Royal Task Force on Substance Dependence.

McLellan AT, Grissom G, Brill P. In press. Improved outcomes from treatment service "matching" in substance abuse patients: A controlled study. *Archives of General Psychiatry.*

Miller WR, Hester RK. 1986. Inpatient alcoholism treatment: Who benefits? *American Psychologist* 41:794-805.

Miller WR, Taylor CA, West JC. 1980. Focused versus broad-spectrum behavior therapy for problem drinkers. *Journal of Consulting and Clinical Psychology* 48:590-601.

Miller WR, Benefield RG, Tonigan JS. 1993. Enhancing motivation for change in problem drinking: A controlled comparison of two therapist styles. *Journal of Consulting and Clinical Psychology* 61:455-461.

Miller WR, Zweben A, DiClemente CC, Rychtarik RG. 1994. *Motivational Enhancement Therapy Manual: A Clinical Research Guide for Therapists Treating Individuals With Alcohol Abuse and Dependence.* Rockville, MD: National Institute on Alcohol Abuse and Alcoholism.

Moos RH. 1974. *Evaluating Treatment Environments.* New York: Wiley.

Moos RH. 1987. *The Social Climate Scales: A Users Guide.* Palo Alto, CA: Consulting Psychologists Press.

Moos RH, Moos B. 1984. The process of recovery from alcoholism. III: Comparing family functioning in alcoholic and matched control families. *Journal of Studies on Alcohol* 45:111-118.

Moos RH, Finney JW, Cronkite RC. 1990. *Alcoholism Treatment: Context, Process and Outcome.* New York: Oxford University Press.

Najavits LM, Weiss RD. 1994. Variations in therapist effectiveness in the treatment of patients with substance use disorders: An empirical review. *Addiction* 89(6):679-688.

Naranjo CA, Sellers EM, Chater K, Iversen P, Roach C, Sykora K. 1983. Nonpharmacologic intervention in acute alcohol withdrawal. *Clinical Pharmacology and Therapeutics* 34:214-219.

O'Brien CP, McLellan AT. 1996. Myths about the treatment of addiction. *Lancet* 347:237-240.

O'Farrell TJ, Cutter HS, Floyd FJ. 1985. Evaluating behavioral marital therapy for male alcoholics: Effects on marital adjustment and communication from before to after treatment. *Behavior Therapy* 16(2):147-167.

ONDCP (Office of National Drug Control Policy). 1995. *Pulse Check: National Trends in Drug Abuse.* Washington, DC: U.S. Government Printing Office.

O'Malley SS, Jaffe AJ, Chang G, Schottenfeld RS. 1992. Naltrexone and coping skills therapy for alcohol dependence: A controlled study. *Archives of General Psychiatry* 49:881-887.

Pettinati HM, Belden PP, Evans BD, Ruetsch CR, Meyers K, Jensen JM. In press. The natural history of outpatient alcohol and drug abuse treatment in a private health care setting. *Alcoholism: Clinical and Experimental Research.*

Platt JJ. 1995. Vocational rehabilitation of drug abusers. *Psychological Bulletin* 117:416-435.

Powell BJ, Pennick EC, Othemer E, Bingham SF, Rice AS. 1982. Prevalence of additional psychiatric syndromes among male alcoholics. *Journal of Clinical Psychiatry* 43:404-407.

Prochaska JO, DiClemente CC, Norcross JC. 1992. In search of how people change: Applications to addictive behaviors. *American Psychologist* 47(9):1102-1114.

Project MATCH Research Group. In press. Matching alcoholism treatments to client heterogeneity. Project MATCH posttreatment drinking outcomes. *Journal of Studies on Alcohol.*

Robinson GM, Sellers EM, Janecek E. 1981. Barbiturate and hypnosedative withdrawal by a multiple oral phenobarbital loading dose technique. *Clinical Pharmacology and Therapeutics* 30:71-76.

Roman P. 1988. Growth and transformation in workplace alcoholism programming. In: Galanter M, ed. *Recent Developments in Alcoholism*. Vol.11. New York: Plenum. Pp. 131-158.

Rounsavile BJ, Weissman MM, Crits-Christoph K, Wilber C, Kleber H. 1982. Diagnosis and symptoms of depression in opiate addicts: Course and relationship to treatment outcome. *Archives of General Psychiatry* 39:151-156.

Rounsaville BJ, Glazer W, Wilber CH, Weissman MM, Kleber H. 1983. Short-term interpersonal psychotherapy in methadone-maintained opiate addicts. *Archives of General Psychiatry* 40:630-636.

Rounsaville BJ, Dolinsky ZS, Babor TF, Meyer RE. 1987. Psychopathology as a predictor of treatment outcome in alcoholics. *Archives of General Psychiatry* 44:505-513.

Satel SL, Price LH, Palumbo JM, McDougle CJ, Krystal JH, Gawin F, Charney DS, Heninger GR, Kleber HD. 1991. Clinical phenomenology and neurobiology of cocaine abstinence: A prospective inpatient study. *American Journal of Psychiatry* 148:1712-1716.

Schonberg SK, ed. 1988. *Substance Abuse: A Guide for Health Professionals*. Elk Grove Village, IL: American Academy of Pediatrics.

Schuckit MA.. 1985. The clinical implications of primary diagnostic groups among alcoholics. *Archives of General Psychiatry* 42:1043-1049.

Schuckit MA, Monteiro MG. 1988. Alcoholism, anxiety and depression. *British Journal of Addiction* 83:1373-1380.

Schuckit MA., Irwin M, Brown SA. 1990. History of anxiety symptoms among 171 primary alcoholics. *Journal of Studies on Alcohol* 51:34-41.

Sells SB, Simpson DD. 1980. The case for drug abuse treatment effectiveness, based on the DARP research program. *British Journal of Addiction* 75:117-131.

Senay EC, Dorus W, Showalter CV. 1981. Short-term detoxification with methadone. *Annals of the New York Academy of Science* 362:16-21.

Simpson D, Savage L. 1980. Drug abuse treatment readmissions and outcomes. *Archives of General Psychiatry* 37:896-901.

Simpson DD, Sells SB. 1982. Effectiveness of treatment for drug abuse: An overview of the DARP research program. *Advances in Alcohol and Substance Abuse* 2:7-29.

Simpson DD, Joe GW, Lehman WEK, Sells SB. 1986. Addiction careers: Etiology, treatment, and 12-year follow-up outcomes. *Journal of Drug Issues* 16:107-121.

Stanton MD. 1979. The client as family member. In: Brown BS, ed. *Addicts and Aftercare*. New York: Sage Publications.

Stanton MD, Todd T. 1982. *The Family Therapy of Drug Abuse and Addiction*. New York: Guilford Press.

Stewart RG, Ware LG. 1989. *The Medical Outcomes Study*. Santa Monica, CA: The RAND Corporation Press.

Stockwell T, Bolt E, Hooper J. 1986. Detoxification from alcohol at home managed by general practitioners. *British Medical Journal* 292:733-735.

Stockwell T, Bolt L, Milner I, Puch P, Young I. 1990. Home detoxification for problem drinkers: acceptability to clients, relatives, general practioners and outcome after 60 days. *British Journal of Addiction* 85:61-70.

Stockwell T, Bolt L, Milner I, Russell G, Bolderston H, Hugh P. 1991. Home detoxification from alcohol: Its safety and efficacy in comparison with inpatient care. *Alcohol and Alcoholism* 26:645-650.

Strain EC, Stitzer ML, Liebson IA, Bigelow GE. 1993. Dose-response effects of methadone in the treatment of opioid dependence. *Annals of Internal Medicine* 119:23-27.

Strain EC, Bigelow GE, Liebson IA, Stitzer ML. 1996. *Moderate Versus High Dose Methadone in the Treatment of Opioid Dependence*. Poster session presented at the annual meeting of the College on Problems of Drug Dependence. San Juan, Puerto Rico. June.

Timko C, Moos RH, Finney JW, Moos BS. 1994. Outcome of treatment for alcohol abuse and involvement in Alcoholics Anonymous among previously untreated problem drinkers. *Journal of Mental Health Administration* 21:145-160.

Transdermal Nicotine Study Group. 1991. Transdermal nicotine for smoking cessation. *Journal of the American Medical Association* 266:3133-3138.

Vaillant GE. 1996. *The Natural History of Alcoholism*. Cambridge, MA: Harvard University Press.

Valle S. 1981. Interpersonal functioning of alcoholism counselors and treatment outcome. *Journal of Studies on Alcohol* 42:783-790.

Volpicelli JR, Alterman AI, Hayashida M, O'Brien CP. 1992. Naltrexone in the treatment of alcohol dependence. *Archives of General Psychiatry* 49:876-880.

Weddington WW. 1992. Cocaine abstinence: "Withdrawal" or residua of chronic intoxication? *American Journal of Psychiatry* 149:1761-1762.

Weisner C. 1993. Toward an alcohol treatment entry model: A comparison of problem drinkers in the general population and in treatment. *Alcoholism: Clinical and Experimental Research* 17(4): 746-752.

Weisner CM, Greenfield TK, Room R. 1995. Trends in treatment for alcohol problems in the US general population, 1979-1990. *American Journal of Public Health* 85(1):55-60.

White Paper. 1995. *Effectiveness of Substance Abuse Treatment*. Washington, DC: U.S. Department of Health and Human Services.

Whitfield CL, Thompson G, Lamb A, Spencer V, Pfeifer M, Browning-Ferrando M. 1978. Detoxification of 1024 alcoholic patients without psychoactive drugs. *Journal of the American Medical Association* 239:1409-1410.

Wilsnack SC, Wilsnack RW. 1991. Epidemiology of women's drinking. Special issue: Women and substance abuse. *Journal of Substance Abuse* 3:133-157.

Wilsnack SC, Wilsnack RW. 1993. Epidemiological research on women's drinking: Recent progress and directions for the 1990s. In: Gomberg ESL, Nirenberg TD, eds. *Women and Substance Abuse*. Norwood, NJ: Ablex Publishing Corporation. Pp. 62-99.

Woody GE, Luborsky L, McLellan AT, O'Brien CP, Beck AT, Blaine J, Herman I, Hole A. 1983. Psychotherapy for opiate addicts: Does it help? *Archives of General Psychiatry* 40:639-645.

Woody GE, McLellan AT, Luborsky L. 1984. Psychiatric severity as a predictor of benefits from psychotherapy. *American Journal of Psychiatry* 141(10):1171-1177.

Woody GE, McLellan AT, Luborsky L, O'Brien CP. 1987. Twelve-month follow-up of psychotherapy for opiate dependence. *American Journal of Psychiatry* 144:590-596.

Woody GE, McLellan AT, Luborsky L, O'Brien CP. 1995. Psychotherapy in community methadone programs: A validation study. *American Journal of Psychiatry* 152(9):1302-1308.

Zanis DA, Metzger DS, McLellan AT. 1994. Factors associated with employment among methadone patients. *Journal of Substance Abuse Treatment* 11:443-447.

C

Consumer Outcomes and Managed Behavioral Health Care: Research Priorities

Donald M. Steinwachs

Center for Research on Services for Severe Mental Illness, Health Services Research and Development Center, Department of Health Policy and Management, Johns Hopkins School of Hygiene and Public Health

The growth in managed care and managed behavioral health care, with their incentives to reduce costs, has raised concerns that active management of utilization may lead to poorer quality of care and to poorer outcomes for persons with mental illness. The current evidence suggests that substantial cost savings are being achieved by managed care, but with patient outcomes that are no worse than those in the fee-for-service system (Iglehart, 1996). However, many concerns are being raised about the potential for adverse consequences as managed behavioral health care expands to cover more seriously ill and disabled populations (Mechanic et al., 1995). It is the purpose of this paper to review what is known about the impact of managed care on the outcomes of care for persons with mental illness and to suggest issues that should be given priority in future research. In one sense this is relatively easy to accomplish. The current literature on mental illness treatment and outcomes in managed care is limited in scope and depth, although it is expanding (Mechanic et al., 1995; Wells et al., 1995). This suggests that much more needs to be known, but provides little insight into the relative importance of different areas of mental health outcomes research and evaluation.

The discussion of information needs and priorities for research uses the quality-of-care paradigm of structure, process, and outcome. The incentives inherent in managed care capitation payment systems versus traditional indemnity fee-for-service (FFS) payment systems are explored to focus on a series of hypotheses regarding differences in structure, process, and outcomes. In this context, the existing research evidence and its limitations are discussed. This leads into a discussion of the author's view of research priorities and strategies for filling the current gaps in knowledge.

BACKGROUND

The growth in the 1990s of managed health care has exceeded all previous expectations. Federal policy actively promoted capitated and comprehensive health care for the first time with the passage of the 1973 Health Maintenance Organization (HMO) Act. The growth in HMO enrollment in the 1970s and 1980s was substantial, but HMOs remained a source of health care for a small proportion of Americans (Luft, 1987). During the 1980s new forms of managed care emerged, including the preferred provider organization (PPO). This added to the penetration of managed care and gave it recognition as a significant and growing sector of the health care system.

The failure of health care reform in 1994-1995 did more to accelerate the implementation of managed care than any federal initiative had previously achieved. This should not be surprising. Over the previous 10 years, elements of managed care had been progressively adopted by major payers to control the growth in utilization and costs. These elements include precertification of elective hospital admissions, concurrent review of length of stay or use of per-case payment, substitution of ambulatory surgery and diagnostic testing for inpatient services when appropriate, and other controls including limiting the use of emergency rooms, establishment of drug formularies, and organizational control over the selection of the practitioners included in networks or group practices (Payne, 1987; Weiner and de Lissovoy, 1993). The literature suggests that these actions can individually and collectively reduce health care costs below the levels found in FFS practice and even more so for mental health care (Frank et al., 1995).

The utilization control strategies used in managed medical care have been applied to mental health and substance abuse services (Mechanic et al., 1995). Among an estimated 185.7 million people with private insurance in 1994, 106.6 million were enrolled in plans that offered some form of managed behavioral health care (Iglehart, 1996). One difference, however, is that the tradition of HMO and indemnity insurance coverage for mental illnesses has not been comparable to the coverage for somatic health problems. Historically, the treatment of chronic mental illness has not been covered by HMOs, and indemnity insurance has restricted mental health benefits such that persons with chronic and disabling illnesses would be likely to use services in excess of the available coverage (McFarland, 1994). The reasons for this distinction between mental and somatic illnesses were numerous, including uncertainty that mental illnesses could be cured or medically managed and the role of the states and the public sector as the last provider of mental health services, particularly for persons with severe and persistent mental illnesses (Grob, 1991). Also, significant stigma has been associated with mental illness, which has tended to suppress the demand for services and for expanding coverage. Another reason for limiting coverage was to limit costs, which became a major topic of debate during health care reform deliberations (Arons et al., 1994; Frank et al., 1992).

Significant changes that have occurred over the past two decades are likely to lead to greater comparability in coverage between mental and somatic disorders. The biological basis of many mental illnesses has been established, and the efficacies of drug and other treatments have been demonstrated for many disorders. Even so, the stigma associated with mental illness continues, but it appears that this may be slowly changing too. Laws to guarantee parity of benefits for mental illness have been passed in several states and were considered recently by the U.S. Congress. Parity legislation can be expected to shift more of the cost burden for the treatment of severe and disabling mental illness from the public sector to the private health insurance system. How this will affect persons with severe mental illness is uncertain. Many of these individuals are deprived of the ability to work and gain income, leaving them in poverty and reliant on welfare and publicly supported health insurance, under Medicare or Medicaid. However, it is clear that managed care will be involved. One of the more recent trends has been the movement of Medicaid programs to managed care. By June 1994, 7.8 million Medicaid beneficiaries were enrolled in some form of managed care, double the number in the previous year (Essock and Goldman, 1995; Iglehart, 1996).

SPECIALIZED MANAGED CARE: MANAGED BEHAVIORAL HEALTH CARE

As managed care grew in the 1980s and grew at an accelerated rate in the 1990s, specialized managed behavioral health care networks emerged (England and Vaccaro, 1991). Managed behavioral health care companies sell managed care services, ranging from utilization review to accepting capitated risk as a provider of specialty mental health services. A new terminology emerged to describe *carve-outs* and *carve-ins* as means of integrating managed behavioral health care services into a network of managed health care services. Managed care organizations are created through a series of contractual arrangements with primary care providers, specialty providers, hospitals, utilization managers, and behavioral health firms (Gold et al., 1995a). This is quite different from the HMO concept embodied in the 1973 HMO Act that stimulated the growth of group practice and independent practice association HMOs. The newer forms of managed care include PPOs, physician-hospital organizations, and point-of-service plans. Although there are growing numbers of variations on the HMO concept, they share most of the elements common to HMOs: they offer a limited choice of practitioners, they make efforts to control the use of high-cost services and to substitute lower-cost services when appropriate, they provide comprehensive coverage, and they require low out-of-pocket payments for services.

MANAGING MENTAL HEALTH CARE

The need for information on managed care is elevated by policy concerns at the state and federal levels. Questions have been raised regarding how treatment and patterns of care received under the managed behavioral health care system differ from those received under the indemnity insurance system. To the extent that patterns of care differ, how is this affecting patient outcomes? The previous discussion suggests a range of hypotheses that derive from financial incentives and organizational differences between the managed care and traditional indemnity insurance systems. These hypotheses are organized around the quality-of-care framework presented by Donabedian (1993) that organizes quality into three areas: structure, process of care, and outcomes of care.

Structure and Access to Care

Choice of Practitioner

In concept, indemnity insurance has made it possible to go to any practitioner in the community. This is largely true for well-insured, middle-class Americans. However, for those with more limited incomes, practitioners who do not accept Medicare and Medicaid payments or who bill their patients for the amounts that are not covered by Medicare or Medicaid may have out-of-pocket costs so high that many people cannot afford them (Berk et al., 1995). For persons covered under medical assistance programs (Medicaid), the level of payment to participating practitioners may be so low that many practitioners will not accept patients with this coverage. Yet, most Americans continue to perceive that indemnity coverage makes it possible to choose any practitioner. In contrast, managed care offers the patient a defined panel of providers, with the size of the panel varying from few to most community providers. In POS and PPO managed care plans, any practitioner can be chosen, but the cost of going outside of the preferred panel is a substantial deductible and coinsurance comparable to those under indemnity coverage. On the basis of these characteristics, the following is hypothesized:

Hypothesis 1A: Managed care leads to the concentration of patient services among a more limited set of providers than occurs under indemnity insured care.

It is clear that the managed care system uses organizational and financial incentives to limit the choice of providers (Gold et al., 1995a), but the literature does not appear to include any studies evaluating the impact of managed care on the number and type of providers seen for specific health problems, including mental illness.

Access and Availability of Services

Another aspect of the structure of health care concerns the availability of services. In each community there are limits on the availability of health services, but additional limits that are not present under indemnity insurance plans are likely to be imposed by managed care plans. Even though managed care plans control the availability of physician services, they provide 24-hour access and have financial incentives to provide accessible urgent care during off hours instead of having enrollees go to hospital emergency rooms (Gold et al., 1995a). A study of Medicare beneficiaries found them to be more satisfied with waiting times for an appointment under the managed care system than under the FFS system (Rossiter et al., 1989); however, these results were not specific to mental health care services. This leads to the following hypothesis:

Hypothesis 1B: Delays in receiving nonurgent care will be less in the managed care system than in the indemnity covered care system; urgent care will be more accessible in the managed care system.

Access and Unmet Need

Important differences exist between indemnity insurance and managed care plans in the use of coverage limits and out-of-pocket payments to control utilization and costs. Indemnity insurance coverage has relied on limiting coverage and imposing significant deductibles and coinsurance to reduce utilization and costs. The effects of deductibles and coinsurance were evaluated in the RAND Corporation's Health Insurance Experiment in the 1970s (Manning et al., 1986). The study found that persons were less likely to seek treatment when faced with significant out-of-pocket payments, but when treatment was sought, the pattern of treatment did not substantially differ by level of deductible or coinsurance (Keeler and Rolph, 1988; Keeler et al., 1986). This was found for both mental and somatic disorders.

In contrast, HMOs and other managed care organizations offer comprehensive coverage (except for specialty mental health services) and impose few or no deductibles and small or no copayments. When there are higher copayments for mental health care, these have comparable effects on reducing utilization (Simon et al., 1994). With the implementation of a managed behavioral health care carve-out in the Massachusetts Medicaid program in 1992, the results from the first year found a higher proportion of enrollees receiving mental health care under managed care (Stroup and Dorwart, 1995). Here changes in access would not have been related to out-of-pocket costs but may have involved changes in other organizational and provider characteristics. In McFarland's (1994) review of previous research on HMO services provided for mental illness, he found a "pattern in which HMO members are as likely as or more likely than non-HMO members to visit a mental health provider but tend to have fewer contacts with that provider after the initial visit." The net effect of lower access barriers in managed care should be greater accessibility of services for those with a need for care. This leads to the following hypothesis:

Hypothesis 1C: Unmet need for care will be higher under indemnity coverage than under managed care.

Provider Participation

One of the complexities in evaluating the impact of managed care, and particularly managed mental health care, is the range and complexity of organizational and financial arrangements (Gold et al., 1995b). Individual practitioners may be paid on a fee-for-service basis but at a reduced rate or may share risk through a full or partial capitation. Since a practitioner sees patients covered under different insurers, the financial incentives may vary substantially from one patient to the next. Thus, practitioners would be expected to respond to incentives in a way that would maximize their practice and income preferences. Little is known regarding how practitioners make choices regarding joining a managed care network and how they respond to a complex array of incentives arrangements when they are part of multiple managed care organizations.

At the same time, managed care organizations make choices regarding which practitioners to ask to participate in their network. This choice may involve the use of practitioner profiles (Salem-Schatz et al., 1994) that identify higher-cost practitioners and that exclude them from the network. Initially, efforts to market managed care organizations in new geographic areas may give priority to market penetration and may include as many participating practitioners as possible. Over time, however, the managed care organization may wish to concentrate its enrollees among a more limited set of practitioners whose practices are consistent with managed care organization expectations. These dynamics are complex and lead to the following hypothesis:

Hypothesis 1D: Practitioner participation in managed care organization networks is jointly determined by practitioner preferences, practice characteristics, and managed care organization market strategies.

The structure of managed care organizations is evolving and changing as organizations seek to learn through experience what works and how to improve on existing organizational and financial incentives. As a result, there are unusual opportunities for research, but some opportunities may be time-limited and may require access to privileged management information.

Process of Care Screening and Treatment

Detection and Diagnosis

The process of care may involve screening, diagnosis, treatment, follow-up, and maintenance care, plus rehabilitation in some instances. Under the managed care system some would argue that the financial incentive is not to diagnose new problems because this adds to costs. However, the mental health research on cost offsets indicates that failure to diagnose and treat mental and emotional problems does not prevent future utilization and costs, and may make utilization more costly (Fiedler, 1989). One example is Northern California Kaiser Permanente Medical Care Program, which has reported savings of medical costs by upgrading its behavioral health care benefit (Iglehart, 1996).

In contrast, the financial incentives under indemnity coverage are to provide more services that might increase rates of detection and follow-up care. The Medical Outcomes Study (MOS) of the diagnosis, treatment, and outcomes of one mental illness, depression, found somewhat lower rates of detection under the prepaid care system, primarily related to the greater use of primary care practitioners, who have substantially lower detection rates than mental health specialists (Wells, 1989; Wells and Sturm, 1995). However, the Massachusetts Medicaid managed behavioral health care carve-out appears to have led to higher rates of specialty care, possibly associated with higher rates of detection and referral (Stroup and Dorwart, 1995). Since there are complex incentives arrangements affecting care-seeking and mental illness recognition, it is uncertain which direction a hypothesis should be stated; however, the following hypothesis is provided:

Hypothesis 2A: The probability of detection and diagnosis of mental and emotional problems will be the same under the managed care system as under the indemnity insurance system.

Use of Hospitals and Specialty Care

Although there is some uncertainty regarding the direction of potential differences in detection and diagnosis rates, there are clear incentives for managed care plans to provide less intensive services for the treatment of mental and emotional problems, as reflected by the lower level of use of inpatient psychiatric services. This usually involves a process for preadmission certification. Wickizer et al. (1996) found little reduction (less than 2 percent) in admissions. In the Massachusetts Medicaid managed behavioral health care carve-out, there was a 22 percent reduction in overall mental health costs in the first year and a 30 percent reduction in inpatient psychiatric services (Stroup and Dorwart, 1995). The structure of incentives leads to the following hypothesis:

Hypothesis 2B: The probability of hospitalization for a mental illness will be lower under the managed care system than under the indemnity insurance system, as will the probability of referral to a mental health specialist, except when there are fiscal incentives for primary care providers to refer a patient to mental health specialty providers.

Duration of Treatment

Another way to control the cost of treatment is to control the duration of treatment. Under the indemnity insurance system, the incentive is to continue to treat mental illness until the coverage limits are reached or the patient decides that no more treatment is desired. Under the managed behavioral health care system, there is active utilization review to assess the need for continuing services in inpatient and outpatient settings. In inpatient settings, one recent study found precertification and continuing stay review led to 16.8 days of stay approved out of 23.5 days requested (Wickizer et al., 1996). In a study of admissions for affective disorders, Frank and Brookmeyer (1995) found both short-term and longer-term savings from preadmission certification programs that came from fewer admissions, even though readmission rates were somewhat higher, and shorter lengths of stay. In the Massachusetts Medicaid managed behavioral health care carve-out there were reductions in length of stay of from 9.7 to 8.7 days in the first year, and for persons with severe mental illness, the reductions were from 22.5 to 17.8 days (Stroup and Dorwart, 1995). In an evaluation of PPOs, Wells et al. (1992) found lower rates of ambulatory services use in the PPO than in the indemnity insurance system, but access was comparable. As a result, it would be expected that:

Hypothesis 2C: The duration of treatment episodes under the managed care system will be shorter than the duration of treatment episodes under the indemnity insurance system.

Prescription Patterns

There does not appear to be much research on the patterns of medication use for mental illness in managed care settings. In a study of general prescription practices, Weiner et al. (1991) found that practitioners at managed care plans were more likely to use generic drugs than practitioners under the indemnity insurance system, but that practitioners under both systems were equally likely to use newer and frequently high-cost medications. The MOS found that the HMO patients were less likely to receive the clinically recommended dose of the prescribed antidepressant than patients receiving care under the indemnity insurance system, but the difference was largely ascribed to the greater use of primary care physicians in the HMO compared with the use of greater numbers of specialists in the indemnity insurance system (Wells and Sturm, 1995). It is not known to what extent managed care organizations have responded to this finding and have encouraged the use of the appropriate dosage that has been found to contribute to better outcomes. The differences that are likely to persist will be those that relate to controlling costs, leading to the following hypothesis:

Hypothesis 2D: Treatment with medications will be the same between the managed care and indemnity insurance systems, but practitioners at managed care plans will be more likely to use generic substitutes and other lower-cost alternatives.

This discussion has reviewed some of the findings related to differences in the use of services between managed care plans and the indemnity insurance system. These differences reflect the differences in financial incentives between capitation and fee-for-service payment plans. In general, managed care plans use less intensive and lower-cost services, with uncertain implications for the quality of care.

Quality of Care

Quality-of-care studies among HMOs in the 1950s to the 1970s found that the prepaid group practice and staff model HMOs provided care of equal or higher quality compared with that provided by other community providers (Luft, 1987; McFarland, 1994). Few studies have been conducted since the rapid growth of managed care organizations. Currently, the Schizophrenia and Depression Patient Outcome Research Team projects are examining quality-of-care issues and the impact of quality of care on patient outcomes. The MOS found process of care differences, with lower rates of diagnosis and appropriate treatment in the HMO, but this was largely explained by a greater reliance placed on primary care physicians than physicians in the FFS practice setting, with greater reliance on mental health specialists (Wells and Sturm, 1995). Under different carve-in and carve-out arrangements, there may be substantial variations in the use of specialty services among managed care organizations. As a result of these uncertainties, the following hypothesis is suggested:

Hypothesis 2E: Adherence to quality-of-care criteria for the diagnosis and treatment of mental illness will be equal under the managed care and indemnity insurance systems, but it will be greater when mental specialists are providing care.

Outcomes of Care: Clinical, Health Status, Satisfaction, and Costs

It is easier to develop hypotheses regarding access to services and patterns of use than to hypothesize the presence and direction of differences in outcome. The hypothesized differences in structure and treatment process discussed above are unlikely to equally affect outcomes. Those likely to have greater impacts are the following:

1. Better access to primary care and preventive services for individuals in managed care settings than for individuals with indemnity insurance coverage may reduce unmet need for services.

2. Reduced access to specialty services for individuals in managed care settings may lead to less adequate treatment and poorer outcomes than for individuals who are covered by indemnity insurance.

3. The provision of less intensive services of shorter duration in managed care settings than in settings covered by indemnity insurance may lead to equal or poorer outcomes.

There is some evidence to support the contribution of specialty care to better mental health outcomes, as found in the MOS for depression (Wells and Sturm, 1995). The receipt of specialty care was less likely in HMOs. The MOS examination of depression treatment and outcomes across fee-for-service and HMO practice settings is unique (Wells, 1989). Although one may want to draw conclusions regarding the impact of the managed care system on mental illness treatment and outcomes, it is important to remember that HMOs are not representative of the range of today's managed care plans and that most fee-for-service practitioners are now practitioners for one or more different managed care plans (Gold et al., 1995b). Studies of the impact of capitation payment in both public and private systems have been conducted (Lurie et al., 1992), with mixed or uncertain findings regarding outcomes. The traditional indemnity coverage is disappearing, with Medicare beneficiaries and a small proportion of privately insured individuals remaining. Thus, the available evidence is stronger for differences in outcomes between specialists and generalist practitioners than between managed care and other settings covered by indemnity insurance.

Hypothesis 3A: Clinical status, health status, and satisfaction outcomes will be better for those receiving specialty care, no matter whether this is under the managed care or the indemnity insurance system, but the costs of specialty care will be higher than primary care.

The expectations that access to primary medical care is better in managed care organizations than in settings covered by indemnity insurance, plus the MOS findings comparing HMO and FFS practice settings, lead to the following hypothesis:

Hypothesis 3B: Population-based outcomes will be better in the managed care setting than in settings covered by indemnity insurance; greater access to primary care services and utilization of preventive and screening services will lead to lower levels of unmet need, although more limited access to specialty services in the managed care setting will contribute to poorer outcomes among those treated.

Unfortunately, there do not appear to be any studies that can support or refute this hypothesis. This requires the linkage of epidemiological studies comparing the need for care with utilization data and outcomes assessment. The methodology might build on the work of Shapiro et al. (1985), who linked indicators of need for mental health services to consumer-reported use of services using the National Institute of Mental Health (NIMH) Epidemiologic Catchment Area Study (Baltimore). The missing elements include indicators of the quality of care received and a strategy for measuring outcomes.

Past studies of Medicare beneficiaries and their satisfaction with care under the HMO and FFS systems have found no overall difference in satisfaction. However, there was greater satisfaction with waiting times and claims processing in HMOs and greater satisfaction with practitioner competence and practitioner willingness to discuss problems in the FFS system (Rossiter et al., 1989). Current work by the Center for Mental Health Services (CMHS) to standardize a consumer-oriented satisfaction survey will aid in understanding these relationships for behavioral health care. Consideration of the incentives and what is known leads to the following hypothesis:

Hypothesis 3C: Patient satisfaction with waiting times, financial arrangements, and out-of-pocket costs will be greater in managed care plans; whereas satisfaction with choice of practitioner and practitioner communication will be greater in settings covered by indemnity insurance.

The financial incentives and the success of managed mental health care in reducing hospitalizations suggest that the costs of care should be lower in managed care.

Hypothesis 3D: The costs of care covered by indemnity insurance will be higher than costs in the managed care system after adjusting for the severity and mix of patients treated.

The literature does not appear to contain studies on the cost of mental illness that rigorously compare services between the managed care and indemnity insurance systems. Case mix adjustment is a key feature of such a comparison.

Summary

The incentives inherent in managed care plans versus those in settings covered by indemnity insurance ensure that there will be important differences in access and treatment patterns, and these may lead to significant differences in outcomes. Neither form of financing and organization is inherently better, but managed care brings a population focus that is critically important in any effort to improve the health of all Americans.

Overall, managed care may provide better access to care for most Americans and will likely provide less costly and intensive services. The value of intensive services varies, and their impacts on outcomes are uncertain. A desirable goal for research on consumer outcomes is to ensure that the potential of managed care to make a positive difference in health outcomes is achieved. There appears to be little question that it is achieving its objective to control or reduce health care costs.

ROLE OF CONSUMER OUTCOMES RESEARCH

The expectations have been very high that research using information on patient outcomes can clarify what is appropriate treatment, for whom, and under what circumstances. Outcomes are broadly conceptualized to include disease or clinical measures, health status (physical, mental, and social functioning), quality of life (satisfaction with health status), and satisfaction with the care process. Also, the costs of care are sometimes included. When the U.S. Congress established the Agency for Health Care Policy and Research in 1989, it specifically directed it to establish a research program on the effectiveness of health care on the basis of patient outcomes. The initial focus was on the Medicare population and the conditions in which a high degree of variability in treatment patterns could be documented and for which costs were high (Wennberg, 1987). This focus has been broadened to other population groups, and the focus on outcomes research has been adopted by other agencies, including NIMH, the U.S. Department of Veterans Affairs, and others.

The experience in outcomes research to date has provided important insights and some valuable lessons. The available statistical methods and measurement tools are being pushed to their limits in efforts to link treatment variations to outcomes in naturalistic (quasiexperimental) study designs. Both need to be improved. Outcomes are multidimensional, and some dimensions may improve while others decline. Relatively little is known about patient, family, practitioner, payer, and society's preferences for different dimensions, but investigators are trying to learn (Kleinman, 1995). Lastly, treatment efficacy trials, which look for significant mean differences in one or more clinical outcomes, are much less ambitious than effectiveness research, which looks for the best match of a treatment to patient characteristics to maximize outcomes for an individual consumer.

Outcomes research must be viewed as a long-term investment in reorienting the health and mental health care systems to place greater value on their most important output: maintenance and improvement of functional status and health-related quality of life. Achieving this goal will require improvements in preventive, treatment, and rehabilitative services for behavioral health problems. Outcomes and effectiveness research is one means for identifying opportunities for improvement in services by providing new insights into the critical managed care question: how can services be organized and provided to defined populations to maintain and improve health outcomes at a reasonable cost? To ensure the relevance and application into practice of the findings of outcomes research, a close alignment between outcomes research priorities and the issues facing managed care will be needed.

RESEARCH PRIORITIES

The challenge of setting priorities in an area of health care that is rapidly changing and that is relatively poorly understood by researchers is significant. Research has traditionally required long-term investments to produce information that can be used by policymakers, practitioners, regulators, consumers, and other users. Maximization of the value of a long-term investment strategy, and at the same time responsiveness to more immediate demands for information, suggest the need for an integrated strategy in which key elements of managed care are characterized and efforts are made to stimulate researchers to examine these elements in a variety of settings. The long-term research question to be addressed is the following: how can health and mental health care be better managed (organized, financed, and delivered) to achieve the full range of outcomes desired by payers, practitioners, consumers, and the public? In a rapidly changing environment, priority may be given to using research to assess the adverse risks of change on quality of care and patient outcomes. This is an important priority and should be pursued. At the same time, a changing environment opens opportunities for innovation that may not be found at other times. Now is a time to encourage researchers to conceptualize and evaluate innovative strategies for providing health care that break from tradition. Health services researchers should be asking the question, "If American health care were being redesigned from the bottom up, what type of health care system should be developed to meet the needs of persons with behavioral health problems?" This might involve a very different mix of health care practitioners and might redefine the roles of patients, families, and practitioners.

In the following discussion a simple framework for examining mental health care management and outcomes will be used to suggest research topics and priorities related to patient outcomes. A caution is offered, however, in listing specific issues: the attention tends to be focused on system components and not the overall system structure. Both need to be addressed in outcomes research.

Assumptions

In an effort to focus on specific priorities, assumptions concerning care for a mental illness and the overall care management process will be made. The first

TABLE C.1   Managing Care: Elements of the Process

Access to care: Consumer, family, and practitioner roles
- Recognition of problem
- Recognition of need for care
- Decision to seek/provide care
- Barriers to receiving/providing care

Diagnosis and treatment
- Diagnostic criteria
- Practitioner—primary care or specialty care (physician or nonphysician)
- Treatment guidelines
- Follow-up arrangements to ensure continuity and maintenance
- Utilization controls
- Financial incentives to practitioner and patient
- Limits of coverage
- Role of family, employer, and self-help groups

Rehabilitation
- Assessment of need for services
- Limits of coverage
- Cost and utilization controls
- Follow-up arrangements
- Role of family, employer, and self-help groups

---

assumption is that mental illness is frequently recurrent or chronic in nature, and its care should be approached from a perspective of long-term management and the prevention of a recurrence. The importance of this assumption is that it suggests that the patient and family need to be full participants in the management of the care and in decision-making processes, or the goals of preventing recurrences and maximizing long-term outcomes are less likely to be achieved.

The second assumption is that managing care involves managing access; diagnosis, treatment, and maintenance; and rehabilitative care. In Table C.1, there is an effort to identify some of the elements used in managing these three stages in the care process. These will be discussed more fully as specific priority recommendations are made.

A third assumption is that research on the care of persons with the greatest needs should be given higher priority, as should research on preventing the worst outcomes of mental illness.

By using these assumptions and the elements in Table C.1, the potential for managed care to improve the delivery of mental health care will be examined to identify priority topics for research.

Population-Based Mental Health Outcomes: Opportunities for Improvement

Under the managed care system, there is a need to address both population- and patient-based outcomes. Population- and patient-based outcomes have not been addressed in the indemnity insurance system. Three observations from the literature regarding mental illness care provide the basis for discussing opportunities for improvements of population-based outcomes. First, mental illnesses tend to go undiagnosed and untreated, leading to high levels of unmet needs for care (Shapiro et al., 1985). These tend to be higher than those for somatic disorders. When diagnosed, mental illnesses are frequently inadequately or inappropriately treated, as is true of many somatic health problems. Even when treatment is initiated, many patients fail to continue treatment, fail to complete referrals, and are lost to follow-up, maintenance, and rehabilitative care. This, too, is true of the care for many chronic somatic disorders. Taken together, population-based outcomes are driven by the combination of unmet needs for care, inadequately or inappropriately met needs when services are received, and a lack of effective long-term maintenance strategies to maximize long-term outcomes.

For example, in the early days of the National Heart, Lung, and Blood Institute National High Blood Pressure Education Program, it was noted that 50 percent of those with high blood pressure knew it, 50 percent of those who knew it were receiving care for high blood pressure, and 50 percent of those who were receiving care had their blood pressures under adequate control. From a population-based perspective, 12.5 percent were achieving the desired clinical outcome. This low rate of effective care for a population with a specific health problem may be quite similar to the current situation in the treatment of behavioral health problems. Efficacious treatments are available for most mental illnesses. The challenge is to bring those who can benefit from treatment under effective and ongoing clinical management.

How can research on managed care accelerate the development and implementation of effective strategies for addressing these three major determinants of poorer health outcomes? The following are suggested elements in a strategy for achieving this goal. In each of these elements, there is the issue of the cost of care and the need to identify efficient service strategies to achieve good outcomes.

Structure of Managed Care

The observation that managed care is rapidly changing and evolving is taken as a truism. For this reason, the study of managed care as an entity is not as relevant as it was in the previous two decades when HMOs were relatively stable and were compared with FFS medicine. Hence, it becomes important to understand the impacts of the specific mechanisms used to manage care and how combinations of these mechanisms affect access, processes of care, and outcomes. As yet, there is little research on specific mechanisms beyond capitation payment (Mechanic et al., 1995) and the need for precertification for inpatient services (Frank and Brookmeyer, 1995).

Another reason for focusing research on managed care mechanisms and their impacts on outcomes of care is the increasing difficulty of identifying opportunities to compare managed care with "unmanaged" or settings covered by indemnity insurance without some managed care features. The current research opportunities are evolving toward comparisons of populations that receive care under different managed care mechanisms that may be applied with varying degrees of rigor and consistency.

An example of managing care for persons with severe and disabling mental illness is the Program for Assertive Community Treatment (PACT). This has been evaluated over the past two decades and has demonstrated positive outcomes at a cost comparable to or less than that for long-term hospitalization (Stein and Test, 1985). Recent work is showing a relationship of outcomes to the degree of fidelity to the PACT model (McGrew et al., 1994). Similarly, research is needed to measure the relationship between managed behavioral health care strategies and outcomes.

Problem Recognition

Population-based health care needs efficient strategies for recognizing behavioral health problems. Multiple foci should be explored, including enhancing practitioners' abilities to recognize behavioral health problems and provide them with incentives to diagnose such problems, examining the role of the employer (e.g., employee assistance programs), and examining the role of the family and consumer. However, recognition of a behavioral health problem is not sufficient. Research is needed on effective strategies to decrease the stigma associated with behavioral health problems and to make consumers and families more willing to enter care. This could involve research on strategies for public education and opportunities for consumers to assess their own problems by having access to screening instruments and referral guidelines. The question is how can the unmet needs of enrolled populations be more effectively addressed at a reasonable cost?

Entering the Care Process

As the managed behavioral health care system grows, many questions are being raised. Are there new models for engaging consumers with behavioral health problems in the care process? What is the role of the primary health care system, in which the majority of patients are treated for behavioral health problems? How can outcomes measurement strategies encompass both those who enter care and those who do not? One of the major concerns is whether it will be known if the managed care system is reducing the number of individuals with unmet needs. An example of a research and demonstration strategy is being implemented by the Mental Health Outcomes Roundtable. It is testing the feasibility of using complementary strategies to measure population- and patient-based outcomes using a population survey and patient questionnaires (Flynn and Steinwachs, 1995). One concern is whether or not there are measurement tools and strategies that can do this at a reasonable cost. The National Committee for Quality Assurance's (NCQA's) Health Plan Employer Data and Information Set (HEDIS) report cards have pushed managed care organizations to be concerned with population-based measures of access for preventive care; comparable measures are needed for behavioral health care.

Choice of Provider: Cost and Effectiveness

As indicated above, the PACT model of team care has been the subject of extensive research on cost and effectiveness. As the managed behavioral health care system attempts to put together provider panels and teams to care for the full spectrum of mental illness and substance abuse problems, there will be questions regarding what makes a cost-effective team, when a team approach is needed, and how mental health professionals should be trained in the future to participate in managed care. In many ways very little is known about staffing and organizational options and how they contribute to consumer outcomes and costs. This issue also touches on the structure of medical practice (e.g., prescription privileges), self-care and consumer-organized care (e.g., clubhouses), and the roles of the different professional groups now providing mental health care. There appears to be little research on how to put together the managed care team for population-based management, and this is critically important to the future of managed care.

Treatment Strategy

Mental health is beginning to adopt practice guidelines and promote quality-of-care research that is comparable to research on medical and surgical conditions. The general impression is that mental health has lagged behind medicine in efforts to move toward explicit quality-of-care criteria (guidelines). Yet, the efficacies of treatments for mental illnesses are in many ways better established than the efficacies of treatments for many medical problems (NIMH, 1993). Using the results of efficacy studies and effectiveness research, the process of developing quality-of-care criteria needs to be accelerated if the information needed to assess quality of treatment under any and all forms of managed care is to be available. Mental health quality-of-care research needs to recognize the special roles of consumers and families in the care of individuals with chronic and recurring illnesses. There are effective ways to involve the family in the care process to improve outcomes, and these should be part of high-quality care (Lehman, 1995).

Individuals may not receive high-quality care for many reasons. Failures may occur in the system, the practitioner may not diagnose the illness or prescribe medications consistent with quality standards, and the patient may not adhere to the practitioner's directions. In research, special attention also needs to be given to the consumer's incentives to be a full participant in the care process, not just the practitioner's incentives to diagnose and treat the consumer effectively. High proportions of patients are reported to drop out of treatment and to stop taking medications. It appears that relatively little is known about how to engage consumers and families in the long-term process of chronic disease management. Essentially, research into ways to support consumers and families in integrating the care process into their daily lives is needed.

Targeting High-Risk, High-Cost Patients

The success of many health care interventions lies in the capacity to efficiently identify high-risk cases and intervene effectively. It is not clear that there has been sufficient progress in developing useful criteria for identifying high-risk or high-cost patients that can be used by managed care plans to target individuals and groups for outreach and active case management. Complicating the problem is the frequent observation that high-risk and high-cost patients have multiple morbidities (comorbidity) and may require specially integrated treatment systems. Current research on cost-effective models for integrated treatment of comorbidities appears to be lacking. If cost-effective strategies to manage high-cost patients are not tested and evaluated, the incentives of managed care may lead to minimal maintenance strategies that attempt to contain costs and that may not maximize outcomes.

Priorities Among Elements of Managed Care

Other elements in care management will need to be examined critically if there is to be a truly managed health care system that respects the consumer and family roles and achieves goals related to outcomes of care and costs. A potentially effective strategy for developing a full research agenda on managed care outcomes would be to bring together all the stakeholders in managed behavioral health care, including consumers and families, payers, regulators, practitioners, policymakers, and researchers. The objective would be to define the long list of researchable issues and to identify priorities. The product could be a national plan that could serve the very useful role that the NIMH National Plan to Improve Care for Persons with Severe and Persistent Mental Illness did in the early 1990s (NIMH, 1990). The purpose of the plan would be to focus research resources and researchers on key issues in the rapidly changing system.

STRATEGIES FOR FILLING THE GAPS IN KNOWLEDGE

Substantial gaps in knowledge related to behavioral health care exist, and the system is in a process of change that does not allow the leisure of relying solely on long-term research strategies if the direction of change is to be influenced through research. This suggests that a mix of strategies may be needed if current demands for better information are to be met and if the long-term needs for information to improve treatment and service systems are to be ensured.

Secondary Data Strategies, Health Statistics, and Report Cards

One of the highest priorities for research should be the development and testing of measures of population-based behavioral health care performance that could be incorporated into report cards. HEDIS and NCQA have begun the process, but measures of mental health care are less well developed than some of those for preventive services and other chronic diseases (e.g., diabetes).

A range of research issues is involved, including quality-of-care measurement (i.e., what care predicts good outcomes), population-oriented as well as patient-oriented measures, and valid and reliable strategies for obtaining measures at reasonable costs. Work by CMHS has provided measures of satisfaction, and the Mental Health Outcomes Roundtable is testing disease-specific modules for depression and schizophrenia plus population-based survey strategies (Flynn and Steinwachs, 1995). The Managed Behavioral Health Association is developing and testing its report card. This work needs to be accelerated and substantially expanded. It should include both public and private initiatives. Notable is the absence from almost all report cards of outcomes measures except in the area of satisfaction. This limitation of current report cards urgently needs to be addressed.

Attention needs to be given to national survey strategies in the new managed care world. The traditional tracking of specialty practitioners and services by CMHS needs to be reconsidered, and ways to incorporate measures of quality and consumer outcomes need to be examined. This may be the only way to track trends over time and to produce timely information on changes in the overall system.

Strategies for Outcomes Management Systems

Increasingly, managed care organizations are attempting to track outcomes and link this information to costs (Burlingame et al., 1995). As early experience suggests (Steinwachs et al., 1994), the routine collection of outcomes information is not simple, and the interpretation of this information for quality improvement is frequently uncertain and can be a complex task. This is an excellent area in which the use of considering multisite outcomes tracking and quality improvement efforts should be considered. No single organization may be able to invest the time and resources needed to adapt research instruments to everyday use and the analytic expertise to analyze and interpret the results. Furthermore, no single organization can know how well it is doing compared with the performance of other practitioners (e.g., benchmarking). The model of outcomes data collection being developed by the Managed Health Care Association Consortium on Outcomes Management, the Mental Health Outcomes Roundtable, and the Foundation for Accountability needs to be examined critically and could become part of a national research demonstration agenda. The goal would be quality improvement, and the products would include report card strategies for ensuring accountability.

Focusing on Mechanisms for Managing Care

The focus on research into the impact of mechanisms for managing care on consumer outcomes will require new partnerships between researchers and managed care organizations. There has been limited experience in developing these partnerships from either the researcher or the managed care perspective. One way to accelerate this process may be to address two fundamental concerns. First, well-developed models (including model contracts) that protect the interests of both the researcher and the managed care organization are needed. Second, funding sources need to be available to promote joint research, much as there has been NIMH funding to promote mental health research in the public sector. A key factor toward success is likely to be the choice of research topics that can bring together the interests of the two parties and that do not involve high levels of risk for either party.

Research on the long-term role of consumers and their families in the successful management of care is also going to be important and may involve working with family and consumer groups, since people switch insurance and managed care plans. Collaborations with consumer and family groups could also benefit from similar investments in developing models for productive relationships and providing targeted support.

Research and Demonstrations on Improved Systems for Mental Health Care

Managed care is making changes, some of which are considered radical, but most are on the margins of current medical practice. One potential drawback of incremental change is that it may not lead to real innovation in treatment and improvement in consumer outcomes. This can result from a series of incremental changes that do not lead to a well-defined vision of what the future health care system should be. There needs to be an effort to solicit the best thinking of researchers and the managed care system regarding innovative models for managed behavioral health care. These could be funded under research and demonstration authority if they were related to the Medicare or Medicaid programs. The key is to attempt to move the research agenda to address issues that are in front of where managed care is making its changes today. Otherwise, the danger is that researchers will too easily focus their energies on evaluating the changes introduced by managed care and not think creatively about what managed care should be. Research and demonstration initiatives should target innovative models that break from tradition by testing alternative ways to manage care, provide services, and monitor outcomes.

SUMMARY AND CONCLUSIONS

The growth of managed behavioral health care is making this one of the most interesting times in U.S. health care, yet it is placing many consumers at considerable risk when existing care arrangements are disrupted. Without systems for measuring quality of care and patient outcomes, the documentation of the impact of change may be no more than a series of anecdotal stories. There is an urgent need to develop and improve measurement tools (quality of care, access, and outcomes) and to refine research designs that can make it possible to monitor and evaluate the end results of health care, that is, consumers' health outcomes. The proposed research focus on how to manage care effectively and efficiently is a long-term agenda. An evaluation of each new type of managed care organization would appear to be of limited value since these organizations usually change consequentially by the time the results become available. There is value in focusing on the specific mechanisms used to manage care and their consequences for consumer outcomes.

The promise of managed care needs to be more clearly conceptualized than it has been. The research agenda needs to examine critically mechanisms and strategies for achieving positive outcomes for consumers through a population-based focus on health and mental health care. Although the challenges for outcomes research are great, the potential to improve consumer health outcomes and control costs will only succeed if there is an ever growing base of information that links the processes of behavioral health care to the outcomes valued by consumers.

REFERENCES

Arons BS, Frank RG, Goldman HH, McGuire TG, Stephens S. 1994. Mental health and substance abuse coverage under health reform. *Health Affairs* 13(1):192-205, Spring.

Berk ML, Schur CL, Cantor JC. 1995. Ability to obtain health care: Recent estimates from the Robert Wood Johnson Foundation National Access to Care Survey. *Health Affairs* 14(3):139-146, Fall.

Burlingame GM, Lambert MJ, Reisinger CW, Neff WM, Mosier J. 1995. Pragmatics of tracking mental health outcomes in a managed care setting. *Journal of Mental Health Administration* 22(3):226-236.

Donabedian A. 1993. The role of outcomes in quality assessment and assurance. *Quality Review Bulletin* 19(3):78.

England MJ, Vaccaro VA. 1991. New systems to manage mental health care. *Health Affairs* 10(4):129-137.

Essock SM, Goldman HH. 1995. States' embrace of managed mental health care. *Health Affairs* 14(3):34-44.

Fiedler JL. 1989. *The Medical Offset Effect and Public Health Policy: Mental Health Industry in Transition.* New York: Praeger.

Flynn L, Steinwachs D. 1995. Special report: Outcomes roundtable includes all stakeholders. *Health Affairs* 14(3):269-270.

Frank RG, Goldman HH, McGuire TG. 1992. A model mental health benefit in private insurance. *Health Affairs* 11(3):98-117.

Frank RG, Brookmeyer R. 1995. Managed mental health care and patterns of inpatient utilization for treatment of affective disorders. *Social Psychiatry and Psychiatric Epidemiology* 30:220-223.

Frank RG, McGuire TG, Newhouse JP. 1995. Risk contracts in managed mental health care. *Health Affairs* 14(3):50-64.

Gold M, Nelson L, Lake T, Hurley R, Berenson R. 1995a. Behind the curve: A critical assessment of how little is known about arrangements between managed care plans and physicians. *Medical Care Research and Review* 52(3):307-341.

Gold MR, Hurley R, Lake T, Ensor T, Berenson R. 1995b. A national survey of the arrangements managed-care plans make with physicians. *The New England Journal of Medicine* 333:1678-1683.

Grob GN. 1991. *From Asylum to Community: Mental Health Policy in Modern America.* Princeton, NJ: Princeton University Press.

Iglehart JK. 1996. Health policy report: Managed care and mental health. *The New England Journal of Medicine* 334(2):131-135.

Keeler EB, Rolph JE. 1988. The demand for episodes of treatment in the Health Insurance Experiment. *Journal of Health Economics* 7(4):301-322.

Keeler EB, Wells KB, Manning WG, Rumpel JD, Hanley JM. 1986. *The Demand for Episodes of Mental Health Care.* Santa Monica, CA: RAND.

Kleinman L. 1995. *Preferences for Outpatient Mental Health Treatment.* Doctoral Thesis. Baltimore, MD: Johns Hopkins School of Hygiene and Public Health.

Lehman AF. 1995. Measuring quality in a reformed health system. *Health Affairs* 14(3):90-101.

Luft HS. 1987. *Health Maintenance Organizations: Dimensions of Performance.* New Brunswick, NJ: Transaction Books.

Lurie N, Moscovice I, Finch M, Christianson J, Popkin M. 1992. Does capitation affect the health of the chronically mentally ill? Results from a randomized trial. *Journal of the American Medical Association* 267:3300-3304.

Manning WB, Wells KB, Duan N, Newhouse JP, Ware JE. 1986. How cost sharing affects the use of ambulatory mental health services. *Journal of the American Medical Association* 256(14):1930-1934.

McFarland BH. 1994. Health maintenance organizations and persons with severe mental illness. *Community Mental Health Journal* 30(3):221-242.

McGrew JH, Bond GR, Dietzen L, Salyers M. 1994. Measuring the fidelity of implementation of a mental health program model. *Journal of Consulting and Clinical Psychology* 62:670-678.

Mechanic D, Schlesinger M, McAlpine DD. 1995. Management of mental health and substance abuse services: State of the art and early results. *The Milbank Quarterly* 73(1):19-55.

NIMH (National Institue of Mental Health). 1990. *National Plan to Improve Care for Persons with Severe Mental Illness.* Report of the National Advisory Mental Health Council. Washington, DC: National Institute of Mental Health.

NIMH. 1993. *Health Care Reform for Americans with Severe Mental Illness.* Report of the National Advisory Mental Health Council. Washington, DC: National Institute of Mental Health.

Payne SM. 1987. Identifying and managing inappropriate hospital utilization. *Health Services Research* 22(5):709-769, December.

Rossiter LF, Langwell F, Wan TH, Rivnyak. 1989. Patient satisfaction among elderly enrollees and disenrollees in Medicare health maintenance organizations. *Journal of the American Medical Association* 262(1):57-63.

Salem-Schatz S, Moore G, Rucker M, Pearson SD. 1994. The case for case-mix adjustment in practice profiling. *Journal of the American Medical Association* 272(11):871-874.

Shapiro S, Skinner EA, Kramer M, Steinwachs DM, Regier DA. 1985. Measuring the need for mental health services in a general population. *Medical Care* 23(9):1033-1043.

Simon GE, VonKorff M, Durham ML. 1994. Predictors of outpatient mental health utilization by primary care patients in a health maintenance organization. *American Journal of Psychiatry* 151(6):908-913, June.

Stein LI, Test MA. 1985. *The Training in Community Living Model.* San Francisco: Jossey-Bass.

Steinwachs DM, Wu AW, Skinner EA. 1994. How will outcomes management work? *Health Affairs* 14(3):153-162.

Stroup TS, Dorwart RA. 1995. Impact of a managed mental health program on Medicaid recipients with severe mental illness. *Psychiatric Services* 46(9):885-889, September.

Weiner JP, de Lissovoy G. 1993. Razing a tower of Babel: A taxonomy for managed care and health insurance plans. *Journal of Health Politics and Law* 18(1):75-103.

Weiner JP, Lyles A, Steinwachs DM, Hall KC. 1991. Impact of managed care on prescription drug use. *Health Affairs* 10(1):140-154.

Wells KB, Astrachan BM, Tischler GL, Unutzer J. 1995. Issues and approaches in evaluating managed mental health care. *The Milbank Quarterly* 73(1):57-75.

Wells KB, Hosek SD, Marquis MS. 1992. The effects of preferred provider options in fee-for-service plans on use of outpatient mental health services by three employee groups. *Medical Care* 30(5):412-427, May.

Wells KB, Sturm R. 1995. Care for depression in a changing environment. *Health Affairs* 14(3):78-89, Fall.

Wells KB. 1989. The functioning and well being of depressed patients: Results from the Medical Outcomes Study. *Journal of the American Medical Association* 262(7):914-919

Wennberg JE. 1987. Population illness rates do not explain population hospitalization rates. *Medical Care* 25:354-359.

Wickizer TM, Lessler D, Travis KM. 1996. Controlling inpatient psychiatric utilization through managed care. *American Journal of Psychiatry* 153(3):339-345, March.

D

Public Workshop Agendas and Participants

INSTITUTE OF MEDICINE
NATIONAL ACADEMY OF SCIENCES

Committee on Quality Assurance and Accreditation Guidelines
for Managed Behavioral Health Care

PUBLIC WORKSHOP AGENDA
April 18, 1996

Cecil and Ida Green Building
2001 Wisconsin Avenue, NW, Room 104
Washington, DC

9:00   Welcome and Introductions
        Jerome Grossman, Committee Chair
        Constance Pechura, Director, IOM Division of Neuroscience and
        Behavioral Health
        Margaret Edmunds, Study Director

Invited Speakers

9:15   Building Accountability Systems for Quality in Managed Behavioral
Health Care
     Margaret O'Kane, President, National Committee for Quality
Assurance, Washington, DC

9:30   Discussion

9:40   Implementation of the ASAM Patient Placement Criteria
     David Mee-Lee, Medical Director, Community Systems, Castle
Medical Systems, Honolulu, HI, and Co-Author, Patient Placement
Criteria for the Treatment of Psychoactive Substance Abuse
Disorders American Society of Addiction Medicine

9:55   Discussion

10:05   Ensuring Meaningful Participation of Consumers in Program
Evaluation, Quality Assurance, Service Provision, and Rights
Protection Under Managed Care
     Daniel Fisher, Director, National Empowerment Center, and
Medical Director, Eastern Middlesex Human Services, Wakefield,
MA

10:20   Discussion

10:30   Break

10:45   PERMS: The American Managed Behavioral Health Care Association
(AMBHA)
     John Bartlett, Executive Vice President for Quality Improvement,
Magellan Health Services, Atlanta, GA, and Chair, AMBHA
Committee on Quality Improvement and Clinical Services

11:00   Discussion

11:10   Measurement of HMO Performance with Behavioral Health Standards
     Susan Goldman, Manager of Behavioral Health Services, John
Hancock Mutual Life Insurance Company, Boston, MA

11:25   Discussion

11:35   Accreditation of Managed Behavioral Health Care
     Paul Schyve, Senior Vice President, Joint Commission on
Accreditation of Healthcare Organizations, Chicago, IL

11:50   Discussion

12:00   Quality Activities and the Health Care Financing Administration (HCFA)
        Robert Valdez, Deputy Assistant Secretary for Health and Director of Interagency Health Policy, HCFA, Washington, DC

12:15   Discussion

12:25   Lunch

1:00   **Public Statement Session**
        Time slots appear in 15-minute intervals to allow for a 10-minute presentation followed by a 5-minute discussion period

1:00   **Ron Manderscheid,** Substance Abuse and Mental Health Services Administration, Center for Mental Health Statistics, Rockville, MD

1:15   **Geoffrey Reed,** American Psychological Association, Washington, DC

1:30   **Mark Parrino,** American Methadone Treatment Association, New York, NY

1:45   **Linda Kaplan,** National Association of Alcoholism and Drug Abuse Counselors, Arlington, VA

2:00   **Rita Vandivort,** National Association of Social Workers, Washington, DC

2:15   **Raphael Metzger,** National Coalition of Hispanic Health and Human Services Organizations, Washington, DC

2:30   **Sarah Stanley,** American Nurses Association, Washington, DC

2:45   **William Dennis Derr,** Mobil Corporation EAP, Princeton, NJ

3:00   **Gwen Rubinstein,** Legal Action Center, Washington, DC

3:15   Break

3:30   **Elizabeth Edgar,** National Alliance for the Mentally Ill, Arlington, VA

3:45   **Donald Galamaga,** Rhode Island Department of Retardation, Mental Health and Hospitals, Providence, RI

4:00   **Elizabeth Hadley,** National Association of Insurance Commissioners, Washington, DC

4:15   **Linda Bresolin,** American Medical Association, Chicago, IL

4:30   **Sybil Goldman,** National Technical Assistance Center for Children's Mental Health, Georgetown University Child Development Center, Washington, DC

4:45   **Golnar Simpson,** National Federation of Societies for Clinical Social Work, Inc., Boston, MA

5:00   **Michael Faenza,** National Mental Health Association, Alexandria, VA

5:15   **Ray Bridge,** Northern Virginia Mental Health Consumers Association, Falls Church, VA

5:30   Closing Comments

       Reception

INSTITUTE OF MEDICINE
NATIONAL ACADEMY OF SCIENCES

Committee on Quality Assurance and Accreditation Guidelines for Managed Behavioral Health Care

PUBLIC WORKSHOP
April 18, 1996

WORKSHOP PARTICIPANTS

John Bartlett, Executive Vice President for Quality Improvement, Magellan Health Services, Atlanta, GA

Linda Bresolin, Director, Department of Women's and Minority Health, American Medical Association, Chicago, IL

Ray Bridge, Chair, Northern Virginia Mental Health Consumer's Association, Falls Church, VA

Jackie Bryan, Director of Health Policy, Association of State and Territorial Health Officials, Washington, DC

Jeff Buck, Acting Director, Office of Policy and Planning, Center for Mental Health Statistics, Substance Abuse and Mental Health Services Administration, Rockville, MD

Mady Chalk, Director of Managed Care Initiatives, Center for Substance Abuse Treatment, Substance Abuse and Mental Health Services Administration, Rockville, MD

William Dennis Derr, Manager, Employee Assistance Program, Mobil Corporation, Member, Employee Assistance Professionals Association, Princeton, NJ

Elizabeth Edgar, State Issues Coordinator, National Alliance for the Mentally Ill, Alexandria, VA

Michael Faenza, President and CEO, National Mental Health Association, Alexandria, VA

Daniel Fisher, Director, National Empowerment Center, Lawrence, MA

Susan Fitzpatrick, Training Coordinator, On Our Own of Maryland, Inc., Baltimore, MD

Donald P. Galamaga, Executive Director, Division of Integrated Mental Health Services, Rhode Island Department of Mental Health and Retardation and Hospitals, Cranston, RI

Don Galvin, President, Commission on Accreditation of Rehabilitation Facilities, Tucson, AZ

Robert W. Glover, Executive Director, National Association of State Mental Health Program Directors, Alexandria, VA

Nancy Goetschius, Health Insurance Specialist, Health Care Financing Administration, Baltimore, MD

Susan Goldman, Manager of Behavioral Health Services, John Hancock Mutual Life Insurance Company, Boston, MA

Sybil Goldman, Associate Director, National Technical Assistance Center for Children's Mental Health, Georgetown University, Washington, DC

John Gustafson, Executive Director, National Association of State Alcohol and Drug Abuse Directors, Washington, DC

Elizabeth Hadley, Associate Counsel for Health Policy, National Association of Insurance Commissioners, Washington, DC

Jeff Harris, Senior Policy Analyst, Health Policy Studies Division, National Governors' Association, Washington, DC

Judith Hines, Interim Co-Director, Council on Accreditation of Services for Families and Children, New York, NY

Robert Huebner, Chief, Health Services Research, National Institute on Alcohol Abuse and Alcoholism, Rockville, MD

Corinne Husten, Medical Officer, Office on Smoking and Health, Centers for Disease Control and Prevention, Atlanta, GA

Marcia Jones, Health Care Attorney, Division of Health Policy, American Foundation of State, County and Municipal Employees, Washington, DC

Linda Kaplan, Executive Director, National Association of Alcoholism and Drug Abuse Counselors, Arlington, VA

Nancy Kennedy, Managed Care Coordinator, Center for Substance Abuse Prevention, Substance Abuse and Mental Health Services Administration, Rockville, MD

Kenneth A. Kessler, President, American Psych Systems, Bethesda, MD

Chris Koyanagi, Director of Government Affairs, Bazelon Center for Mental Health Law, Washington, DC

Beverly B. Long, President, World Federation for Mental Health, Atlanta, GA

Bob Lubran, Chief, Quality Assurance and Evaluation Branch, State Programs Division, Center for Substance Abuse Treatment, Substance Abuse and Mental Health Services Administration, Rockville, MD

Irene Lynch, Collaborative Support Programs, Aleppos Foundation, NJ

Ron Manderscheid, Chief, Survey and Analysis Branch, Center for Mental Health Statistics, Substance Abuse and Mental Health Services Administration, Rockville, MD

Thomas McLellan, Professor, Department of Psychiatry, School of Medicine, University of Pennsylvania, Philadelphia, PA

David Mee-Lee, Medical Director, Community Systems, Castle Medical Center, Honolulu, HI

Raphael Metzger, General Counsel, National Coalition of Hispanic Health and Human Services Organizations, Washington, DC

J. Peter Nixon, Senior Policy Analyst, Service Employees International Union, Washington, DC

Margaret O'Kane, President, National Committee for Quality Assurance, Washington, DC

Mark Paris, Senior Policy Analyst, Mental Health Quality, Directorate of Quality Management, Office of the Assistant Secretary of Defense, U.S. Department of Defense, Washington, DC

Mark W. Parrino, President, American Methadone Treatment Association, Inc., New York, NY

Lee Partridge, Director of Health Policy Unit, American Public Welfare Association, Washington, DC

Linda Peltz, Medicaid Analyst, Medicaid Bureau, Health Care Financing Administration, Baltimore, MD

Natan Polster, Adolescent Medicine Newsletter, Washington, DC

Lane Porter, DC Health Law Consultant, Washington, DC

Lucille Pritchard, National Mental Health Association, Alexandria, VA

Susan Probyn, Senior Manager, Quality Improvement Initiatives, American Association of Health Plans, Washington, DC

Dan Quinn, Media Associate, Office of News and Public Information, National Academy of Sciences, Washington, DC

Geoffrey Reed, Assistant Executive Director for Professional Development, American Psychological Association, Washington, DC

Annette U. Rickel, Clinical Psychiatry Professor, Department of Psychiatry, Georgetown University, Washington, DC

Larry Robertson, Consultant to the Center for Substance Abuse Treatment, Substance Abuse and Mental Health Services Administration, Johnson, Bassin and Shaw, Silver Spring, MD

Gail Robinson, Mental Health Policy Resource Center, Washington, DC

E. Clarke Ross, Executive Director, American Managed Behavioral Health Care Association, Washington, DC

Gwen Rubinstein, Health Policy Associate, Legal Action Center, Washington, DC

Jenny Schnaier, Health Research Policy Analyst, Research Triangle Institute, Washington, DC

Paul Schyve, Senior Vice President, Joint Commission on Accreditation of Healthcare Organizations, Oakbrook Terrace, IL

Claire Sharda, National Committee for Quality Assurance, Washington, DC

Golnar Simpson, National Federation of Societies for Clinical Social Work, Inc., Arlington, VA

Sarah Stanley, Director of Nursing Practice, American Nurses Association, Washington, DC

Tom Stantis, National Association of State Alcohol and Drug Abuse Directors, Washington, DC

Robert Valdez, Deputy Assistant Secretary for Health, Interagency Health Policy, U.S. Department of Health and Human Services, Washington, DC

Rita Vandivort, Senior Staff Associate for Mental Health and Addiction, National Association of Social Workers, Washington, DC

Linda R. Wolf Jones, Executive Director, Therapeutic Communities of America, Washington, DC

Anne Young, Center for Mental Health Statistics, Substance Abuse and Mental Health Services Administration, Rockville, MD

INSTITUTE OF MEDICINE
NATIONAL ACADEMY OF SCIENCES

Committee on Quality Assurance and Accreditation Guidelines for Managed Behavioral Health Care

PUBLIC WORKSHOP AGENDA
May 17, 1996

The Arnold and Mabel Beckman Center of the National Academy of Sciences
100 Academy Drive, Lecture Room
Irvine, CA

9:00   Welcome and Introductions
           Jerome Grossman, Committee Chair
           Margo Edmunds, Study Director

Invited Speakers

9:15   Council on Accreditation (COA): A Unique Combination of Generic
           Standards and Service-Specific Standards for the Full Array
           Judith Hines, Executive Director, Council on Accreditation of
           Services for Families and Children, New York, NY

9:30   Discussion

9:40   Commission on Accreditation of Rehabilitation Facilities (CARF)
           Accreditation Process and Standards in Behavioral Health Care
           Tim Slaven, National Director, Behavioral Health Division,
           Commission for the Accreditation of Rehabilitation Facilities,
           Tucson, AZ

9:55   Discussion

10:05   Utilization Review Accreditation Commission (URAC) Accreditation
           Randall Madry, President, Utilization Review Accreditation
           Commission, Washington, DC

10:20   Discussion

10:30   Break

10:45   Behavioral Health Care Industry Perspectives on Proposed
        Performance Indicators
        Tom Trabin, Vice President, Informatics and Outcomes Initiatives,
        CentraLink, Tiburon, CA

11:00   Discussion

11:10   Implementing Quality Improvement Programs
        Peter Panzarino, Medical Director, Vista Behavioral Health Plans,
        San Diego, CA

11:25   Discussion

11:35   Purchasers' Perspectives on Quality
        Catherine Brown, Senior Project Manager, Pacific Business Group
        on Health, San Francisco, CA

11:50   Discussion

12:00   Lunch

 1:00   Quality Issues as Seen by Benefits Consultants
        Michael J. Jeffrey, Associate, William M. Mercer, Inc., Baltimore,
        MD

 1:15   Discussion

 1:25   County Perspectives on Performance Measurement
        Robert Egnew, Director, Behavioral Health Division, Monterey
        County Health Department, Salinas, CA

 1:40   Discussion

 1:55   Managed Care, Public-Sector Style
        Ann Froio, Director of Quality Management, ComCare, Phoenix,
        AZ

 2:10   Discussion

 2:20   Technical Challenges for Outcomes Researchers in Health
        Departments
        Don Austin, Oregon Health Division and Centers for Disease
        Control and Prevention, Atlanta, GA

 2:35   Discussion

 2:45   Closing Comments

 3:00   Adjourn

INSTITUTE OF MEDICINE
NATIONAL ACADEMY OF SCIENCES

Committee on Quality Assurance and Accreditation Guidelines for Managed Behavioral Health Care

PUBLIC WORKSHOP
May 17, 1996

WORKSHOP PARTICIPANTS

Don Austin, Oregon Health Division, Portland, OR

Catherine Brown, Pacific Business Group on Health, San Francisco, CA

Robert Egnew, President, National Association of County Managed Behavioral Health Directors, Behavioral Health Division, Salinas, CA

Ann Froio, Director of Quality Management, ComCare, Phoenix, AZ

Mary Graham, Director, Office of Economic Affairs and Practice Management, American Psychiatric Association, Washington, DC

Judith Hines, Executive Director, Council on Accreditation of Services for Families and Children, Inc., New York, NY

Michael Jeffrey, Associate, William M. Mercer, Inc., Baltimore, MD

Marcia Jones, Health Care Attorney, American Federation of State, County, and Municipal Employees, Washington, DC

Randall Madry, President, Utilization Review Accreditation Commission, Washington, DC

Joan McCrea, Corporate Manager, Hughes Aircraft Company, EAP, Corporate Human Resources, Los Angeles, CA

Mary Cesare Murphy, Director, Behavioral Health Accreditation Services, Joint Commission on Accreditation of Health Care Organizations, Oakbrook Terrace, IL

Peter Panzarino, Medical Director, Vista Health Plan, San Diego, CA

Gail Shultz, California Society of Addiction Medicine, Oakland, CA

Tim Slaven, National Director, Behavioral Health Division, Commission for the Accreditation of Rehabilitation Facilities, Tucson, AZ

Tom Trabin, Vice President, Informatics and Outcomes Initiatives, CentraLink, Tiburon, CA

Nancy Young, Children and Family Futures, Irvine, CA

INSTITUTE OF MEDICINE
NATIONAL ACADEMY OF SCIENCES

Committee on Quality Assurance and Accreditation Guidelines for Managed Behavioral Health Care

FOURTH COMMITTEE MEETING AGENDA
June 25-26, 1996

The Foundry Building
1055 Thomas Jefferson Street, NW, Room 2004
Washington, DC

8:30   Continental Breakfast

9:00   Welcome and Introductions
       Jerome Grossman, Committee Chair
       Constance Pechura, Director, IOM Division of Neuroscience and Behavioral Health
       Margo Edmunds, Study Director

Invited Speakers

9:15   Concerns of Mental Health Consumers and Family Members in Managed Care
       Laura Lee Hall, Deputy Director of Policy and Research, National Alliance for the Mentally Ill, Arlington, VA

9:30   Discussion

9:40   Managed Care and Populations With Special Health Care Needs: Child and Family Mental Health
       Robert Cole, Director, Washington Business Group on Health, Washington, DC

9:55   Discussion

10:05   Perspectives on Quality Management and Managed Care in the Department of Defense
       Mark Paris, Senior Policy Analyst, Mental Health Quality, Office of the Assistant Secretary of Defense, Washington, DC

10:20   Discussion

10:30   Break

10:45   Quality Issues in Managed Care for Seniors
      Sarah Gotbaum, Director, Managed Care Project, United Seniors
      Health Cooperative, Washington, DC

11:00   Discussion

11:10   Cultural Competence in Health Care
      Julia Puebla Fortier, Director, Resources for Cross-Cultural Health
      Care, Silver Spring, MD

11:25   Discussion

11:35   Coordination of Services for Native Americans
      Reginald Cedar Face, Public Affairs Specialist, Pine Ridge
      Hospital, Indian Health Service, Pine Ridge, SD

11:50   Discussion

12:00   Culturally Appropriate Managed Care for Asians and Pacific Islanders
      Grace Wang, Medical Consultant, Association of Asian Pacific
      Community Health Organizations, Oakland, CA

12:20   Discussion

12:30   Closing Remarks

INSTITUTE OF MEDICINE
NATIONAL ACADEMY OF SCIENCES

***Committee on Quality Assurance and Accreditation Guidelines
for Managed Behavioral Health Care***

FOURTH COMMITTEE MEETING
June 25, 1996

PARTICIPANTS LIST

Reginald Cedar Face, Public Affairs Specialist, Pine Ridge Hospital, Indian
Health Service, Pine Ridge, SD
Robert Cole, PhD, Director, Washington Business Group on Health,
Washington, DC
Sarah Gotbaum, PhD, Director, Managed Care Project, United Seniors Health
Cooperative, Washington, DC

Lieutenant Commander Mark Paris, PhD, Senior Policy Analyst, Mental Health Quality, Directorate of Quality Management, Office of the Assistant Secretary of Defense (Health Affairs), Washington, DC

Julia Puebla Fortier, Director, Resources for Cross-Cultural Health Care, Silver Spring, MD

Laura Lee Hall, Deputy Director of Policy and Research, National Alliance for the Mentally Ill, Arlington, VA

Grace Wang, MD, MPH, Medical Consultant, Association of Asian and Pacific Community Health Organizations, New York, NY

Observers:

Jon Gold, Public Health Analyst, Managed Care Initiatives, Center for Substance Abuse Treatment, Substance Abuse and Mental Health Services Administration, Rockville, MD

Robert Valdez, PhD, Deputy Assistant Secretary for Health, U.S. Department of Health and Human Services, Washington, DC

Joy Midman, Executive Director, National Association of Psychiatric Treatment Centers for Children, Washington, DC

IOM Staff

Margo Edmunds, PhD, Study Director
Constance Pechura, PhD, Division Director
Eugene Lee, Student, MIT/IOM Intern
Terri Scanlan, Administrative Assistant
Thomas Wetterhan, Project Assistant/Research Assistant
Amelia Mathis, Project Assistant

E

Liaison Panel Members to the Committee on Quality Assurance and Accreditation Guidelines for Managed Behavioral Health Care

PRIVATE SECTOR

Affiliation	*Panel Member*
Academic Health Centers	
Georgetown University School of Medicine, Department of Biomathematics and Department of Biostatistics	Gary Chase
George Washington University, Department of Psychiatry	Annette Rickel
New York Hospital, Cornell Medical Center	Gary Tischler
University of Wisconsin, Department of Family Medicine	Richard L. Brown
Accreditation Organizations	
Council on Accreditation of Services for Families and Children (COA)	Joe Frisino
	Judith Hines
Joint Commission on Accreditation of Healthcare Organizations (JCAHO)	Mary Cesare Murphy
	Paul Schyve
	Margaret Van Amringe
National Committee for Quality Assurance (NCQA)	Margaret O'Kane
	Claire Sharda

| Rehabilitation Accreditation Commission (CARF) | Don Galvin
Tim Slaven |
| Utilization Review Accreditation (URAC) Commission | Garry Carneal |

Associations—Health Care Industry

American Association of Health Plans (AAHP)	Susan Probyn Liza Greenberg
American Managed Behavioral Healthcare Association (AMBHA)	Clarke Ross
Health Insurance Association of America (HIAA)	Joseph O'Hara
National Association of Health Data Organizations (NAHDO)	Barbara Kurtzig
National Business Coalition on Health (NBCH)	Catherine Kunkle
Pacific Business Group on Health (PBGH)	Catherine Brown
Washington Business Group on Health (WBGH)	Veronica Goff Robert Cole

Associations—Professional

American Academy of Addiction Psychiatry (AAAP)	Jeanne Trumble
American Academy of Family Physicians (AAFP)	Jacqelyn Admire
American College of Preventive Medicine (ACPM)	Donna Grossman
American Medical Association (AMA)	Linda Bresolin
American Methadone Treatment Association (AMTA)	Mark Parrino
American Nurses Association (ANA)	Sarah Stanley
American Psychiatric Association	Mary Graham
American Psychological Association	Russell Newman Geoffrey Reed
American Society of Addiction Medicine (ASAM)	James Callahan David Mee-Lee
California Society on Addiction Medicine (CSAM)	Gail Jara
National Association of Alcoholism and Drug Abuse Counselors (NAADAC)	Linda Kaplan
National Association of Social Workers (NASW)	Rita Vandivort
National Federation of Societies for Clinical Social Work (NFSCSW)	Ann Kilguss Golnar Simpson
Therapeutic Communities of America (TCA)	Linda Wolf Jones
World Federation for Mental Health (WFMH)	Beverly Long

Associations—State and County

American Public Welfare Association (APWA)
Association of State and Territorial Health
Officials (ASTHO)
National Association of County and City Health
Officials (NACCHO)
National Association of County Managed
Behavioral Health Directors (NACMBHD)
National Association of Insurance Commissioners
(NAIC)
National Association of State Alcohol and Drug
Abuse Directors (NASADAD)
National Association of State Mental Health
Program Directors (NASMHPD)
National Governors' Association (NGA)

Lee Partridge
Cheryl Beversdorf
Jackie Bryan
Grace Gorenflo

Robert Egnew

Elizabeth Hadley
Mary Beth Senkewize
John Gustafson
Tom Stantis
Colette Crose
Robert Glover
Jeff Harris

Behavioral Health Care Companies and Consultants

American Psych Systems
Blue Cross-Blue Shield of New Hampshire
CentraLink
ComCare

Eastern Carolina Health Network
Health Law Consultant
Human Systems and Outcomes
Institute for Behavioral Healthcare (IBH)
Magellan Health Services
Medco Behavioral Care Corporation
Open Minds
Principal Behavioral Health Care
Qualifacts Systems
United Behavioral Systems, Inc.
Value Behavioral Health
VISTA Behavioral Health Plan
William M. Mercer, Inc.

Ken Kessler
John Bunker
Stewart Bloom
Ann Froio
Pamela Hyde
Randall Madry
Lane Porter
Ivor Groves
Tom Trabin
John Bartlett
Robert Reiser
Monica Oss
Kelley Phillips
James Spicer
Bruce Bobbitt
Ian Schaffer
Peter Panzarino
Michael Jeffrey

Business and Industry

Ameritech
Digital Equipment Corporation
Hughes Aircraft Company
John Hancock Mutual Life Insurance Company
Mobil Corporation

Alan Peres
Bruce Davidson
Joan McCrea
Susan Goldman
William Dennis Derr

Children and Families

Child Guidance Center	Dennis Mohatt
Federation of Families for Children's Mental Health	Barbara Huff
National Association of Psychiatric Treatment Centers for Children	Joy Midman
National Technical Assistance Center for Children's Mental Health, Georgetown University	Sybil Goldman

Consumer Organizations

Alcohol and Drug Abuse Association	Anne Tafe
Center for the Study of Services, CHECKBOOK Magazine	Robert Krughoff
Consumer Managed Care Network	Laura Van Tosh
DC Consumer League	Nancy Lee Head
Legal Action Center	Gwen Rubenstein
Mental Health Consumers Association	Ray Bridge
National Alliance for the Mentally Ill (NAMI)	Elizabeth Edgar
	Laurie Flynn
	Laura Lee Hall
National Empowerment Center (NEC)	Daniel Fisher
National Mental Health Association (NMHA)	Michael Faenza
	Lucille Pritchard
On Our Own of Maryland, Inc.	Michael Finkle
	Susan Fitzpatrick
Technical Assistance Collaborative	Martin Cohen
The Information Exchange	Burt Pepper
United Seniors Health Cooperative	Sarah Gotbaum

Diversity

Association of Asian Pacific Community Health Organizations (AAPCHO)	Grace Wang
National Coalition of Hispanic Health and Human Service Organizations (COSSHMO)	Jane Delgado
	Raphael Metzger
Pine Ridge Reservation	Reginald Cedar Face
Resources for Cross-Cultural Health Care	Julia Puebla Fortier

Policy Research

Bazelon Center for Mental Health Law	Claudia Schlosberg
	Chris Koyanagi
Center for the Advancement of Health	Jessie Gruman

Employee Benefits Research Institute
Intergovernmental Health Policy Project

Mental Health Policy Resource Center

Research Triangle Institute (RTI)

Science Applications International Corporation (SAIC)

Paul Fronstin
Lee Dixon
Molly Stauffer
Leslie Scallet
Gail Robinson
Kathleen Lohr
James Lubalin
Judith Emerson

Publications

Adolescent Medicine
Advances
Health Affairs
Mental Health Report

Natan Polster
Harris Dienstfrey
John Iglehart
Patrick Cody

Unions

American Federation of State, County, and
    Municipal Employees
Service Employees International Union

Marcia Jones
Ann Kempski
Peter Nixon

PUBLIC SECTOR

Affiliation   **Panel Member**

Federal Government

U.S. Department of Health and Human Services
    Agency for Health Care Policy and Research
    Centers for Disease Control and Prevention

Health Care Financing Administration (HCFA)

Lisa Simpson
Julie Fishman
Jeffrey Harris
Corinne Husten
Yvonne Lewis
Suzanne Smith
Clarke Cagey
Peggy Clark
Nancy Goetschius
James Hadley
Linda Peltz
Sally Richardson

National Institute on Alcohol Abuse and Alcoholism (NIAAA)

Office of the Assistant Secretary for Health

Substance Abuse and Mental Health Services Administration (SAMHSA)

    Center for Mental Health Services (CMHS)

    Center for Substance Abuse Prevention (CSAP)

    Center for Substance Abuse Treatment (CSAT)

U.S. Department of Defense (DOD)

    Office of the Assistant Secretary of Defense

    U.S. Navy

U.S. Department of Veterans Affairs (VA)

Faye M. Calhoun
Robert Huebner

Robert Valdez

Eric Goplerud

Jeff Buck
Paolo del Vecchio
Ron Manderscheid
Anne Young

Nancy Kennedy

Mady Chalk
Bob Lubran

Mark Paris
Beverly Paige-Dobson

Thomas B. Horvath

State Governments

Department of Mental Health and Addiction Services, State of Connecticut

Department of Mental Health, Retardation, and Hospitals, State of Rhode Island

Department of Public Health, Commonwealth of Massachusetts

Mental Hygiene Administration, State of Maryland

Nebraska Department of Health

State of Oregon Health Division

Texas Department of Health

Texas Department of Mental Health and Mental Retardation

Susan Essock

Donald P. Galamaga
A. Kathyrn Power

David H. Mulligan

John Allen
Mark B. Horton
Don Austin
David R. Smith
H. Ed Calahan
Vijay Ganju

F

Organizations That Submitted Written Materials to the Committee

Organization	**Contact Person**
American Managed Behavioral Healthcare Association	E. Clarke Ross
American Medical Association	Linda Bresolin
American Methadone Treatment Association	Mark Parrino
American Nurses Association	Sarah Stanley
American Psych Systems	Kenneth Kessler
American Psychological Association	Geoffrey Reed
American Society on Addiction Medicine	David Mee-Lee
	Michael Miller
Association of Asian Pacific Community Health Organizations	Grace Wang
Council on Accreditation of Services for Children and Families	Judith Hines
Employee Assistance Professionals Association	William Dennis Derr
Federation of Families for Children's Mental Health	Sybil Goldman
Institute for Behavioral Health Care	Tom Trabin
John Hancock National Account Services	Susan Goldman
Joint Commission on Accreditation of Healthcare Organizations	Paul Schyve
	Carol Newcomb
Legal Action Center	Gwen Rubinstein
Medstat Group	Leigh Ann Albers

National Alliance for the Mentally Ill	Elizabeth Edgar
National Association of Alcoholism and Drug Abuse Counselors	Linda Kaplan
National Association of Insurance Commissioners	Elizabeth Hadley
National Association of Social Workers	Rita Vandivort
National Coalition of Hispanic Health and Human Services Organizations	Raphael Metzger
National Committee for Quality Assurance	Margaret O'Kane
	Claire Sharda
National Empowerment Center	Daniel Fisher
National Federation of Societies for Clinical Social Work	Anne Kilguss
	Golnar Simpson
National Mental Health Association	Michael M. Faenza
National Technical Assistance Center for Children's Mental Health	Sybil Goldman
Northern Virginia Mental Health Consumers Association	Ray Bridge
Rehabilitation Accreditation Commission	Tim Slaven
University of Wisconsin at Madison	Richard Brown
Utilization Review Accreditation Commission	Randall Madry
Vista Health Plans	Peter Panzarino

Public Sector

Center for Mental Health Services, Substance Abuse and Mental Health Services Administration	Jeff Buck
	Ronald Manderscheid
Center for Substance Abuse Treatment	Mady Chalk
Centers for Disease Control and Prevention	Corinne Husten
Rhode Island Department of Mental Health, Retardation, and Hospitals	A. Kathryn Power
	Donald Galamaga

Index

A

Access to care
  barriers to, 169-171
  for children and adolescents, 152-153, 154
  concerns about managed care, 168-169, 316-317
  cultural competency as factor in, 174
  definition, 171
  gender differences, 175
  measures of, 4-5, 142, 171-174, 175, 178-180
  need for care and, 174-175, 178
  negative effects of limiting, 170
  as quality assessment component, 168
  racial/ethnic considerations in, 175-176, 248
  for special populations, 249
  universal coverage and, 171
  wraparound services, 136-138
Accountability
  consensus on quality for, 199
  employer coalitions for, 191
  in evolution of behavioral health care, 189-190
  for outcomes, 237-238
  in primary care, 87
  public reporting systems for, 198
  quality of care and, 184-186
  through credentialing and privileging, 187
Accreditation
  and clinical practice guidelines, 252-253
  cost issues, 214-215
  effect on quality of care, 54, 186
  findings, 243-244
  goal of, 203
  government role in, 218-219, 246
  of Indian Health Service health centers, 158
  for monitoring contracts, 7-8
  for monitoring quality of care, 6, 186
  organizations for, 32, 204, 214. See also Accreditation organizations
  process, 215-216
  quality improvement program requirements, 64
  recommendations for, 6-9, 244-247
  requirements for, 214
  scope of, 186
  trends, 203-204, 214-215

See also Certification and licensure
Accreditation organizations
    Council on Accreditation of Services
        for Families and Children, 23, 204-
        205
    Joint Commission on Accreditation of
        Healthcare Organizations, 32, 158,
        204, 218
    National Committee for Quality
        Assurance, 190-191, 202, 205-213
    Rehabilitation Accreditation
        Commission, 32, 204
    Utilization Review Accreditation
        Committee, 32, 213-214
Adverse selection, 51-52
Advocacy, consumer, 23-24
Affective disorders, 77
    risk among children, 153
Agency for Health Care Policy and
        Research
    activities, 203
    recommendations for, 9, 11, 12, 14,
        247, 250, 253, 254
Alcohol abuse/dependence, 77
    co-occurring disorders, 176-177
    detoxification, 276-277, 278
    disease model, 106
    drunk driving, 112
    evolution of treatment system, 104-107
    measures of local prevalence, 178
    mortality, 157
    suicide and, 78
    treatment effectiveness, 84
    trends in insurance coverage, 90-91
    See also Substance abuse
Alcohol, Drug Abuse, and Mental Health
        Administration, 107, 111. *See also*
        Substance Abuse and Mental
        Health Services Administration
Alcoholics Anonymous, 105, 114, 293
Alternative/innovative healing practices,
        10, 248
American Managed Behavioral Healthcare
        Association, 141-142, 174
    quality standards, 190-191
Anxiety disorders, 77, 177, 191
Auditing activities, 187-188, 245

B

Behavioral health problems
    among seniors, 156
    co-occurring, 176-177
    cost of care trends, 141
    historical development of treatment
        system, 96, 103
    negative effects of restricted access, 170
    prevalence and incidence, 1, 15, 77
    public perception/understanding, 20-
        21, 23-24, 170
    risk among children, 153
    service needs, 80-84
    social costs, 77-78, 84
    social stigma, 170
    suicide and, 78
    terminology, 22
    underdiagnosed/underestimated, 3, 76,
        78-80, 170
    utilization patterns, 28
Benefits consulting, 31-32

C

Capitated payments
    as barrier to access, 168, 169
    definition, 46
    in Medicaid, 47
    prevalence, 46
    role of, 46
    soft, 48
Carve-in arrangements, 45, 49
Carve-outs, 45, 49, 88
Case management, 49
Center for Mental Health Services, 201-
        202, 247
Center for Substance Abuse Prevention,
        201
Center for Substance Abuse Treatment,
        85, 112-113, 201
Centers for Disease Control and
        Prevention, 11, 250
Certification and licensure
    credentialing and privileging, 123, 187
    peer review for, 186
    quality of care issues, 57-58

state activities, 54-56, 186-187
for substance abuse counselors, 58-59,
294-295
substance abuse treatment, 57-58
transition of public services into
managed care, 59
types of practitioners, 123
Child abuse, 153
Child and Adolescent Service System
Program, 154
Children and adolescents
adolescent treatment issues, 155
findings, 251-252
health screening, 153
with impaired parents, 152-153
mental health care trends, 141
military health services for, 149-150,
151
prevalence of behavioral health
problems, 77
principles of care for, 154
program financing, 153-154
recommendations regarding, 11-12, 252
risk for abuse, 153
risk for mental health problems, 153
school-based intervention, 153
service needs, 152-153
substance abuse, 77, 155, 177
Civilian Health and Medical Program of
the Uniformed Services, 148, 149-
150, 151, 152, 189
Clinical outcomes information system,
230, 233
Clinical practice
alternative/innovative techniques, 10,
248
coverage design/limitations and, 26
credentialing and privileging, 123, 187
cultural competence in, 159-162
duration of treatment, 319-320
effectiveness of, 84-85
findings, 252-253
focus of outcomes research, 84
in managed behavioral health care,
318-320
peer review, 186
prescription patterns, 320

recommendations for, 12-13, 253
standardization, 26-27
state licensure and effectiveness of, 57-
58
structural measures of quality, 122
substance abuse counselors, 26, 58-59,
123, 294-295
terminology, 22
types and characteristics of
practitioners, 25-26, 123
use of hospitals, 319
Clinical practice guidelines
as accreditation issue, 252-253
current extent of use, 60
current limitations, 252
outcomes research and, 235
potential effects, 60-61
role of, 60, 188-189
Cocaine, 276, 277-278
Community Mental Health Centers Act
of 1963, 103, 104
Comprehensive Alcohol Abuse and
Alcoholism Prevention, Treatment,
and Rehabilitation Act. *See* Hughes
Act
Comprehensive Drug Abuse Prevention
and Control Act of 1970, 110
Confidentiality, 35
in carve-outs, 88
concerns, 67-68
in substance abuse treatment, 68
Consultants
health benefits, 188
for regulatory compliance, 144-145
See also Benefits consulting
Consumer protection, 2
confidentiality rights, 67-68
government role in, 8-9, 219, 245-246
in managed care system, 241
meaning of, 21
patient autonomy, 69
recommendations for, 8-10, 245-246,
248
strategies, 241-242
structural/process models, 219
Consumers and families
advocacy efforts by, 23-24

definition, 21-22, 247
diversity, 25
involvement in health care system,
        247-248
Consumer satisfaction
    with access, 171, 175
    measurement of, 9-10, 201-202
    as measure of quality, 189, 245
    media dissemination of findings, 189
Continuity of care/coverage, 6, 93, 245
Contracts/contracting
    public sector-managed care, 48-49
    quality assessment provisions, 29
    quality of care and, 66
    recommendations for, 7-8, 245
    scope of coverage, 66-67
    soft capitation, 48
Cost of care
    adverse selection effects, 51-52
    behavioral health problems, 77-78, 80
    behavioral health trends, 141
    concerns about quality of care, 16-17,
        312
    financing of child and adolescent
        programs, 153-154
    indirect costs, 80-84
    integration of service systems for, 146
    managed care containment strategies,
        42-45, 168
    preventive interventions in workplace
        to reduce, 147
    regional disparities, 176
    spending trends, 28
    substance abuse treatment
        expenditures, 28, 135
    for substance-abusing criminal
        offenders, 113-114
Cost shifting, 53, 93
Council on Accreditation of Services for
        Families and Children, 32, 204-205
Coverage design/limitations
    adverse selection effects, 51
    benefits consultants, 31-32
    competition for enrollees, 45-46
    current status, 91
    effect on quality of care, 54
    employer-sponsored plans, 94, 184-185

historical limitations on mental health
        services, 313-314
    legislative efforts, 24, 25
    Medicaid, 128-129
    Medicare, 130-131
    parity, 24, 170-171, 314
    private sector trends, 93-95
    purchaser influence, 28-29
    to restrict access, 169-170
    substance abuse counseling, 26
    treatment planning and, 26
    trends, 90, 314
    universal coverage, 171
Criminal justice system
    alcoholism intervention, historical
        development of, 105-106
    cost of behavioral health problems,
        78
    drug abuse intervention, historical
        development of, 107-109, 112
    implications of limiting access to care,
        170
    managed care contracts, 114
    public addiction treatment system and,
        112
    substance abuse by criminals, 112-113,
        114
    substance abuse treatment in, 113-114
Cultural competence
    as ethical issue, 254
    findings, 248
    meaning of, 159
    military health services, 150
    models for practice, 160
    need for, 159
    recommendations for, 10, 248
    resource networks, 162
    threshold issues, 160-161

D

Data collection and management
    admissions/discharge forms, 236
    claims data, 217, 236
    clinical outcomes information system,
        230
    confidentiality issues, 67-68

Mental Health Statistics Improvement
Program, 201-202
for outcomes measurement, 233, 236-
237
private sector quality standards, 191-
199
public sector performance standards,
199-200
for quality improvement, 64
for quality measurement, 217-218
for report cards, 66
research priorities, 331
shortcomings of, 217-218
Defense, Department of, 4, 189
historical development of mental
health care, 148-149
managed care services in, 151-152
TriCare program, 151-152
See also Military programs
Deinstitutionalization, 103
Delivery system
alcoholism intervention, historical
development of, 104-107
behavioral health disability
management plans, 145
challenges to, 3, 77
components of, 3, 122-123
in criminal justice system, 113-114
current functioning, 76-77
drug abuse intervention, historical
development of, 107-111
employee assistance programs, 114-115
fragmented nature of, 76-77, 80, 96,
153-154, 163
historical development, 96, 103-111
Indian Health Service, 157-159
integration of public-private services,
49, 59, 115-116
managed care, 29-31
military managed care programs, 151-
152
organizational interactions, 4
primary care in, 87-89
for rural areas, 162-163
service sector boundaries, 91-93
for special populations, 10
state level, 95-96

structural measures of quality, 122
wraparound services, 138-139
Demand management, 147
Depression/depressive disorders
among seniors, 156
primary care treatment, 87, 89
Disability
access to care, 249
behavioral, management of, 145
Medicare coverage, 130
substance abuse-related, 25
Drug Abuse Office and Treatment Act of
1972, 110
Drug Abuse Prevention, Treatment, and
Rehabilitation Act, 68

E

Employee assistance programs, 114-115,
143-144, 146
Employee Retirement Income Security
Act of 1974, 90-91
Employer-sponsored health plans
behavioral health disability
management, 145
control of competition in, 45-46
cost of coverage, 46, 94
coverage design, 94
current status, 27-28
employer coalitions for quality
accountability, 191
enrollment patterns, 46, 93-94
historical development, 184-185
mechanisms to restrict access in, 169-
170
as purchasers of behavioral health care,
190-191
See also Workplace service systems
Enabling services. *See* Wraparound
services
Enrollment patterns
behavioral health care, 20-21
employee assistance programs, 115
employer-sponsored plans, 46, 93-94
health maintenance organizations, 31
indemnity insurance, 46

insured population, 28
managed behavioral health care, 1, 15, 45, 313
managed care, 1, 15, 31, 41-42
market influences, 45-46
Medicaid, 129, 202, 314
Medicare, 129, 131, 156-157, 202
private insurance, 31
substance abuse programs, 134-135
Ethical concerns, 71
confidentiality, 67-68
findings, 254
patient autonomy, 69
recommendations for, 13-14, 254
therapeutic relationship, 69-70

F

Families
with impaired parents, 152-153
military programs for, 149, 150
as substance abuse rehabilitation outcome factor, 290
Federal government
confidentiality regulations for substance abuse treatment, 68
consumer advocacy for behavioral health care, 24
consumer protection role for, 8, 9, 219, 245-246
current regulation of managed behavioral health care, 89-90
funding for substance abuse treatment, 135
historical development of alcoholism treatment, 104-107
historical development of delivery system, 96, 103, 104, 148
historical development of drug abuse treatment, 107-111
parity legislation, 24, 170-171, 314
recommendations for, 8, 9, 245-246
regulatory compliance by employers, consultants for, 144-145
research role, 249

role in quality assurance, 218-219
state level implementation, 95, 96
Foundation for Accountability, 191-198

G

Gender differences, 175

H

Harrison Narcotic Act, 107-108
Health Care Financing Administration, 29, 128
auditing activities, 187-188
quality management activities, 202
recommendations for, 14, 254
responsibilities and authorities, 202
Health maintenance organizations
accreditation requirements, 214
behavioral health care in, 45, 314
characteristics, 42
current regulation, 89-90
enrollment trends, 31
staff model, 45
Health Plan Employer Data and Information Set, 171-174, 198, 202, 217
Health Resources and Services Administration, 9, 11, 12, 247, 250, 252
Healthy People 2000, 200-201
Homeless mentally ill, 103
Housing, 83
Hughes Act, 57, 68, 106-107, 114-115

I

Indemnity insurance
enrollment trends, 46
in managed care system, 31
reimbursement system, 41
Independent practice associations, 42
Indian Health Service, 157-159
Infant mortality, 157
Institute for Behavioral Healthcare, 142

J

Job training, 83
Joint Commission on Accreditation of
    Healthcare Organizations, 32, 158,
    204, 218

K

Kassebaum-Kennedy bill, 24, 170-171

L

Legal issues, 188
Length of stay, 319-320

M

Managed behavioral health care
    advantages of, 27, 48
    adverse selection, 51
    barriers to effective primary care,
        88-89
    choice of practitioner in, 315-316
    clinical practice in, 318-320
    competition, 50
    conceptual approach to, 33-35
    concerns about access, 169, 316-317
    concerns about quality, 17, 47-48, 241,
        312, 321
    cost shifting, 53, 93
    cultural competence issues, 160-161
    current coverage, 91
    current regulatory environment, 89-90
    demands for quality, 53
    effectiveness of, 50, 241, 242
    employee assistance programs
        integrated with, 144, 146
    enrollment, 1, 15, 313
    ethical issues, 71
    goals, 47
    health promotion programs, 56-57,
        146-147
    historical growth, 31, 45, 314
    integration of public-private services,
        49-50, 59, 115-116

mechanisms to restrict access in, 169-
    170
in military health services, 151-152
moral hazard. *See* Adverse selection
outcomes of care, 321-324
performance measurement, 141-142
population needs assessment, 174-175
practitioner resistance to, 27
practitioners, 25-27, 123
principal issues, 19-20
quality improvement programs, 65
quality monitoring mechanisms, 41, 45
quality standards in private sector, 191-
    199
research priorities, 325-330
service sector boundaries, 91-93
skimming, 53
spending, 141
system trends, 41, 314
treatment planning in, 26
treatment trends, 15-16
Managed care
    accreditation, 186
    carve-outs, 45, 49, 88
    challenges to confidentiality, 67-68
    concerns about access, 168-169
    consumer concerns, 24
    cost management strategies, 42-45, 168
    enrollment trends, 15, 28, 31, 41-42
    evolution of structure, 42
    financial incentives in, 46
    goals, 1, 15, 40
    historical growth, 42, 313
    in Indian Health Service programs,
        158-159
    industry stakeholders, 31-32
    influence on health care system, 40,
        90-91
    insurance industry in, 31
    measuring local needs and access, 178-
        179
    outcome studies, 229
    patient autonomy and, 69
    quality of care concerns, 16-17, 312
    in rural areas, 162-163
    structure and operations, 29-31, 41-45
    terminology, 21

therapeutic relationship in, 69-70
See also Managed behavioral health
    care
Medicaid, 4, 92-93, 128
    administrative structure, 129, 202
    auditing activities, 188
    capitated payment system in, 47
    child health screening, 153
    cost containment in, 129
    coverage design, 128-129, 169
    enrollment trends, 129
    funding, 128
    managed behavioral health care in, 94
    managed care enrollment, 45, 128,
        129, 202, 314
    mental health care expenditures, 129
    performance assessment, 130
    recipients, 128
    spending trends, 129
    structure and operations, 128
    in system of behavioral health care, 80,
        104
Medicare, 4, 130
    auditing activities, 188
    benefit design, 130-131
    costs, 131
    disabled population, 130
    enrollment, 31, 129, 131, 156-157, 202
    managed care plans, 31, 129, 131, 202
    mental health care provisions, 131
    performance assessment, 130
    quality improvement program, 64
Mental Health Statistics Improvement
    Program, 201-202
Methadone treatment, 109, 110
Military programs
    child and adolescent services, 149-150,
        151
    coordination of treatment in, 149
    cultural competence, 150
    family services, 149
    historical development, 148-149
    older adult services, 150
    services for chronic relapsing
        conditions, 150
    See also Defense, Department of;
        Veterans Affairs, Department of

N

Narcotic Addict Rehabilitation Act of
    1966, 109
Narcotics Anonymous, 293
National Alliance for the Mentally Ill,
    246
National Association for Research on
    Schizophrenia and Depression, 246
National Committee for Quality
    Assurance, 190-191, 202, 205-213
National Depressive and Manic
    Depressive Association, 246
National Drug and Alcohol Treatment
    Utilization Survey, 131-133, 134
National Institute of Mental Health
    alcohol abuse research, 106, 111
    Community Support Program, 103-104
    drug abuse research, 110, 111
    historical development, 103
    recommendations for, 9, 11, 247, 250,
        252
National Institute on Alcohol Abuse and
    Alcoholism, 106, 114-115
National Institute on Drug Abuse, 110-
    111, 250, 252
National Institutes of Health, 9, 11, 12,
    247, 250, 252
National Mental Health Association, 246

O

Obsessive-compulsive disorder, 177
Older adults/senior citizens
    coordination of services for, 156
    as health care consumers, 156-157
    health perceptions of, 156
    military health services for, 150
    risk for chronic conditions, 156
    risk for mental health problems, 156
    substance abuse patterns, 177
Opiate addiction/detoxification, 277, 278
Outcomes measurement/research
    accountability for findings, 237-238
    analytical framework for, 231-232
    clinical outcomes information system,
        230

clinical practice guidelines and, 235
criteria for evaluating, 235-236
data sources, 236-237, 245
effect on quality of care, 54
efficacy/effectiveness assessments, 234
employee assistance program
   performance, 143-144
general measures, 230-232
indicators of access, 173-174
limitations of, 5, 84, 85, 233-234, 238-
   239, 249
long-term and short-term objectives,
   228-229
in managed behavioral health care,
   321-323
managed care research, 142, 229
as measure of quality, 3, 61, 198
multidimensional context, 226, 228
new approaches, 229-230
performance indicators for, 233
population-based, 327
practitioner characteristics, 123
process variables, 232
prospects for, 237-238
public dissemination of findings,
   237
public expectations for treatment and,
   227-228
quality improvement and, 234-235
quality indicators, 272-274
significance of, 5-6, 226, 232, 239, 324-
   325
stakeholder perspective as factor in,
   20
standardized instruments for, 230, 236
structural variables, 232
substance abuse findings, 271-272
substance abuse rehabilitation
   indicators, 282-287
substance abuse treatment, 84-85
substance abuse treatment quality
   indicators, 272-273, 299-304
treatment effectiveness, current
   understanding of, 84-85
treatment goals and, 226-227
treatment setting as variable, 230

P

Parity, 24, 170-171, 314
Peer review, 186
Performance-Based Measures for Managed
   Behavioral Healthcare, 174, 217
Pharmacotherapy
   prescription patterns in managed care,
      320
   prospects, 85
   for substance abuse rehabilitation, 281-
      282, 295-297
Physician-patient relationship, 69-70
   cultural resource networks, 162
Planning Systems Development Program,
   154
Point-of-service plans, 15, 42, 44
Preferred provider organizations, 15, 42,
   43
President's Commission on Mental
   Health, 101
Preventive intervention(s), 56-57
   with children in schools, 153
   cultural competence in, 160
   demand management as, 147
   educational, in workplace, 147
   health promotion plans, 56-57, 146-
      147
   opportunities in workplace, 142-143
Primary care
   barriers to behavioral health
      assessment, 88, 170
   child/adolescent behavioral problems
      in, 153
   definition, 87
   in delivery of behavioral health care, 3,
      76, 87
   diagnostic accuracy in, 87
   findings, 253
   in integration of services, 87, 116
   practitioners, 25
   quality assurance in, 89
   quality of behavioral health care in,
      76
   recommendations for, 13, 253
   utilization, 87
   vs. managed care carve-outs, 88

Private systems of care
  accountability, 184-186
  alcoholism intervention, historical
    development of, 105
  coverage trends, 93-95
  in delivery of behavioral health care, 3,
    4
  drug abuse intervention, historical
    development of, 109
  employee assistance programs,
    historical development of, 115
  health benefits consultants, 188
  measures of quality in, 5, 184, 190-191
  public sector services and, 91-93
  quality standards, 191-199
  strengths and limitations of, 94
Process measures of quality, 3, 5, 61
  as outcome variables, 232
Provider inclusion
  determinants of, 317-318
  managed care practice, 46, 168
  recommendations for, 9, 246-247
Public Health Service, 200-201
Public perception/understanding
  of behavioral health care, 20-21, 23-24
  as factor in outcomes measurement,
    227-228
  of mental illness, 170
Public services
  characteristics of substance abuse
    treatment programs, 133-134
  for children and adolescents, 153-154
  concerns with managed care contracts
    for, 47-48, 49-50
  contracting with managed care
    organizations for, 47-49, 67, 94
  criminal justice system and, 112
  eligibility criteria for mental health
    services, 169
  funding for, 76, 80, 111, 122, 242-243
  historical development of alcoholism
    treatment, 104-107
  historical development of delivery
    system, 96, 103-104
  historical development of drug abuse
    intervention, 107-111

  integration with private services, 49,
    59, 115-116
  measures of quality in, 5, 184
  mental health care expenditures, 80
  mental health treatment system, 135-
    136
  performance measurement for, 199-200
  private sector insurance boundaries,
    91-93
  state-federal relationship, 95, 96
  substance abuse screening, 56-57
  substance abuse treatment program
    funding, 135
  in system of behavioral health care, 3,
    4, 76, 80, 91
  wraparound services, 138-139
Purchasers, group
  adverse selection effects, 51-52
  assessments of access by, 179-180
  competition for enrollees, 45-46
  employer coalitions, 191
  influence of, 28-29
  potential for savings, 48
  price sensitivity, 51-52
  purchasing alliances, 28
  quality of care as issue for, 53
  state governments as, 47
  See also Employer-sponsored plans

Q

Quality assessment
  access to care as measure for, 168
  auditing for, 187-188, 245
  challenges to, 6, 18, 19-20
  conceptual variables, 3, 61
  consensus on measurement of, 199
  consumer involvement in, 9-10, 17-18,
    189, 219, 248
  contract provisions, 29
  by corporate purchasers, 190-191
  in Department of Defense TriCare
    program, 152
  of employee assistance programs, 143-
    144
  framework for, 2-3, 33, 232

goals of, 199
historical development in behavioral
    health care, 189-190
information infrastructure for, 217-218
managed care industry activities, 32-
    33, 141-142
managed care monitoring mechanisms,
    41, 45
Medicaid, 130
Medicare, 131
methods, 186-187
participants, 6
private sector quality standards, 191-
    199
in public sector, 199, 202, 203
stakeholder perspective as factor in, 19-
    20, 21, 184
Quality assurance, 61
good program qualities, 223
government role, 218-219
limitations of, 62
in primary care, 89
Quality control, 61
Quality improvement, 72
applications in behavioral health care,
    65
applications in health care, 64-65
goals, 53
outcome measurement and, 234-235
principles of, 62-64
recommendations for, 7, 245
role of, 35
tools for, 64
Quality indicators
definition, 272
good qualities of, 273-274
for substance abuse detoxification, 278-
    279
for substance abuse rehabilitation, 287-
    298
for substance abuse treatment, 272-
    273, 299-304
Quality of care
accountability and, 184-186
competition and, 95
components, 35-36

concerns about managed care, 16-17,
    47-48, 312, 321
consumer advocacy for, 24-25
contracting and, 66-67
definition, 17
determinants of, 21
goals, 33
legal considerations, 188
management trends, 189-190
market forces, 53
measurement approaches, 2-3, 5, 17-18
in primary care settings, 76
purchaser standards, 28-29
recommendations for monitoring, 7,
    244-245
responsibility for, 54
role of accreditation systems, 6
system determinants, 54
treatment setting as variable in, 87

R

Race/ethnicity
patterns of substance abuse, 175-178
See also Cultural competence
Reagan administration, 103-104
Rehabilitation Accreditation
    Commission, 32, 204
Rehabilitation medicine, 83
goals for substance abuse, 279-282
outcome indicators for substance abuse
    rehabilitation, 282-287
quality indicators for substance abuse
    rehabilitation, 287-298
Report cards
data collection for, 66, 331
market demands, 198
public sector initiatives, 201-202
role of, 66
standardization of, 66
Research
child and adolescent interventions,
    155
choice of provider, 329
current status, 249
population-based outcomes, 327

priorities, 325-330
problem recognition, 328
recommendations for, 10-11, 250
strategies for, 331-333
structure of managed care, 327-328
targeting high-risk patients, 330
on treatment strategy, 329-330
See also Outcomes measurement/
    research
Risk sharing, 50
Rural areas, 162-163, 176

S

Screening policies
for adults, 56-57
for children, 153
Skimming, 53
Social Security Disability Income, 25
Special Action Office for Drug Abuse
    Prevention, 110
Special populations
access issues, 175-178, 249
cultural competence issues, 159-162
findings, 249
goals for, 35
recommendations regarding, 10, 249
rural services, 162-163
See also Children and adolescents
State government
alcoholism treatment requirements, 90
certification and licensure activities,
    54-56, 186-187
current regulation of managed
    behavioral health care, 89-90
federal action and, 95, 96
funding for mental health treatment,
    136
funding for substance abuse treatment,
    135
historical development of alcoholism
    treatment, 106-107
historical development of behavioral
    health care, 104
historical development of drug abuse
    treatment, 110, 111

integration of public-private services,
    116
Medicaid administration, 128, 129
as purchaser of managed care services,
    47
recommendations for, 8-9, 246
role in quality assurance, 218-219
shortcomings of behavioral health care
    delivery, 96
structure of delivery system, 95
substance abuse treatment regulation,
    57-58
support for purchasing alliances, 28
Structure of behavioral health care system
access to care as component of, 168
accreditation review, 214
for child and adolescent services, 153-
    154
components, 122-123, 232
findings, 242-243
fragmented nature of, 163
as measure of quality, 3, 61, 122
mental health treatment, 135-136
military, 148-149, 151-152
organizational linkages, 3, 76-77
as outcome variable, 232
recommendations for, 6, 243
research needs, 327-328
in rural areas, 162-163
substance abuse service systems, 131-
    135
workplace services, 142-148
wraparound services, 136-139
See also Delivery system
Substance abuse
among children and adolescents, 77,
    177
co-occurring mental health problems,
    176-177
criminal behavior and, 112-113
gender differences, 175
measures of local prevalence, 178-179
by older adults, 177
parental, 152-153
racial/ethnic differences in, 175-178
research needs, 304

risk among children, 153
screening policies, 56-57
social costs, 77-78
See also Alcohol abuse/dependence;
    Substance abuse treatment
Substance Abuse and Mental Health
    Services Administration, 18, 134-
    136
managed care initiatives, 201
Mental Health Statistics Improvement
    Program, 201-202
quality standards, 188, 190-191
recommendations for, 9, 10, 11, 12, 14,
    247, 249, 250, 252, 253, 254
Substance abuse treatment
client characteristics, 134-135
confidentiality regulations for, 68
cost of, 28, 141
counselor practitioners, 26, 58-59, 123,
    294-295
coverage patterns, 169
credentialing of practitioners, 123
detoxification and stabilization, 274-
    279
disparities in delivery, 176
effectiveness of managed care
    programs, 50
effectiveness research, 84
employee assistance programs, 114-115
employment-related outcome factors,
    289-290
family-related outcome factors, 290
future prospects for, 85
goals, 227
historical development of system, 96,
    103, 107-111
long-term and short-term goals, 228-
    229
military service system, 149
outcomes research findings, 271-272
patient-related outcome factors, 285,
    288-289
pharmacotherapy, 281-282, 295-297
program enrollment, 134-135
program funding, 135
psychiatric problems as outcome factor,
    286-287

public sector managed care initiatives,
    201
quality indicators, 272-273, 299-304
rehabilitation goals, 279-282
rehabilitation outcome indicators, 282-
    287
rehabilitation quality indicators, 287-
    298
severity of abuse as outcome factor,
    285-286
state regulation of, 57-58
treatment-related outcome factors,
    290-298
types and characteristics of
    practitioners, 123
types and characteristics of service
    systems, 131-135
wraparound services, 138-139, 251
See also Alcohol abuse/dependence
Suicide
among seniors, 156
behavioral health problems and, 78
prevention among adolescents, 252
Supplemental Security Income, 25
Synanon, 109

U

Uniform Alcoholism and Intoxication
    Treatment Act, 57, 107
Uninsured individuals, 92-93
Universal coverage, 171
Utilization
estimates of, 28
gender differences, 175
measurement of, for quality assessment,
    217
primary care, 87
substance abuse treatment, 133
trends in, 20-21, 23-24
Utilization effect, 50-51
Utilization management
effectiveness of, 190
as mechanism to restrict access, 169-
    170
role of, 46
tools of, 46

Utilization Review Accreditation
  Commission, 32, 213-214

V

Veterans Affairs, Department of, 4
  historical development of mental
    health care, 148-149
  managed care services in, 151
  services for chronic relapsing
    conditions, 150
  See also Military programs

W

Workplace service systems, 4
  behavioral health disability
    management, 145

consultants for regulatory compliance,
    144-145
demand management, 147
findings, 250
health promotion plans, 146-147
health training and education, 147
recommendations for, 11, 250
significance of, 142-143, 147-148
special needs of, 145
See also Employee assistance programs;
    Employer-sponsored health plans
Wraparound services
  findings, 251
  funding, 138-139
  historical development, 136-138
  recommendations for, 11-12, 245, 251
  types and characteristics of, 138-139